Basic Poultry Nutrition

CW01476331

Basic Pediatric Nutrition

Second Edition

Madhu Sharma RD
Diploma in Dietetics
MSc (Food and Nutrition)
Formerly, Senior Dietician
Postgraduate Institute of Medical
Education and Research (PGIMER)
Chandigarh, India

Foreword
BNS Walia

The Health Sciences Publisher
New Delhi | London | Panama

Jaypee Brothers Medical Publishers (P) Ltd

Headquarters
Jaypee Brothers Medical Publishers (P) Ltd
4838/24, Ansari Road, Daryaganj
New Delhi 110 002, India
Phone: +91-11-43574357
Fax: +91-11-43574314
Email: jaypee@jaypeebrothers.com

Overseas Offices

J.P. Medical Ltd
83 Victoria Street, London
SW1H 0HW (UK)
Phone: +44 20 3170 8910
Fax: +44 (0)20 3008 6180
Email: info@jpmedpub.com

Jaypee-Highlights Medical Publishers Inc
City of Knowledge, Bld. 235, 2nd Floor, Clayton
Panama City, Panama
Phone: +1 507-301-0496
Fax: +1 507-301-0499
Email: cservice@jphmedical.com

Jaypee Brothers Medical Publishers (P) Ltd
17/1-B Babar Road, Block-B, Shaymali
Mohammadpur, Dhaka-1207
Bangladesh
Mobile: +08801912003485
Email: jaypeedhaka@gmail.com

Jaypee Brothers Medical Publishers (P) Ltd
Bhotahity, Kathmandu, Nepal
Phone: +977-9741283608
Email: kathmandu@jaypeebrothers.com

Website: www.jaypeebrothers.com
Website: www.jaypeedigital.com

Basic Pediatric Nutrition

First Edition: 2009

Second Edition: **2017**

ISBN 978-93-5270-025-7

Printed at Rajkamal Electric Press, Plot No. 2, Phase-IV, Kundli, Haryana.

Dedicated to

*The memory of my late husband
Professor AC Sharma
whose unseen presence inspired me
to fulfill my dream*

Foreword

Malnutrition is affecting almost half the children the world over. Nutritional deficiencies are widely prevalent, common ones amongst them being protein-energy malnutrition, anemia, vitamin A deficiency and iodine deficiency disorders. All these reflect poor intake of essential nutrients by children, mainly affected by poverty, but also abetted by ignorance regarding what to feed the child at what age.

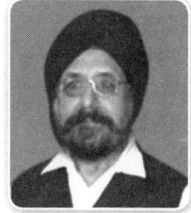

Several attempts by professionals to improve the knowledge base of our population regarding nutritional matters have been made from time to time. Parents can learn about nutritional aspects regarding their children from doctors, nurses, health workers and teachers. All these professionals focus on their main task and hardly ever touch upon the subject of nutrient intake. It may be because they do not know enough to advise or they do not appreciate the preventive value of such advice on the overall survival of a growing child.

Madhu Sharma's book *Basic Pediatric Nutrition* is an attempt to fill that gap by putting together basic facts about nutritional matters into a short textbook. Starting with basic nutrient requirements at different ages and assessment of nutritional status, this book covers numerous important aspects, like diet surveys, functions of different nutrients and result of their deficiencies in a growing child, construction of age appropriate diets and finally how to feed children with different nutritional disorders like anemia, obesity, iron and vitamin A deficiency, chronic diarrhea and food allergies.

The therapeutic management of some common childhood problems have been highlighted in a very simple, straightforward and practical approach for all those involved in child care.

The book succeeds in keeping a style which is readable and simple. The food items advised for various age groups are culturally acceptable and affordable.

The issues regarding breastfeeding and its management adds to the value of this compendium.

BNS Walia
MD FRCPCH (London)
Emeritus Professor
Department of Pediatrics
Formerly, Director
Postgraduate Institute of Medical Education and Research
Chandigarh, India

Preface to the Second Edition

"Many things can wait, the child cannot. Now is the time his bones are being formed, his mind is being developed. To him you cannot say tomorrow; his name is today"

—Gabriela Mistral

Food has always been an important aspect of any living being and humans are no exceptions. Survival of the human being is in fact dependent on food from the moment one is born. Nature has endowed the greatest gift to the newborn, that of breastfeeding by the mother. The needs of the newborn are taken care of by the mother exclusively well up to 6 months of its life. Thereafter, the infant is gradually introduced to other foods besides milk. Knowledge of the right type and quality of food offered to him from this phase is essential, so that adequate growth and development continues uninterrupted. Even if the mother or the caregiver is aware of the importance, it is often observed, that they are unable to implement it successfully, due to various practical problems encountered.

Although there is a plethora of books and material available on various aspects of food, nutrition and diet, a need for some concise and focused guide on the basic knowledge of nutrition related to infants and children in the Indian context was felt by many students and professionals dealing with food and nutrition and dietetics.

An attempt has been made in this book, to outline various aspects of diet, and nutritional needs of the pediatric group right up till the phase of adolescence. Furthermore, the basic practical considerations while dealing with this group of population for the benefit of the young nutritionists and dieticians exposed in a hospital setting has been deliberated upon.

The present edition is an updated version of the first one, with revised guidelines brought out after 2010, besides elaborating in greater detail certain facts and figures like in the chapters of feeding of infants, 0–6 months, and 6–24 months. Keeping in mind the relevance of some basic issues related to child health and nutrition, which were not dealt upon in the first edition, seven new chapters have been added like maternal nutrition in pregnancy and lactation, nutrition for the athlete child, vegetarianism in children, interaction of nutrition and infection, role of other micronutrients, and probiotics.

It is hoped that this book would prove to be of great help and a guide for all professionals, teachers, students (including nursing), dieticians and nutritionists involved in the pediatric care, whether in a hospital or in the community.

Since pediatricians cannot treat a sick child without considering his nutritional status, it can also serve as a useful handy guide for all medical students involved in pediatric training and in their day-to-day practice. Other health workers involved in the community dealing with various child development projects can also find this book as a useful tool in understanding the basic concept of child care.

Madhu Sharma

Preface to the First Edition

Many things can wait, the child cannot. Now is the time when his bones are being formed and his mind is being developed. To him you cannot say tomorrow; his name is today.

—Gabriela Mistral

Food has always been an important aspect of any living being and humans are no exceptions. Survival of the human being is in fact dependent on food from the moment one is born. Nature has endowed the greatest gift to the newborn, that of breastfeeding by the mother. The needs of the newborn are taken care of by the mother exclusively well up to 6 months of its life. Thereafter, the infant is gradually introduced to other foods besides milk. Knowledge of the right type and quality of food offered to him from this phase is essential so that adequate growth and development continues uninterrupted. Even if the mother or the caregiver is aware of the importance, it is often observed that they are unable to implement it successfully, due to various practical problems encountered.

Although there is a plethora of books and material available on various aspects of food, nutrition and diet, a need for some concise and focused guide on the basic knowledge of nutrition related to infants and children was felt by many students and professionals dealing with food, nutrition and dietetics.

An attempt has been made in this book to outline various aspects of diet and nutritional needs of the pediatric group right up till the phase of adolescence. Furthermore, the basic practical considerations while dealing with this group of population for the benefit of the young nutritionists and dieticians exposed in a hospital setting has been deliberated upon.

It is hoped that this book would prove to be of great help and a guide for all professionals, teachers, students (including nursing), dieticians and nutritionists involved in the pediatric care, whether in a hospital or in the community.

Since pediatricians cannot treat a sick child without considering his nutritional status, it can also serve as a useful handy guide for all medical students involved in pediatric training and in their day-to-day practice. Other health workers involved in the community dealing with various child development projects can also find this book as a useful tool in understanding the basic concept of child care.

Madhu Sharma

Acknowledgments

I wish to acknowledge my sincere thanks to Dr BNS Walia, who was the first to inspire me to bring out a book which would be of help to all those involved in the nutritional care of the pediatric population.

My thanks are due to my friends and colleagues, who encouraged and guided me to complete this book.

I also wish to acknowledge the help of my students in the initial typing of the manuscript.

Contents

Functions of Food

BALANCED DIET

"Proper diet can become an instrument for maintaining health and cultivating increased levels of awareness"

—Chinese proverb
—Master Mantak Chia

All of us know and have heard so often of a 'Balanced Diet' and tend to believe it is a healthy diet. But, unfortunately they are actually confusing the two entities—rather use it as synonyms. A 'Balanced Diet' is one which provides us with all the nutrients (present in a wide range of foods) in the right proportion and the right amount. It will also provide a regular supply of vitamins, minerals and other nutrients, ensuring optimum health and vitality. Optimum health means less illness and health complications.

A 'Healthy' diet plan is mainly a consumption of natural, fresh and wholesome foods for each meal of the day. Such food may be low in fats, sodium and refined sugars. The difference is a healthy diet plan provides us with 'some nutrients', but the balanced diet plan provides all 'essential nutrients'.

A combination of both healthy and balanced diet plan can help achieve the following:

- A variety in the diet
- Provide more grain, fresh fruits and vegetables to provide energy
- Low fat intake—especially saturated fats
- Reduce sugar intake
- Lower salt intake
- Provide optimum health and vitality to remain active
- Mental well being
- Ability to withstand ongoing ageing process with minimum functional impairment.

- Ability to combat disease, like
  1. Resisting infections, i.e. providing immunity.
  2. Preventing onset of degenerative diseases and cancer.
  3. Resisting the effect of environmental toxins and pollutants.

There is a wide variety of foods consumed by us over the whole day. Some of them may not be consumed daily or there are some which might be consumed in greater proportions compared to certain other types of food. All these foods have some role to play in our health—directly or indirectly. Based on the functions of various foods and the nutrients provided by them, these can be classified into three main types as given in Table 1.1.[1]

Based on these functions, foods are further classified into groups depending upon the main nutrients provided by them. Some experts have classified them into seven groups, where in fruits were grouped apart from vegetables. Others grouped meat and other animal foods as a separate group from pulses, but grouped fruits with vegetables. But most experts have classified food into five basic groups as given in Table 1.2.[2] These food groups can be used as follows:

1. *Tools for nutritional assessment and screening*: A brief dietary history can give us an idea of the inadequacies of any nutrient from any of the groups and thus provide a hint of the possible deficiency if any.
2. *Tool for nutritional counseling*: It can serve as a guide for nutrition education by any health care providers.
3. *Food labeling and surveillance:* Food groups can be used for food labeling and for nutrition surveillance system.

Table 1.1: Classification of foods based on functions

Food Function	Foods	Other Nutrients
Energy rich foods	*Carbohydrates and fats*	
	Cereals, millets, whole grains	Fiber, minerals, calcium, iron, B complex vitamins
	Oils, butter, ghee	Fat-soluble vitamins, essential fatty acids
	Nuts and almonds	Proteins, vitamins, minerals
	Sugar	Carbohydrates
Body building foods	*Proteins*	
	Pulses, nuts, oilseeds	B complex vitamins, invisible fat, fiber
	Milk and milk products	Calcium, vitamin A, riboflavin, vitamin B_{12}
	Meat, fish, dairy	B complex vitamins, iron, iodine, fat
Protective foods	*Vitamins and minerals*	
	Green leafy vegetables	Anti-oxidants, fiber, carotenoids
	Other vegetables and fruits	Fiber, sugar and anti-oxidants
	Eggs, milk/milk products, flesh foods	Protein and fat

Table 1.2: Food groups and their nutrients

Food groups	Major nutrients
Cereal and millets	Energy, iron and B group vitamins
Pulses and legumes Nuts and oilseeds	Proteins, energy, B group vitamins
Milk, egg and flesh foods	Proteins, calcium, vitamin A
Vegetables and fruits	Vitamins, minerals, fiber
Fats and sugars	Energy, essential fatty acids (fats only)

Cereals and millets like wheat flour, rice, maize, bajra, etc. are basically the staple food item of any Indian meal. Besides providing energy which is their main function, also provides proteins and other minerals and vitamins. These are a good source of fiber too.

Pulses comprise a variety of dals, which are an important component of any Indian diet. These are a rich source of proteins, almost double those of cereals (24%). Soya beans of course are the highest source of proteins amounting to almost 40%. These are also good substitutes for vegetarian diets with respect to protein contents. *Besides these are also rich in certain other important nutrients like phyto oestrogens.*

Pulses and cereals are generally consumed in combination in most Indian households and this is very important in order to enhance the bioavailability of proteins. The amino acid lysine is deficient in cereals but rich in pulses. On the other hand cereals are a good source of methionine but deficient in lysine. Therefore, when consumed in combination, the deficit of each food is complemented by each other, thereby improving the quality of total proteins consumed. The role of pulses is mainly body building with of course good energy content. For nonvegetarians, meat, chicken fish and eggs are an excellent source of high biological value proteins. However, unlike pulses these are poor source of fiber.

Milk and milk products are a group by themselves and rich in proteins besides being a useful source of calcium for all age groups. The proteins of milk (casein) are of high biological value and considered as first class quality. Their basic role is that of body building apart from the protective role by virtue of its being rich in fat-soluble vitamins like A and D.

Green leafy vegetables and fruits are mainly protective foods due to their mineral and vitamin content besides also being a good source of fiber. They are however low in calories and proteins. Vitamins like A, E and C are also considered as anti oxidants, therefore a good helping of these foods in the diet can protect the body from free radical produced consequent to various metabolic actions. Fiber in the diet is a very important component of food to keep the gastrointestinal tract in action and also helps control hyperglycemia and hyperlipidemia.

Fats and oils and sugars are basically high caloric foods used as a part of the ingredients of any food preparation and termed as energy giving foods as they are calorie dense. Fats are twice as high in calories compared to sugars.

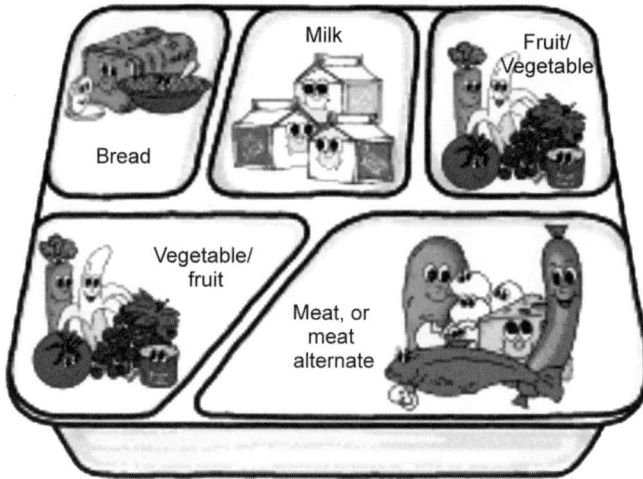

Fig. 1.1: Food groups

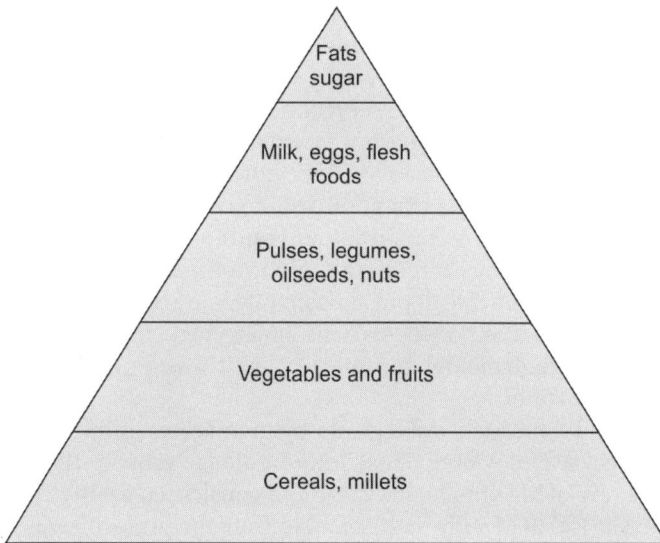

Fig. 1.2: Food pyramid

A judicious use of foods chosen from all the food groups (as per gender and age requirements) will take care of the requirements of all macronutrients, i.e. proteins, fats and carbohydrates, as also the micronutrients which include all vitamins, minerals trace elements and fiber (Fig. 1.1). Figure 1.2 illustrates the typical food pyramid for any healthy individual. The amounts of each food group can vary depending upon the age and gender of the individual. Overall, a balanced diet should provide around 60–70% of total calories from carbohydrates, 10–20% from proteins and 2–25% of total calories from fat as illustrated in the food pyramid (Fig. 1.2).

Table 1.3: Nutrient exchange list for portion size of various food groups

Food groups	g/Portion	Energy (Kcals)	Protein (g)	Carbohydrate (g)	Fat (g)
Cereals/Millets	30	100	3.0	20	0.8
Pulses	30	100	6.0	15	0.7
Egg	50	85	7.0	-	7.0
Meat/Chicken/Fish	50	100	9.0	-	7.0
Milk (toned)	100	70	3.0	5.0	3.0
Roots/Tubers	100	80	1.3	18.0	-
Green leafy vegetables	100	45	3.6	-	0.4
Other vegetables	100	30	1.7	-	0.2
Fruits	100	40	-	10.0	-
Sugar	5	20	-	5.0	-
Fats/Oils	5	45	-	-	5.0

The segments of the pyramid depict the ratio of the different food groups that need to be consumed in any balanced diet. Cereals and millets are shown to be consumed in the maximum ratio followed by vegetables and fruits, pulses and nuts, milk and other flesh foods and lastly the fats and sugars which need to be consumed in the least ratio.

A balanced diet may be planned and calculated using the simple exchange list for portion size and nutrient content of all food groups as given in Table 1.3.[3]

PRINCIPLES OF PLANNING A BALANCED DIET

While planning a balanced diet there are certain important criteria to keep in mind. These apply to the family as a whole, but in the case of a child special points need to be considered:

- *Meeting the nutritional requirements*: A menu providing adequate nutrients from all the food groups, which includes macro- and micronutrients
- *Meal pattern should fulfill family needs*: The menu should be such that members of different age groups and sex need to be accounted for. The requirements of a 5-year-old girl would be different from those of her adolescent sib, which again would differ for another sib who is an adult in the family and perhaps a sports person
- *Meal planning should be time sparing*: Any meal planning should be such that the housewife is not left to spend long hours cooking or the recipes are such that they involve a great deal of effort time and energy
- *Economic considerations*: The meal planned is based on the economic factors to a large extent. Low cost nutritious recipes can be counseled to families with limited resources, like, utilizing the seasonal foods available

judiciously can be healthier than spending more on foods not easily available or difficult to procure

- *Prevention of maximum nutrient losses*: Meal planning should involve recipes and techniques which do not involve excessive nutrient losses; e.g. too much of frying or boiling involved in recipes, though may be delicious, but may result in maximum losses especially of the water-soluble vitamins or fat-soluble vitamins in case of frying for long duration. Cooking methods involving pressure cooking, baking or microwave cooking can save time, nutrient losses and also retain maximum flavor of the food itself. Sprouting, malting or fermenting processes can enhance certain nutrients in the meals
- *Likes and dislikes*: Although meal planning should consider nutrient quality and balance of all nutrients etc., it is equally important to consider the individual likes and dislikes of the child. The recipes can be modified to appeal to their taste or some other substitutes may be offered instead
- *Variety:* Variety is not only the spice of life as is said, but also helps break monotony in the meals from day to day. Recipes may be modified or substituted for equally balanced alternatives so that the interest of the child is maintained. This can specially be of help for 'fussy eaters'
- *Meals should give satiety*: If a meal is prepared taking into account all the food groups, comprising cereals, pulses, fats etc. can provide more satiety than just cereal alone or some vegetables. Spaced out meals are better than one time heavy meals
- *Availability of foods*: Meals should include locally available foods rather than planning off season foods, which are not only expensive but, may also not be fresh, or need more cumbersome procedure for cooking or processing it.

REFERENCES

1. National Institute of Nutrition (ICMR), 2011– Dietary Guidelines for Indians—A manual.
2. Thimayamma BVS, Pasricha S. Balanced diet. In: Textbook of Human Nutrition. Bamji MS, Rao NP, Reddy V (Eds). 1996.
3. Nutrient Requirements and Recommended Dietary Allowances for Indians. A report of the expert group of the Indian Council of Medical Research, 2010.

Nutrient Requirements

INTRODUCTION

Nutrient requirements of any individual are based on their age, sex and activity. These nutrient requirements are met by a combination of various foods obtained from the five food groups discussed earlier.

A detailed list of nutrient requirements for each group including special conditions like pregnancy and lactation have been compiled by the Nutrition Expert Committee, ICMR, India (2010) as given in Table 2.1.[1] These requirements represent the optimum amount of each nutrient provided in a day's diet to support optimum health and maintain good nutrition through each stage of one's life.

Since the life cycle of an infant actually begins from the womb, it would be prudent to first discuss the optimum nutritional requirements of a mother to be, i.e. during the pregnancy stage.

NUTRITIONAL REQUIREMENTS DURING PREGNANCY AND LACTATION

It would not be an exaggeration to state that the foundation of a healthy baby at birth is in fact laid during the adolescent stage of a girl who eventually is going to be the 'future mother'. Therefore, it becomes important that due attention be given to the nutritional requirements of a girl right from her adolescence. However, in this chapter, we shall begin by first discussing the requirements of a woman during pregnancy and lactation.

During the first 8 weeks of prenatal period, the fetal organs are being formed. The second half is crucial because the major gain in weight of the fetus takes place during that period. Consequently, the demands for the building material for new or added tissues steps up markedly. These additional requirements have to be made up by increased/improved diet. The increased dietary requirements also take into account the growth of certain tissues like the mammary glands and accessory tissues supporting the fetus.

Table 2.1: Recommended dietary allowances for Indians

Group	Particulars	Body Wt. kg	Net Energy Kcal/d	Proteins g/d	fat g/d	Cal-cium mg/d	Iron mg/d	Vit. Aug/d Retinol	Vit. Aug/d B-caro tene	Thia-mine mg/d	Ribon-avin mg/d	Niacin mg/d	Pyri-doxine mg/d	Ascorbic acid mg/d	folic acid mg/d	Vit. Bl2 ug/d
Men	Sedenatry Work		2425							1.2	1.4	16				
	Moderate Work	60	2875	60	20	400	28	600	2400	1.4	1.6	18	2.0	40	100	1
	Heavy Work		3800							1.6	1.9	21				
Women	Sedenatry Work		1875							0.9	1.1	12				
	Moderate Work	50	2225	50	20	400	30	600	2400	1.1	1.3	14	2.0	40	100	1
	Heavy Work		2925							1.2	1.5	16				
	Pregnant Woman	50	+300	+15	30	1000	38	600	2400	+0.2	+0.2	+2	2.5	40	400	1
	Lactation			+25							+0.3	+4				
	0–6 months	50	+550	+18	45	1000	30	950	3800	+0.3	+0.2	+3	2.5	80	150	1.5
	6–12 months		+400							+0.2	+0.2					

Contd...

Contd...

Group	Particulars	Body Wt. kg	Net Energy Kcal/d	Proteins g/d	fat g/d	Cal-cium mg/d	Iron mg/d	Vit. Aug/d Retinol	Vit. Aug/d B-caro tene	Thia-mine mg/d	Ribon-avin mg/d	Niacin mg/d	Pyri-doxine mg/d	Ascorbic acid mg/d	folic acid mg/d	Vit. Bl2 ug/d
Infants	0–6 months	5.4	108/kg	2.05/kg						55 ug/kg	65 ug/kg	710 ug/kg	0.1			
	6–12 months	8.6	98/kg	1.65/kg		500		350	1200	50 ug/kg	60 ug/kg	650 ug/kg	0,4	25	25	0.2
Children	1–3 years	12.2	1240	22			12	400	0.6	0.7	8				30	
	4–6 years	19.0	1690	30	25	400	18	400	1600	0.9	1.0	11	0.9	40	40	0.2–1.0
	7–9 years	26.9	1950	41	26			600	2400	1.0	1.2	13	1.6		60	
Boys	10–12 years	35.4	2190	54				34		1.1	1.3	15	1.6	40	70	0.2–1.0
Girls	10–12 years	31.5	1970	57	22	600	19	600		1.0	1.2	13				
Boys	13–15 years	47.8	2450	70			41			1.2	1.5	16				
Girls	13–15 years	46.7	2060	65	22	600	28	600	2400	1.0	1.2	14	2.0	40	100	0.2–1.0
Boys	16–18 years	57.1	2640	78	50	1.3	1.6	17								
Girls	16–18 years	49.9	2060	63	22	500	30	600	2400	1.0	1.2	14	2.0	40	100	0.2–1.0

Source: Indian Council of Medical Research, 2010.

Energy Requirements in Pregnancy

Energy requirements during pregnancy comprise the normal requirement for an adult woman in addition to that required for the fetal growth, besides also the associated increase in body weight of the woman during pregnancy. Most of the additional weight gain occurs during the 2nd trimester and the 3rd trimesters of pregnancy.

The total energy requirement during pregnancy for a woman weighing 55 kg is estimated to be 80,000 K calories, of which 36,000 K cals is deposited as fat, which is utilized subsequently during lactation.[2] Data from developed countries indicate that the optimal pregnancy outcome in terms of birth weight and infant growth and survival is seen when pregnancy weight gain is 12–14 kg.

The weight gained during pregnancy comprises protein, fat and water. Protein is predominantly deposited in fetus (42%), uterus (17%), blood (14%), placenta (10%) and breast (8%). Fat is predominantly deposited in fetus and maternal tissues and contribute significantly to overall energy cost of pregnancy.

For Indian women additional energy requirements has been computed on the basis of the reference Indian woman and pregnancy weight gain of 10–12 kg. based on various factors for Indian women, the following figures can be recommended as additional energy requirement for her, with pre pregnancy weight of 55 kg.[3]

	12 kg	10 kg
1st Trimester	85	70
2nd Trimester	280	230
3rd Trimester	470	390
During 2nd and 3rd Trimester	375	310

So, an average recommendation of 350 Kcals/d through the 2nd and 3rd trimesters, as added requirement during pregnancy for an Indian woman of 55 kg body weight and pregnancy weight gain between 10 and 12 kg, may be advised.

Energy Requirements in Lactation

The daily additional requirement of energy for a woman doing exclusive breast feeding during 7–12 months would be 600 calories and for partial feeding during 7–12 months, it would be 520 calories, as per revised reports published by ICMR 2010.[1] These figures are based on data showing an average milk production of 624 mL was approximately 549 K calories. This would work out to 594 K calories for 722 mL of milk output. Overall energy requirement for lactating woman works out as shown in Table 2.2, during the entire period of 0–12 months. These figures are computed on the basis of the study on energy expenditure of Indian lactating women, which indicated negative energy.

Protein Requirements in Pregnancy

The extra proteins required (at safe level) has been computed to be 0.5, 6.9 and 22.7 g/d during the first, second and third trimesters respectively, as elaborated in Table 2.3.

Table 2.2: Energy requirements during lactation in Indian women

Month post-partum	Mean milk output (g/d)	Gross energy content (kcals/d)	Daily gross energy secreted (kcals/d)	Energy cost of milk production (kcals/d)
1	562	395	494	468
2	634	446	558	520
3	582	409	511	484
4	768	540	675	639
5	778	547	684	648
6	804	566	708	671
Mean	688	483	605	573
Partial breastfeeding				
7	688	484	605	598
8	635	452	565	558
9	516	367	479	453
10	--	--	--	--
11	565	402	563	497
12	511	364	455	449
Mean	583	612	414	517

Source: ICMR, 2010.

Table 2.3: Protein requirements from 1st to 3rd trimesters and safe levels

Trimester	Mid trimester gain (Kg)	Addn. prot. for mainten. (g/d)	Prot. deposition (g/d)	Diet. prot reqd for deposit (g/d)	Mean extra prot. reqd (g/d)	Safe intake (g/d)
1st	0.6	0.4	0.0	0.0	0.4	0.5
2nd	3.5	2.3	1.4	3.3	5.5	6.9
3rd	8.0	5.3	5.4	12.9	18.2	22.7

Source: ICMR, 2010.

Protein Requirements in Lactation

Additional protein requirements of lactating woman works out to be approximately 15 g/d, and a safe level being 18.9 g for the first 6 months of exclusive breastfeeding and approximately 12.5 g/d during the latter 6 months of lactation (Table 2.4). Based on a cereal pulse, Indian dietary pattern, protein with PDCAAS (protein digestibility corrected amino acid score) of 825 would be 2.9 and 15.2 g/d during the 0–6 months and 6–12 months, respectively. This implies a lot of energy and also high-quality protein containing foods, with a high PE ratio.[1] These can be met with a balanced diet with a PE ratio between 12–13%.

Months	Milk output (g/d)	Protein concent. (g/lt)	Mean dietary requirement (g/d)	Safe intake (g/d)
1	699	10.4	16.2	20.2
2	731	9.6	15.6	19.5
3	751	8.8	14.8	18.5
4	780	6.7	14.3	17.9
5	796	6.8	14.4	18.1
6	854	7.3	15.5	19.4
Mean 1–6	768.5	7.1	15.1	18.9
Mean 6–12	550	4.7	10.0	12.5

Table 2.4: Additional protein requirement during lactation

Source: ICMR, 2010.

So, the rounded off high-quality protein for 10 kg gestational weight gain are 1.7 and 23 g/d in first, second and third trimesters, respectively.

This extra protein can be provided from foods with high protein content, e.g. pulses or legumes with a protein efficiency (PR) ratio of 28%, in the form of lentils or whole gram at meal time or even in between meals as snacks. Also increased use of milk and milk products (PE ratio of 15%) or nonvegetarian foods like eggs (PE ratio of 30%) can further increase the protein intake.

Activity level of the pregnant woman will also determine the PE ratio of protein foods. A sedentary lifestyle will need higher PE ratio in the diet (about 13%). A solely vegetarian diet may not be able to provide a PE ratio of 13%, so in order to achieve this, low fat milk (at least 600 mL/d) and a pulse: cereal intake in 1:5 ratio and reducing root vegetables and fats will be required. Nonvegetarian foods can help meet this demand easily.

Fat

The minimum level of fats should be 20% of energy and the accepted macronutrient dietary average (AMDR) is the same as for general population.[1]

To achieve this level, diets of pregnant and lactating women should contain at least 30% of visible fat to be selected for different food applications.[2]

Dietary Fiber

During later stages of pregnancy, there is an increased tendency of developing constipation. It is therefore, very important that the diet in pregnancy be good in fiber sources like green leafy vegetables, whole grains, legumes, fruits and also seeds like flax seeds which are a good source of soluble fiber.

Micronutrients in Pregnancy and Lactation

Calcium

Calcium is an integral component of the skeletal system and naturally routinely prescribed for all pregnant and nursing mothers. As per the ICMR recommendations an extra intake of 600 mgs is advised in addition to that required for normal individuals.[1] This works out to be 1200 mgs/day. The role of adequate calcium also helps minimize problems like osteoporosis in later age among the women, which is so frequently encountered by most in their mid forties. Of course calcium supplement also helps provide adequate stores to the rapidly developing skeletal growth of the fetus.

Calcium-rich dietary sources for pregnant women are milk and milk products like yoghurt and cheese or paneer, sea food like fish, eggs, green leafy vegetables like spinach, mustard leaves, methi leaves, turnip and radish leaves, soya bean products, broccoli, okra, etc. Nuts like almonds, raisins and dried figs and oranges, tomatoes, tender coconut water, oats and legumes, especially sprouts, peanuts are also good sources of calcium. Certain cereals or juices fortified with calcium are also options available but it is best to derive the nutrients from fresh sources. However, to avail the best availability from foods like high fiber cereals or greens, etc., which contain oxalates too, it is best to cook them thoroughly or avoid very high fiber sources along with these foods.

Iron

Iron deficiency anemia is very common among most of the Indian women especially during pregnancy. Very often the mothers to be are already anemic before their conception and if on an already poor reserve of iron in the body, the burden of a pregnancy is thrust upon, the brunt is borne both by the mother herself and also the growing fetus. The mother lands into severe anemia and the fetal growth too is affected resulting in low birth weight babies. Studies have demonstrated that maternal hemoglobin (Hb) levels have been related to perinatal and neonatal mortality.[4] Bhargava et al. have shown that severe anemia is associated with higher Hb and ferritin values in the fetus and a significant decrease in birth weight and gestational age.[5]

The requirements for iron during pregnancy is based on the requirements for fetal growth, expansion of maternal tissue including red cell mass, iron in the placental tissue and the blood loss during parturition, in addition to the basal requirements. Considering an Indian woman having a prepregnancy weight of 55 kg and assuming a gestational weight gain (GWG) of 10 kg and 12 kg, an additional 760 mg of iron is required during the entire period of pregnancy, accounting for all the above mentioned factors (Table 2.5).[1]

Table 2.5: Iron requirements during pregnancy (trimester wise)		
Trimester	Requirement (mg)	
	10 kg GWG	12 kg GWG
1st Trimester	130	138
2nd Trimester	320	372
3rd Trimester	310	351
Total	760	861

Source: ICMR, 2010

Zinc

Low zinc intake during pregnancy increases the risk of delivering a low birth weight baby and may increase risk of birth defects.[6] Zinc requirements are about 50% higher during pregnancy.

Zinc requirement for pregnant Indian women is recommended as 12 mg/d which is about 2 mg higher than for nonpregnant woman.[1]

Dietary source for zinc are foods like milk, good grains, pulses and nuts and animal sources like liver and fish.

Magnesium

Deficiency of magnesium can cause fatigue and muscle cramps and increase risk of premature birth and maternal hypertension. An intake of 400 mg/d is recommended. In a cross-sectional study, birth weight has been shown to be positively co-related to magnesium intakes in early pregnancy.[7]

For Indian pregnant women the requirements are almost similar to that of nonpregnant women.

Iodine

The role of iodine in prevention of hypothyroidism and cretinism is well known especially during pregnancy. This is evident from the fact that following the Iodized Salt Program in India nation wide, the incidence of neonatal hypothyroidism has markedly decreased.[8]

Deficiency of iodine (one of the most common micronutrient deficiencies in India) in the pregnant woman can led to serious implications for the fetal growth and development. A condition called goiter developing subsequent to low levels in the mother's diet can result in abortions, still births, low birth weight, cretinism, mental retardation, hypothyroidism, psychomotor defects and impaired coordination. The minimum recommended amount for pregnant and lactating women is 200 μg/d as compared to 150 μg/d for other adults. A daily intake of 10 g of iodized salt with iodine content of minimum 15ppm provides 150 μg/d besides the amounts present in the foods consumed. These estimates are based on the assumption that some iodine is lost during cooking processes and of the rest available, only about 73.5 μg is absorbed per day.

Fat-soluble Vitamins

During pregnancy there is no extra requirement of vitamin A and is similar to that of a normal adult woman. But during lactation period, the needs are slightly increased, taking into account the content present in breast milk. Hence, an additional 350 μg/d have been recommended.[1]

Water-soluble Vitamins

Deficiency of folic acid can lead to abnormal hemopoiesis and megaloblastic anemia in pregnant women. Another very common major consequence of folic acid deficiency in early stages of conception in Indian woman, is known to be neural tubal defect (NTD) in the neonates. Good stores of folic acid during the pre- and perinatal period helps prevent this defect.[9] Besides, folic acid deficiency is also shown to affect the birth weight of infants.[9] An additional requirement of 300 µg/d and 100 µg/d is recommended during pregnancy and lactation, respectively.[1] Good dietary sources of folic acid are green leafy vegetables, legumes, egg yolk, fortified cereals, fresh beans, sunflower seeds.

REQUIREMENTS OF INFANTS AND CHILDREN

Fluids

Fluid requirements for neonates are as shown in Table 2.6.

For older children the Holiday and Segar formula is used as for energy requirements. In case of an illness associated with fever, the requirements may be increased by 10% for every 10°C of fever.

Energy

The growth pattern of infants during the first year of life (Table 2.7) follows a pattern of rise and fall. It is most rapid during the first 3 months after birth. Then the velocity of weight gain slows down from 4 to 9 months after which there is a gradual rise again till the end of the first year of life.

The energy requirements for normal Indian infants have been adapted by ICMR as per the Consultation Group of FAO/WHO/UNU, who have used the body weights of infants from 0 to 12 months representing both the industrial and the developing countries.

For children and adolescents, the recommendations are based on healthy boys and girls, who have attained 95th percentile of weight for age and have a moderate activity level as given in Table 2.8.

However, there are other authors who have devised more simple and practical formula for calculating the energy requirements of children which is also referred to as 'bedside' estimates for these requirements.[10] This estimate has been based on the assumption that a one year old child requires 1000 calories and then for every increase of age by one year 100 calories are added

Table 2.6: Fluid requirement of neonates	
Day of life	*Fluid volume (mL/kg/d)*
1	60
2	70
3	80
4	90
5	100
6	110
7	Onwards 120

Source: Reference 10

Table 2.7: Recommended energy requirements of infants

Age (Months)	Boys			Girls		
	Weight (kg)	Energy (kcals/d)	kcals/kg/d	Weight (kg)	Energy (kcals/d)	kcals/kg/d
0–1	4.58	520	115	4.35	460	105
1–2	5.50	570	105	5.14	520	100
2–3	6.28	600	95	5.82	550	95
3–4	6.28	570	80	6.41	540	85
4–5	7.48	610	80	6.92	570	80
5–6	7.93	640	80	7.35	600	80
6–7	8.30	650	80	7.71	600	80
7–8	8.62	680	80	8.03	630	80
8–9	8.89	700	80	8.31	650	80
9–10	9.13	730	80	8.55	680	80
10–11	9.37	750	80	8.87	690	80
11–12	9.62	780	80	9.0	710	80

Source: ICMR, 2010.

Table 2.8: Energy requirements of Indian children and adolescents

Age (years)	Boys			Girls		
	Weight (kg)	Energy (kcals/d)	kcals/kg/d	Weight (kg)	Energy (kcals/d)	kcals/kg/d
1–2	10.9	910	85	10.2	830	80
2–3	13.3	1120	85	12.7	1030	80
3–4	15.3	1230	80	15.0	1150	75
4–5	16.5	1290	80	16.0	1200	75
5–6	18.2	1390	80	17.7	1290	75
6–7	20.4	1510	75	20.0	1400	75
7–8	22.7	1630	70	22.3	1510	70
8–9	25.2	1630	70	22.3	1510	65
9–10	28.0	1890	70	27.6	1740	65
10–11	30.8	2030	65	31.2	1880	60
11–12	34.1	2180	65	34.8	2010	60
12–13	38.0	2370	60	39.0	2140	55
13–14	43.3	2580	60	43.4	2260	50
14–15	48.0	2760	60	47.1	2340	50
15–16	51.0	2890	55	49.4	2390	50
16–17	54.3	2980	55	51.3	2430	45
17–18	56.5	3060	55	52.8	2450	45

Source: ICMR, 2010.

Table 2.9: Holiday and Segar formula	
Upto 10 kg	100 calories/kg
10–20 kg	1000+50 Kcal for each kg above 10 kg
Above 10 kg	1500+20 Kcal in excess above 20 kg

Source: Reference 10

on yearly till puberty. This estimate works out to be lower than recommended by ICMR, but then this can be considered as minimum requirement. This implies that beginning from one year if the calorie requirement is 1000, then for every subsequent year it would be 1100, 1200 and so on till twelve years when it would be 2100. After that for adolescent boys it can be taken as 2400 and for adolescent girl it would be 2100 calories.

Another quick way of calculating has been given by Holiday and Segar formula as given in Table 2.9.[10]

Proteins

Protein requirements for infants are derived from the estimate of protein content of breast milk and the volume of milk consumed by healthy infants growing normally. Studies from Gopalan on Indian mothers have shown that this requirement is about 2.0 g/kg during the first two weeks which falls to around 1.1 g/kg at 94 weeks.[11] Beyond 6 months, breast milk is not adequate to sustain normal growth of an infant; supplements in the form of vegetable proteins have to be added to breast milk. Based on this fact, the computed values of protein requirements for infants are as given by ICMR (2010) in Table 2.10.[1]

In case of children, the protein requirements are computed based on figures of actual body weight and ideal body weight. The ICMR Expert Committee therefore recommended intakes based on body weights observed in normally growing well to do children as was done in case of energy requirements. These requirements are based on the assumption that the average quality of protein in Indian diets is considered to have net protein utilization (NPU) of 65%. (Table 2.10).

Fats

Fats are an important component of any Indian diet and provide a major percent of calories. Besides contributing to the calorie density of a diet, fats also help make the food palatable. Fats are made up of fatty acids which are mainly saturated or unsaturated. The unsaturated fats are further classified into mono and polyunsaturated fatty acids. Saturated fats are the ones which solidify at room temperature and include palmitic and stearic acid like ghee, hydrogenated fats and coconut oil. However, these are poor sources of essential fatty acids. The polyunsaturated fatty acids include linoleic acid (omega 6) and linolenic acid (omega 3), both of which are not synthesized in the body and hence have to be provided in the diet. These are termed as essential fatty acids like safflower, sunflower, corn and soya oils and contain almost 50–70 % of the

Table 2.10: Protein requirements and dietary allowances for infants boys and girls

Age group	Requirement[a,b] g protein/kg/d	Body weight g/d	Total daily requirement (g protien/d)	Requirement[a,b] g protein/kg/d	Body weight (kg)	Total daily requirement (g protien/d)
Infants (months)						
6–9	1.69	7.9	13.4			
9/12	1.69	8.8	14.9			
Preschool children (years)	*Boys*			*Girlss*		
1–2	1.47	10.3	15.1	1.47	9.6	14.1
2–3	1.25	12.8	16.0	1.47	12.1	15.1
3–4	1.16	14.8	17.2	1.16	14.5	16.8
4–5	1.11	16.5	18.3	1.08	16.0	17.8
School children (years)	*Boys*				*Girls*	
5–6	1.09	18.2	19.8	1.9	17.7	19.3
6–7	1.15	20.4	23.5	1.15	20.0	23.0
7–8	1.17	22.7	26.6	1.1	22.3	26.1
8–9	1.18	25.2	29.7	1.18	25.0	29.5
9–10	1.18	28.0	33.0	1.18	27.6	32.6
Adolescents (years)	*Boys*				*Girls*	
10–11	1.18	30.8	36.3	1.18	31.2	36.8
11–12	1.16	34.1	39.6	1.15	34.8	40.0
12–13	1.15	38.0	43.7	1.14	39.0	44.5

Contd...

Contd...

Age group	Requirement[a,b] g protein/kg/d	Body weight g/d	Total daily require-ment (g protien/d)	Requirement[a,b] g protein/kg/d	Body weight (kg)	Total daily require-ment (g protien/d)
13–14	1.15	43.3	49.8	1.13	43.4	49.0
14–15	1.14	48.0	54.7	1.12	47.1	52.8
15–16	1.13	51.5	58.2	1.09	49.4	53.8
16–17	1.12	54.3	60.8	1.07	51.3	54.9
17–18	1.10	56.5	62.2	1.06	52.8	56.0

[a] In terms of mixed indian vegetarian diet protein (Annexure 5.1; PDCAAS varying from 77.4 to 79.0% for different age groups, see Table 5.13)
[b] Requirements for each age band taken as the protein requirement for the lower age limit at that age band, see Tables 5.7 and 5.8.
[c] For infants below 6 months, see Table 5.6.
Source: ICMR 2010.

essential fatty acids. Groundnut oil has about 25% essential fatty acids (EFA). An important point to bear in mind is that the omega 6 and omega 3 fatty acids need to be maintained in a desirable ratio of around 5–10. A ratio beyond 10 can produce adverse affects like inflammatory diseases and respiratory problems like asthma. All refined oils are a good source of linoleic acid, but may be too low in linolenic acid, thereby disturbing the ratio. Oils like mustard and ghee have a balanced ratio of omega 6 and omega 3 and hence considered desirable in appropriate ratio. The ideal ratio of the three types of the fats should be one each of saturated fats polyunsaturated fats (PUFA) and monounsaturated fats (MUFA). A normally breast fed infant receives nearly 70 g of fat per day of which 10% is linoleic acid, and 1% is linoenic acid.[1] Thereby taking care of the requirements of EFA of an infant which is about 6% of total energy. The recommendations of fat as given by ICMR are as given in Table 2.11.

Infants: The fat content of human milk is relatively constant at 3–4% by weight and delivers 50–60% of energy. Infant formulae should have fat and individual fatty acid contents {including arachidonic (AA) and docosahexaenoic acid DHA)} similar to levels of human milk. Pre term infants have a higher requirement for AA and DHA.

A typical Indian mixed diet based on cereals, pulses and vegetables provides approximately 10–15% of fat as invisible fat. Based on this fact, the recommended the recommended level of visible fat is restricted to about 20% of total energy provided by the diet. In any case, the total fat intake should not exceed 30% of the total energy due to adverse affects on the cardiovascular system.

By the second half of the first year of life the percent fat can be increased to 35% of energy gradually, depending on the physical activity. Babies can

Table 2.11: Recommended fat requirements for infants and children

Age Group		Min. intake % energy	Invisible fat (foods) % energy	Visible fat % energy	(Cooking oil) g/d
Infants	0–6 months	40–60	Human milk	Human milk	25
	7–24 months	35[a]	10*	25	
Children	3–6 years	25	10	15	25
	7–9 years	25	10	15	30
Boys	10–12 years	25	10	15	35
	13–15 years	25	10	15	45
	16–17 years	25	10	15	50
Girls	10–12 years	25	10	15	35
	13–15 years	25	10	15	40
	16–17 years	25	10	15	35

Source: ICMR 2010.
a. gradually reduce depending on physical activity.
*human milk/infant formula + complementary foods.

derive a mix of breast feeds and complementary foods between 6–24 months which should provide at least 3–4.5% energy. By two years to adolescence (17 years), the fat intake should be approximately 25% of total energy to maintain growth, for which the minimum level of visible fat should range between 25 and 30 grams per day in the diets of children and adolescents (Table 2.11).

Vitamins

Fat-soluble Vitamins

These vitamins are stored in the liver and the body reserves can be utilized from day-to-day. These are not easily destroyed by heat unlike the water soluble vitamins. Generally, it is the deficiency of vitamin A and occasionally vitamin D which are encountered among children in the form of night blindness, Bitot's spots, (vitamin A) or rickets (vitamin D). However, the other two vitamin deficiency and K are not generally seen and hence no specific recommendations are made for different age groups. Recently vitamin E has been emphasized for its role as an anti-oxidant in many disease conditions in therapeutic doses. ICMR has recommended 0.8 mg per g of EFA in food. No such recommendation has been laid down for vitamin K.

Vitamin A: The recommended intake of vitamin A for infants and children in terms of retinol and beta carotene as determined by ICMR are given in Table 2.12. The requirement in early infancy is 50 µg/kg, based on the retinol content of breast milk of well nourished mothers.[12] This requirement is proportional to the growth rate of children at different stages.

Vitamin D: This vitamin is considered as a prohormone in the formation of bones and calcium absorption. The required amount is generally met by adequate exposure to sunlight. Estimates suggest that only 5 minutes of exposure to sunlight is adequate to meet the daily requirements.

Water-soluble Vitamins

As these vitamins are not stored in the body these need to be provided on a daily basis from dietary source.

Table 2.12: Recommended intake of vitamin A for children

Group	Age	Retinol (IU)	B-carotene (µg)*
Infants	0–6 months	350	-
	6–12 months		
Children	1–6 years	400	3200
	7–9 years	600	4800
Adolescents	10–17 years	600	4800

Source: ICMR 2010.
*Conversion ratio of 1:8 is used.

Table 2.13: Recommended intakes for calcium for children			
Group	Age	Calcium (mg/d)	Phosphorous (mg/d)
Infants		800	750
Children	1–9 years	600	600
	10–17 years	800	800

Source: ICMR 2010.

Vitamin C: This vitamin has an important role to play in prevention of scurvy. The recommended doses for infants and children are shown in Table 2.1.

B complex vitamins: This group includes vitamin B_1 (thiamine), B_2 (riboflavin), B_6 (pyridoxine), niacin, B_{12} and folate. Niacin is a derivative from tryptophan, an essential amino acid. 60 mg of tryptophan is equivalent to 1 mg of niacin. The RDA for B_1 and B_2 are computed on the basis of total calorie consumption or ideal calorie requirement as seen in Table 2.1.

Folic acid and B_{12}: These are mainly involved in hemopoesis, the deficiency of which can lead to megaloblastic anemia. The recommended intakes are shown in Table 2.1.

Calcium and Phosphorous

Calcium and phosphorous are an important component of a diet for infants and children due to their role in formation of strong skeletal system besides good dental health. Calcium in ionic form plays a crucial role in transmission of nerve impulses. On the other hand, phosphorous is an important constituent of nucleic acids and phospholipids involved in cellular metabolism. As in the case of EFA ratio, the Ca:P ratio also is important to be maintained at a desirable level of 1:1 in case of children and in infants 1:1.5. Table 2.13 gives the recommended intakes of calcium and phosphorous for children up to 18 years.[1] No recommendation has been fixed for phosphorous on the assumption that a mixed Indian diet can provide sufficient content to cater to the daily body needs.

Iron

The iron needs of an infant are taken care of by the breast milk up to 6 months of life. Beyond that milk, whether breast or cow's milk, both are inadequate to sustain the increasing demands of the child. Though breast milk too is not a very good source of iron, the needs of the infant are taken care of by the maternal reserves deposited during the course of the mother's pregnancy. At birth the infant has about 80 mgs of iron/kg body weight or total of 270 mg. The maternal iron stores are used up by the infant by 6 months after which there is no reserve store until about 2 years. During childhood the iron stores build up to 5 mg/kg, and remain so until menarche in the females. In males there is further increase of 12–15 mg/kg between 15 and 30 years.[1]

After 6 months, if the child is fed exclusively either on breast milk or cow's milk, or even predominantly formula milk, the reserve iron stores get gradually depleted. In this situation if no dietary source is provided, the child begins to show signs of anemia. Therefore, it is very important that from 6 months onwards, the child's feeds are supplemented with cereals, pulses and vegetables gradually over a period of time. Formula-fed babies may have an adequate store of iron as most of the baby milk formulae are fortified with important minerals and vitamins. The RDA for iron requirements of infants and children are as given in Table 2.1.

REFERENCES

1. Nutrient Requirement and Recommended Dietary Allowances for Indians. A Report of the Expert Group of the Indian Council of Medical Research. New Delhi, Indian Council of Medical Research, 2010.
2. Madavapeddi R, Narsinga Rao BS. Energy balance in lactating undernourished women. Eur L Nutr. 1992;46:349-54.
3. Raman L, Shatrugana V. Nutrition in pregnancy and lactation. In: Textbook of human nutrition Ed, Bamji MS, Rao NP, Reddy V. 1996.
4. Rathi S, Khosla A, Sharma N, et al. Pregnancy and outcome in severe anemia. J Obst Gynec India. 1987;4:478-80
5. Bhargava M, Kumar R, Iyer PU, Ramji S, et al. Effect of maternal anemia and iron depletion on fetal iron stores, birth weight and gestation. Acta Pediatr Scand. 1989;78:321-2.
6. Islam MA, Hemalatha P, Bhaskaran P, Ajeya Kumar P. Leucocyte and plasma zinc in maternal cord blood: Their relationship to period of gestation and birth weight. Nutr Res. 1994;14:353-60.
7. Roberts JM, Balk J, Bodnar LM, et al. Nutrition involvement in pre eclampsia. J Nutr. 2003;133(Suppl 2):1684S-1692S.
8. Kochupillai N. The impact of iodine deficiency on human resources development. Prog Food Sci. 1989;122:322-6.
9. MRC Vitamins Study Research Group: Prevention of neural tube defects. Results of the Medical Research Council Vitamin Study. Lancet. 1991:338:131-7.
10. Elizabeth KE. Applied Nutrition. In: Nutrition and Child Development, 3rd ed. Hyderabad: Paras Medical Publishers; 2004.
11. Gopalan C. Protein requirements of breast fed poor infants. J Trop Pediatr. 1956;289.
12. Mahtab S Bamji, Kamla Krishnaswamy, GNV Brahman. Nutrient Requirements. In: Textbook of Human Nutrition, 3rd ed. New Delhi: Oxford and IBH Publishing Co Pvt Ltd; 2010.

Nutritional Assessment of Children

In order to plan any dietary regime for a child or any individual, it is important to first have an idea of his/her preexisting condition. For this, the child is assessed for his nutritional status which may include various parameters depending upon what circumstances and where he is managed. Ideally nutritional assessment is the first step towards the management of a child brought in a hospital. This gives us an idea of his preexisting condition, besides the clinical picture that might be presented to us upon admission or may be in the out patient clinic also. Based on this assessment, the further course of action is planned.

The four main parameters generally used for nutritional assessment of a child in a hospital are as follows:

- Anthropometry
- Dietary
- Clinical
- Biochemical.

Besides these there are other parameters like radiological, morphological and epidemiological which are beyond the scope of present discussion. We shall look into the four parameters listed above in detail.

ANTHROPOMETRY

This is perhaps the first step undertaken when a child is presented for any medical management. The various parameters covered under this give a fair idea of the nutritional status of the child. However, it is important that measurements taken to assess anthropometry be very accurate and done by trained personnel using certain accepted standard techniques. In case of children, the parameters so assessed are compared to standard 'growth charts'. The weights and heights are plotted against the curve on these charts and depending upon where they fall, the level of nutritional status can be evaluated. The equipments used for the measurements also should be precise and free from errors. The tools used to cover anthropometry are as follows:

Weight

Weight is a useful tool to evaluate the nutritional status of children of all age groups, from birth to adolescence. The weighing scale should be accurate. The commonly used scales are the ones using a beam. Care should be taken to set the pointer at zero at resting phase and should be moving freely. The surface where the scale is placed should be flat and even. Readings are taken in kilograms. The accuracy should be to the nearest 500 grams for older children and for smaller children up to 100 grams. Electronic scales are commonly used in many centers and are more accurate. Ideally weight should be taken with minimum clothing and without shoes. Small children can be made to sit on the scale designed for them, while older children can be made to stand on the platform weighing scale.

The weights so measured are compared to some appropriate reference standards for his age, over a period of time which is done using the growth charts (Figs 3.1 to 3.6). The references internationally accepted are those by Combined National Center for Health Statistics (NCHS) and Center for Disease Control (CDS) Task Force, which have been published by WHO in 1983,[1] also referred as WHO standards. The fiftieth centile of Harvard Standards was taken as 100 percent and references are available for weight for age, height for age, weight for height and head circumference separately for boys and girls. Based on these reference standards, a child was classified as normal or malnourished. However, these charts are not much popular now after a new set of new growth charts were brought out in 2000 by the National Center for Chronic Disease Prevention and Health Promotion, referred to as the CDC charts. These are a revised version of the 1977 NCHS growth charts.[2] These charts consist of percentiles related to weight, length and head circumference for infants (0–36 months) and percentiles related to weight, height and BMI for children (2–19 years).

The new CDC charts now include an assessment for BMI (Figs 3.7 and 3.8). These are based primarily on data gathered through National Health and Nutrition Examination Survey (NHANES), the only survey that collects data from actual physical examination on a cross section of people from all over the United States. The new BMI growth charts can be used clinically beginning at 2 years of age, when an accurate stature can be obtained.

In order to revise the growth charts, the NHANES survey conducted from 1988 through 1994, contained more than 8000 children aged 2 months to six years. The data showed that in the past two decades, the number of overweight children and teens has doubled. It was hoped that these new charts will be used to identify overweight children and teens for intervention at an early age. Moreover, the new CDC charts track children through 19 years of age, two years longer than the 1977 NCHS charts. The revised head circumference charts also show some significant differences when compared to the earlier ones. Compared to the original infant charts that were based on primarily formula fed infants, the revised growth charts for infants contain a better mix of both breast and formula fed infants in the US population.

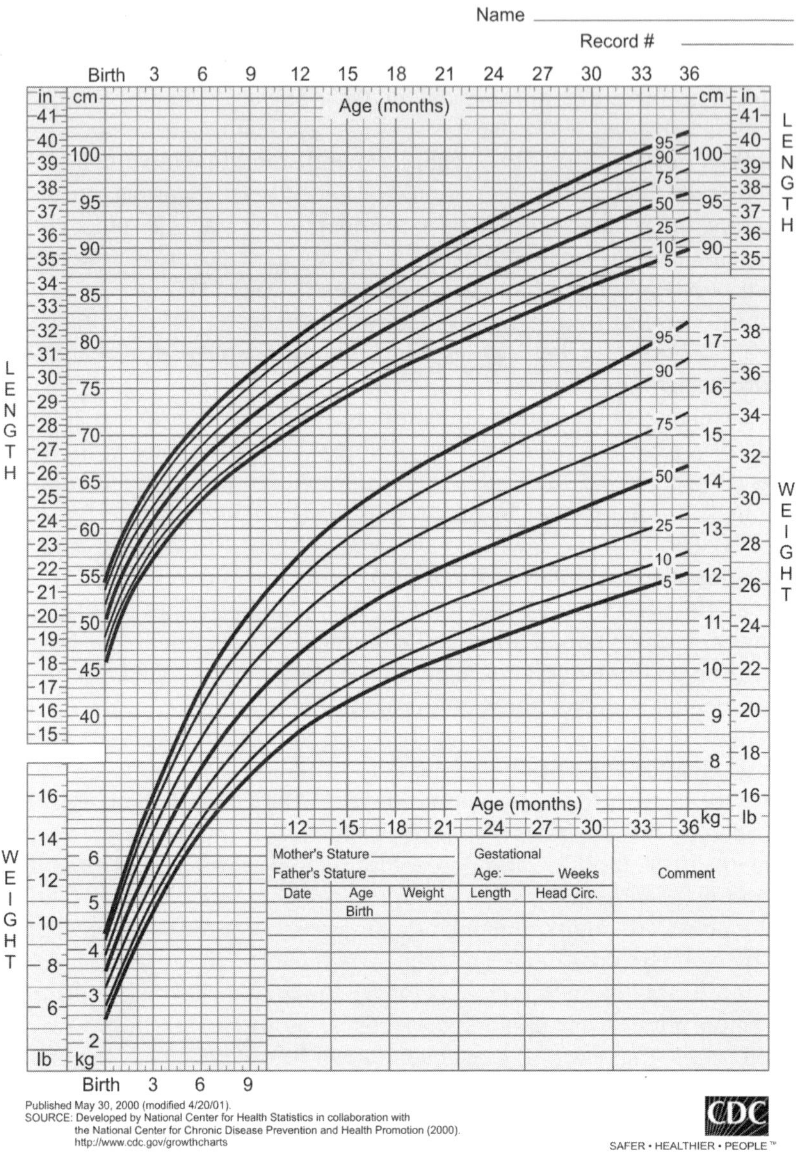

Name _____

Record # _____

Published May 30, 2000 (modified 4/20/01).
SOURCE: Developed by National Center for Health Statistics in collaboration with
the National Center for Chronic Disease Prevention and Health Promotion (2000).
http://www.cdc.gov/growthcharts

CDC

SAFER • HEALTHIER • PEOPLE™

Fig. 3.1: Birth to 36 months: Boys
Length-for-age and weight-for-age percentiles

WHO has published multicentric growth reference standard (MGRS) for 0-60 months boys and girls,[3] based on studies carried out among predominantly exclusively breast fed children for 6 countries (USA, Brazil, Ghana, Norway, Oman and India). The median weights of infants and preschool children (1–3 years) can be taken as reference values even for Indian children (Table 3.1).

Table 3.1: Median weights and lengths of 0–60 months children				
Boys		Age in months	Girls	
Weight (kg)	Length (cm)		Weight (kg)	Length (cm)
3.3	49.9	0	3.2	49.1
4.5	54.7	1	4.2	53.7
5.6	58.4	2	5.1	57.1
6.4	61.4	3	5.8	59.8
7.0	63.9	4	6.4	62.1
7.5	65.9	5	6.9	64.0
7.9	67.6	6	7.3	65.7
8.3	69.2	7	7.6	67.3
8.6	70.6	8	7.9	68.7
8.9	72.0	9	8.2	70.1
9.2	73.3	10	8.5	71.5
9.4	74.5	11	8.7	72.8
9.6	75.7	12	8.9	74.0
10.2	82.3	18	10.2	80.7
12.2	87.8	24	11.5	86.4
13.3	91.9	30	12.7	90.7
14.3	96.1	36	13.9	95.1
15.3	99.9	42	15.0	99.0
16.3	103.3	48	16.1	102.7
17.3	106.7	54	17.2	106.2
18.3	110.0	60	18.2	109.4

Source: Sauberlich Dowdy.[12]

IAP GROWTH MONITORING GUIDELINES (2015)

The growth charts committee of Indian Academy of Pediatrics has revised the growth charts for 5–18 years old Indian children in January 2015 ,as shown in Figs 3.9 and 3.10.[3] In view of the economic and nutritional transition taking over and consequently the growth pattern of Indian children, the last IAP charts of 2007 now seem obsolete and hence, no longer applicable. These new charts were compiled by collating from nine groups and were constructed from total of 87,022 middle and upper socioeconomic families from all five zones of India (Agartala, Ahmedabad, Chandigarh, Chennai, Delhi, Hyderabad, Kochi, Kolkata, Madurai, Mumbai, Mysuru, Pune, Raipur and Surat).

Name _____

Record # _____

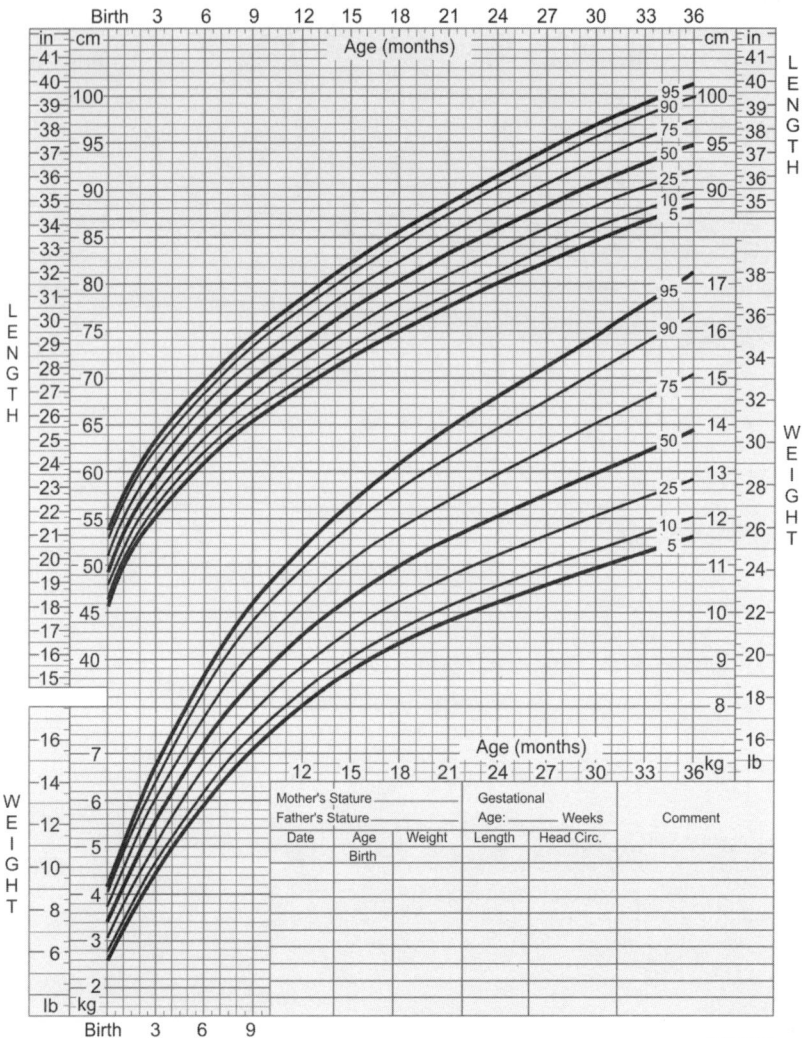

Fig. 3.2: Birth to 36 months: Girls
Length-for-age and weight-for-age percentiles

BODY MASS INDEX (BMI)

This is a measure of body fatness expressed in relation to body weight and height. It is calculated as wt (kg)/ht (m)^2. Certain cut off values have been fixed

Name _____

Record# _____

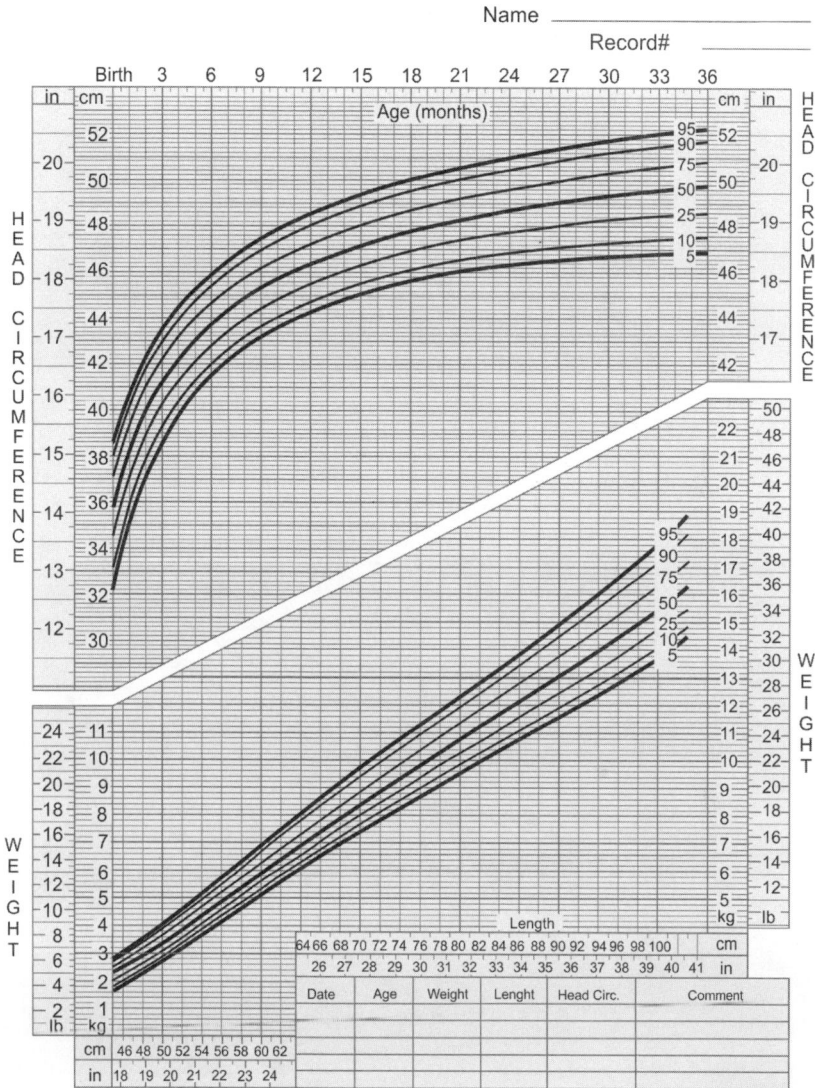

Fig. 3.3: Birth to 36 months: Boys
Head circumference-for-age and weight-for-length percentiles

for defining under nutrition or over nutrition. BMI changes with age. At birth, the median is about 13 kg/m², increasing to 17 at one year and then decreasing to 15 at 6 years and gradually increasing to 21 by adulthood.

In recent years, BMI has received increased attention for pediatric use. In 1994, an expert committee charged with developing guidelines for overweight

Name _____

Record# _____

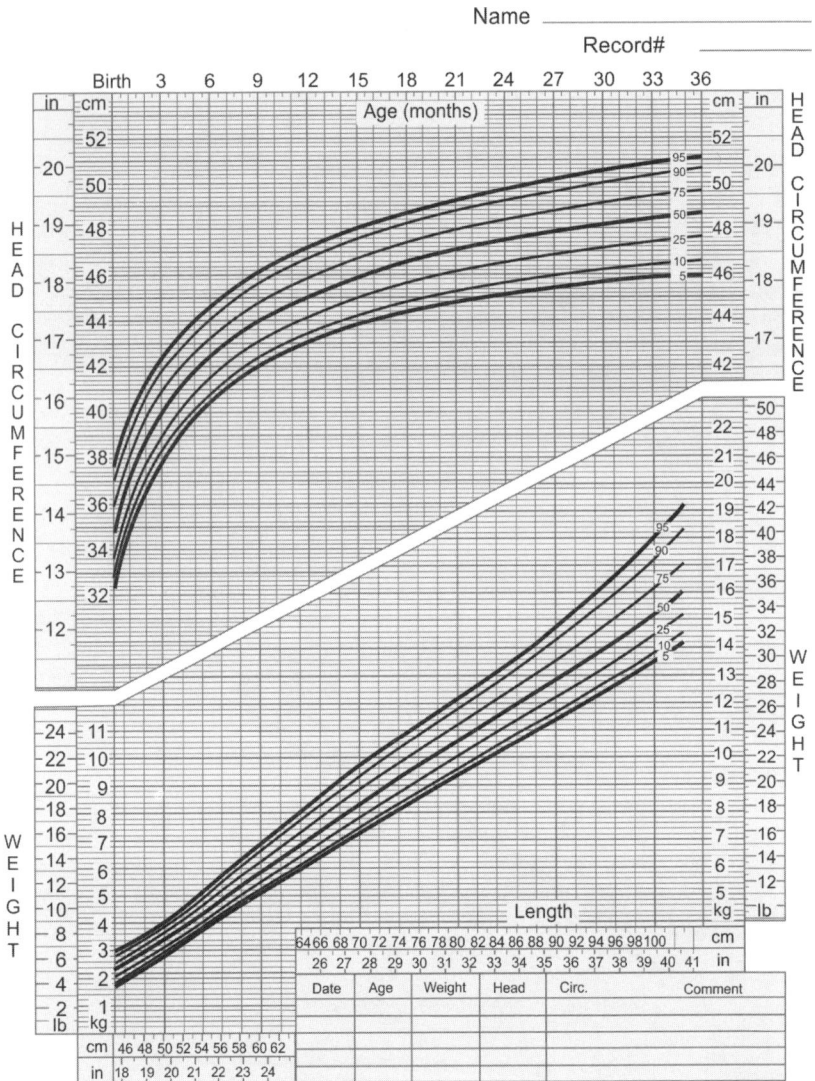

Fig. 3.4: Birth to 36 months: Girls
Head circumference-for-age and weight-for-length percentiles

in adolescent preventive services (ages 11–21 years) recommended that BMI be used routinely to screen overweight adolescents. In addition, in 1997 an expert committee on the assessment and treatment of obesity concluded that BMI should be used to screen for overweight children, ages 2 years and older, using BMI curves from the revised growth charts. BMI can also be

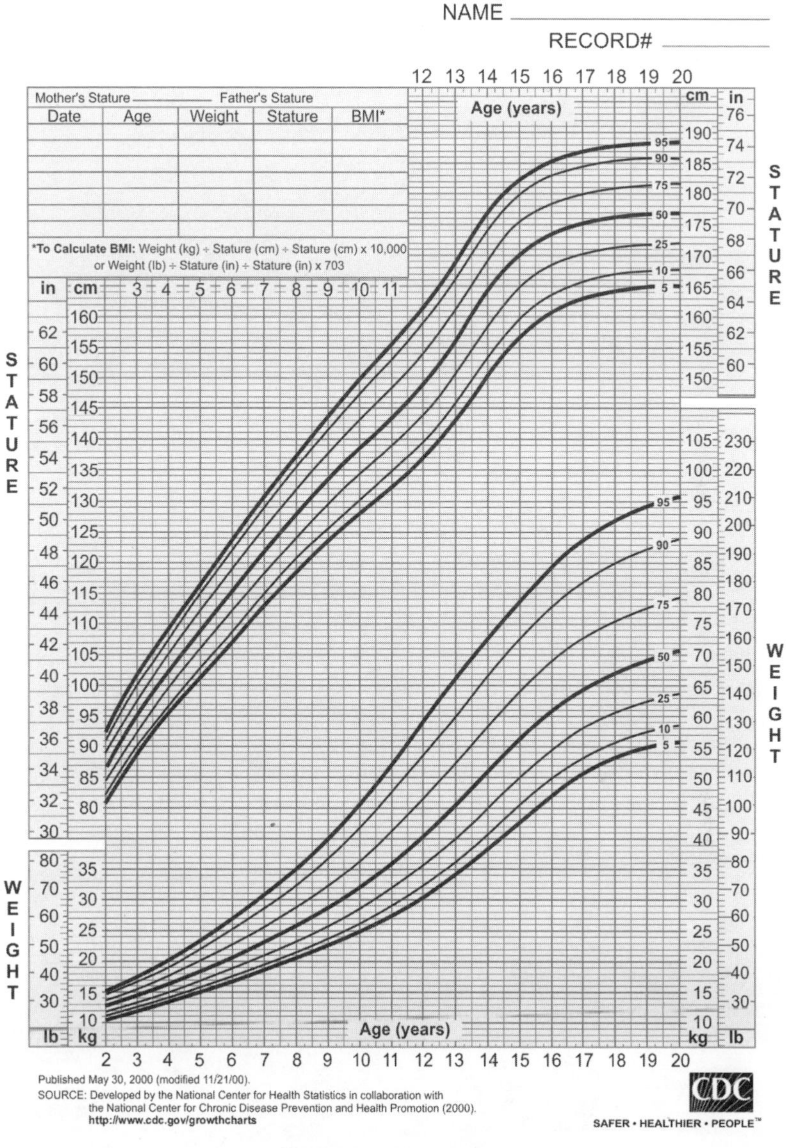

NAME _____

RECORD# _____

Fig. 3.5: 2 to 20 years: Boys
Stature-for-age and weight-for-age percentiles

used to characterize underweight (though no expert guidelines exist for the classification of underweight based on BMI).[4]

However, most studies have shown that even though BMI above 18.5 is regarded as normal, most of our adolescents falling below 13 years have a BMI >18.5. It was felt by certain workers that BMI <15 indicated under nutrition or

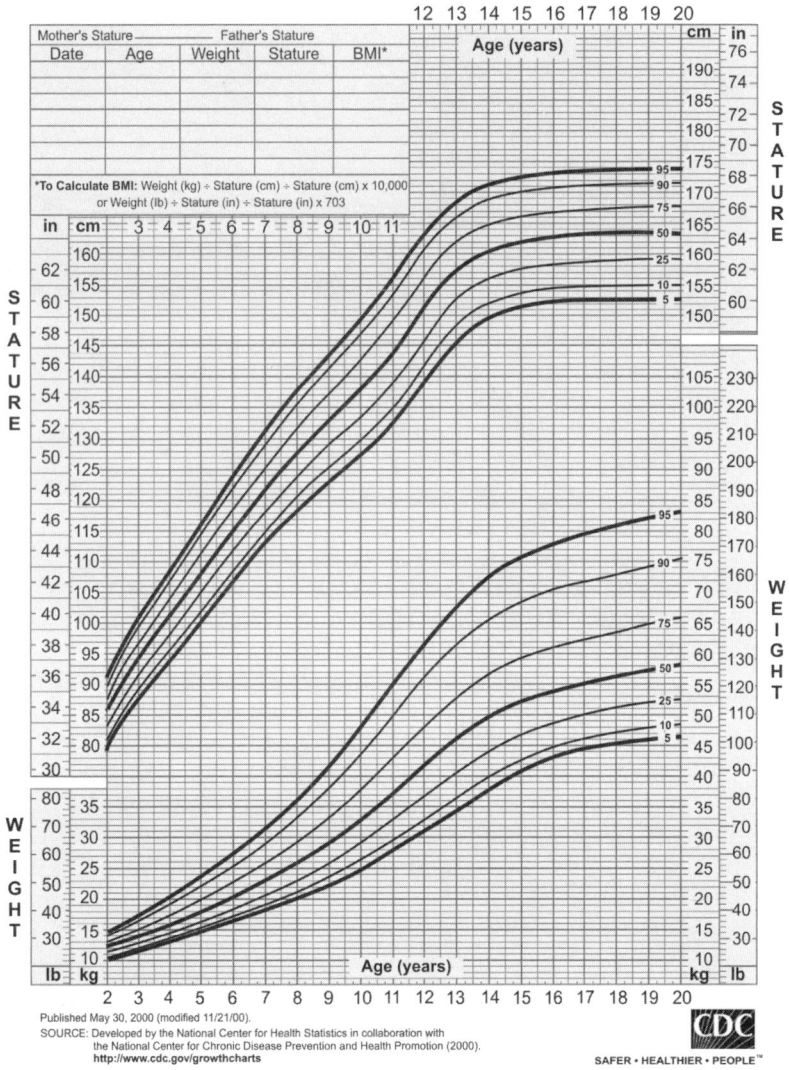

Fig. 3.6: 2 to 20 years: Girls
Stature-for-age and weight-for-age percentiles

chronic energy deficiency (CED) and <13 indicates severe malnutrition. The upper value of 22 has been fixed as cut off for overweight and 25 for obesity in young adolescents during the growth period.

As compared to previous IAP charts, boys and girls were taller at all ages. At 18 years average boy's height was 2.8 cm higher and the 97th percentile was 5 cm higher; for girls these figures were 0.8 cm and 2.6 cm.

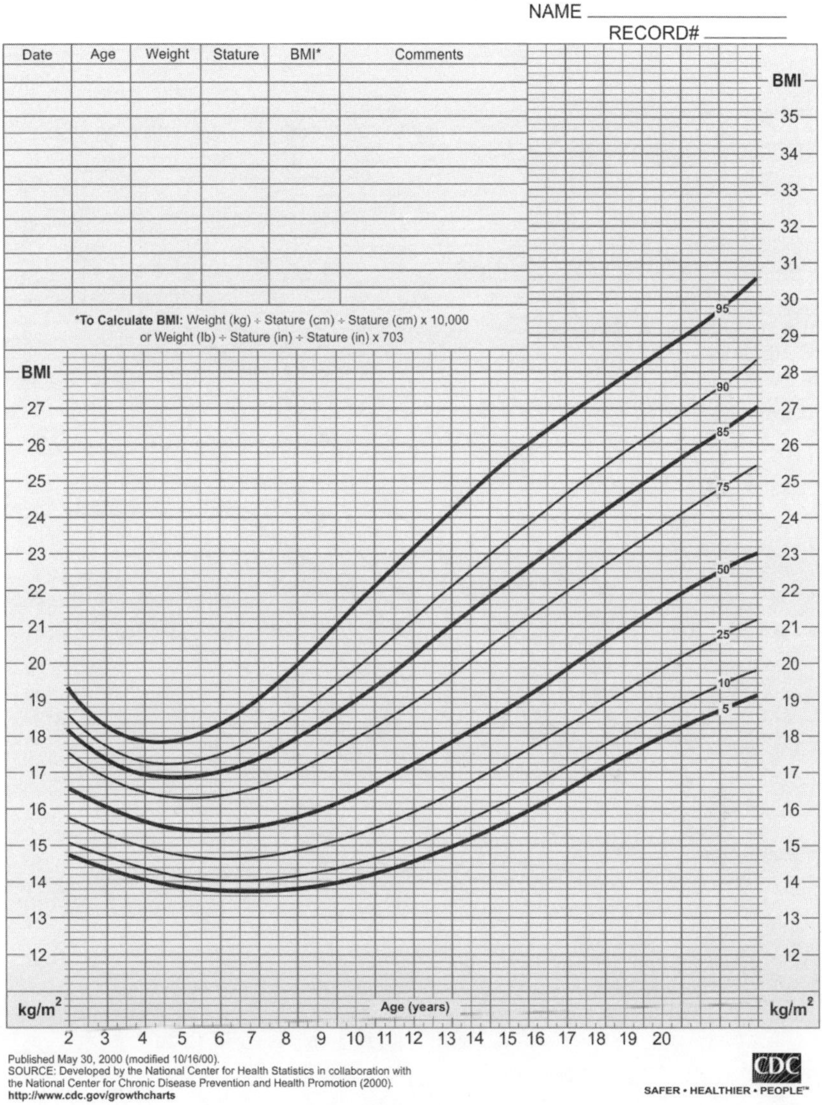
NAME
RECORD#
Date
Age
Weight
Stature
BMI*
Comments
*To Calculate BMI: Weight (kg) ÷ Stature (cm) ÷ Stature (cm) x 10,000
or Weight (lb) ÷ Stature (in) ÷ Stature (in) x 703
BMI
35
34
33
32
31
30
29
28
27
26
25
24
23
22
21
20
19
18
17
16
15
14
13
12
95
90
85
75
50
25
10
5
kg/m2
Age (years)
2 3 4 5 6 7 8 9 10 11 12 13 14 15 16 17 18 19 20
Published May 30, 2000 (modified 10/16/00).
SOURCE: Developed by the National Center for Health Statistics in collaboration with
the National Center for Chronic Disease Prevention and Health Promotion (2000).
http://www.cdc.gov/growthcharts
CDC
SAFER • HEALTHIER • PEOPLE™

Fig. 3.7: 2–20 years: Boys
Body mass index-for-age percentiles

BMI charts as presented in Figs 3.11 and 3.12 are based on those suggested by IOTF.[5]

The 23 and 27 adult equivalent cut off line (for overweight and obesity, respectively) are more appropriate for use in Asian children as Asians are known to have more adiposity and increased cardio-metabolic risk at a lower BMI.[6]

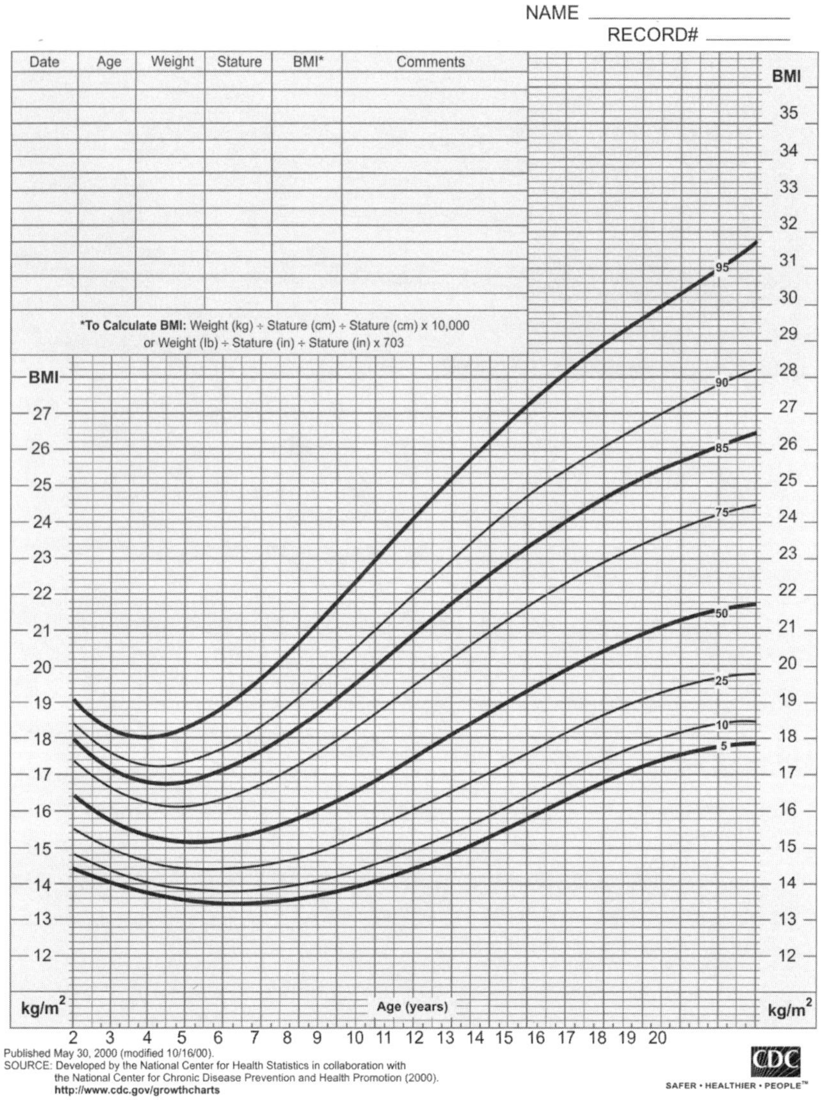
NAME
RECORD#
Date
Age
Weight
Stature
BMI*
Comments
*To Calculate BMI: Weight (kg) ÷ Stature (cm) ÷ Stature (cm) x 10,000
or Weight (lb) ÷ Stature (in) ÷ Stature (in) x 703
BMI
35
34
33
32
31
30
29
28
27
26
25
24
23
22
21
20
19
18
17
16
15
14
13
12
95
90
85
75
50
25
10
5
kg/m2
Age (years)
2 3 4 5 6 7 8 9 10 11 12 13 14 15 16 17 18 19 20
Published May 30, 2000 (modified 10/16/00).
SOURCE: Developed by the National Center for Health Statistics in collaboration with
the National Center for Chronic Disease Prevention and Health Promotion (2000).
http://www.cdc.gov/growthcharts
CDC
SAFER • HEALTHIER • PEOPLE™

Fig. 3.8: 2–20 years: Girls
Body mass index-for-age percentiles

The new IAP 2015 study 23 and 27 adult equivalent cut offs are very close to IOTF's extended 23 ad 27 cut offs in both sexes. These charts show that there is little difference between the stature of Indian children and the Caucasian children until the onset of pubertal years, but beyond that the growth spurt is reduced in Indian children in both sexes, although in girls this effect is more pronounced. The difference in height between the Caucasian and the Indian

5–18 Years : IAP Girls Body Mass Index Charts

Name _____
DOB _____

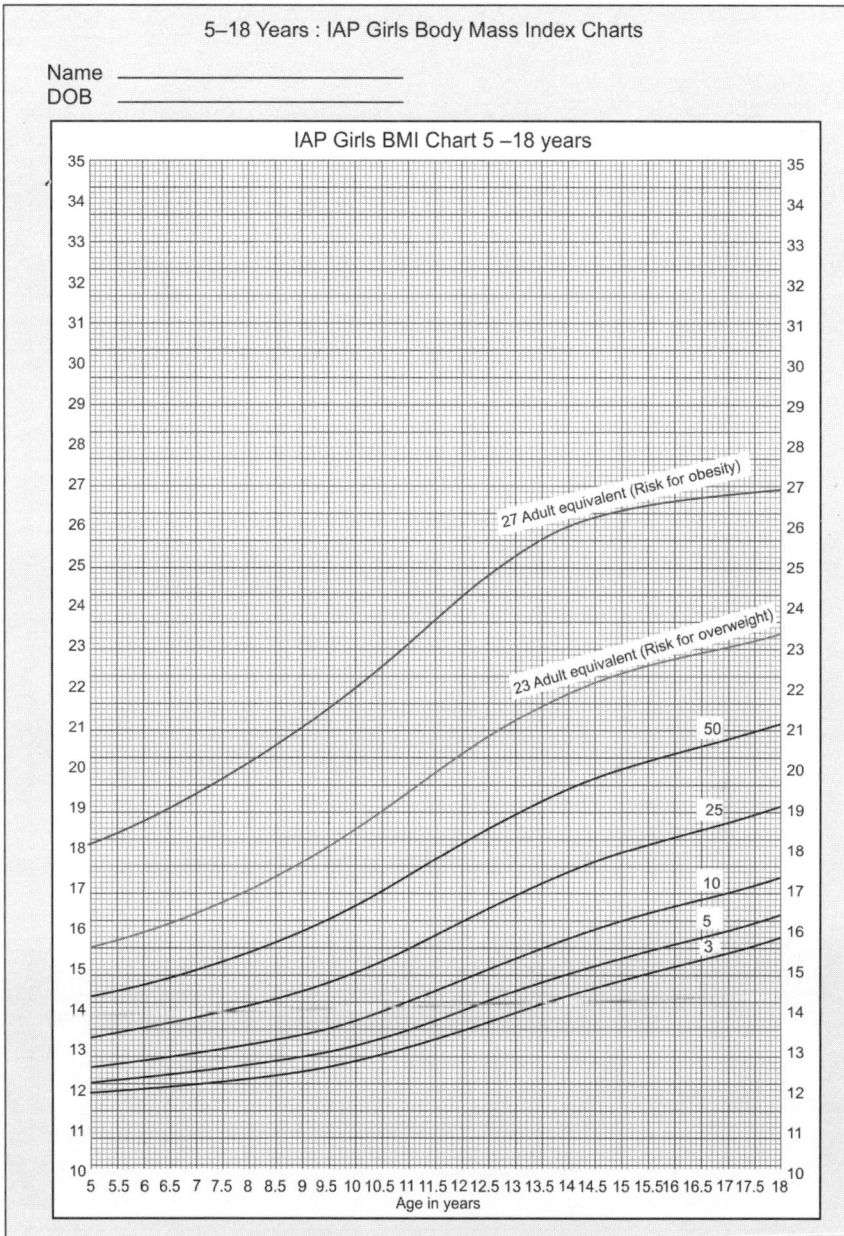

Fig. 3.9: Growth charts (girls) 5–18 years
Refer 3. IAP Growth Charts Committee. Khaldilkar V, Yadav S, et al. Indian Pediatrics. 2015;52:47-55

girls is about 1 cm (ages 5–11 years) but this gap widens to 6 cm at 18 years. In boys too the gap is 1 cm till age 5–12.5 years, but thereafter it becomes 3.5 cm at 18 years.

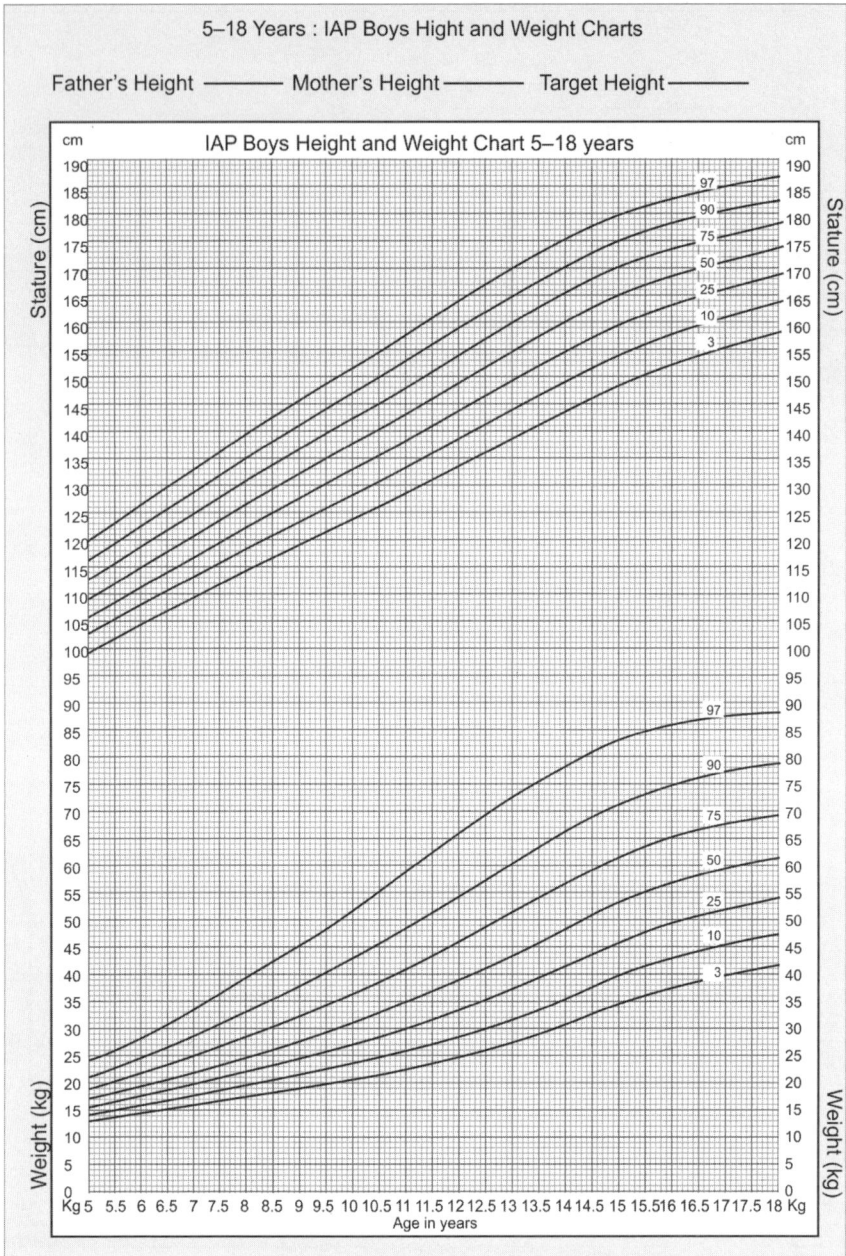

5–18 Years : IAP Boys Hight and Weight Charts

Father's Height ———— Mother's Height ———— Target Height ————

IAP Boys Height and Weight Chart 5–18 years

Fig. 3.10: Growth charts (boys) 5–18 years
Refer 3. IAP Growth Charts Committee. Khaldilkar V, Yadav S, et al. Indian Pediatrics. 2015;52:47-55

These new growth charts can also be relevant to calculate the target height and predicting adult height based on the prediction equations (Figs 3.9 and 3.10).

5–18 Years : IAP Girls Body Mass Index Charts

Name _____

DOB _____

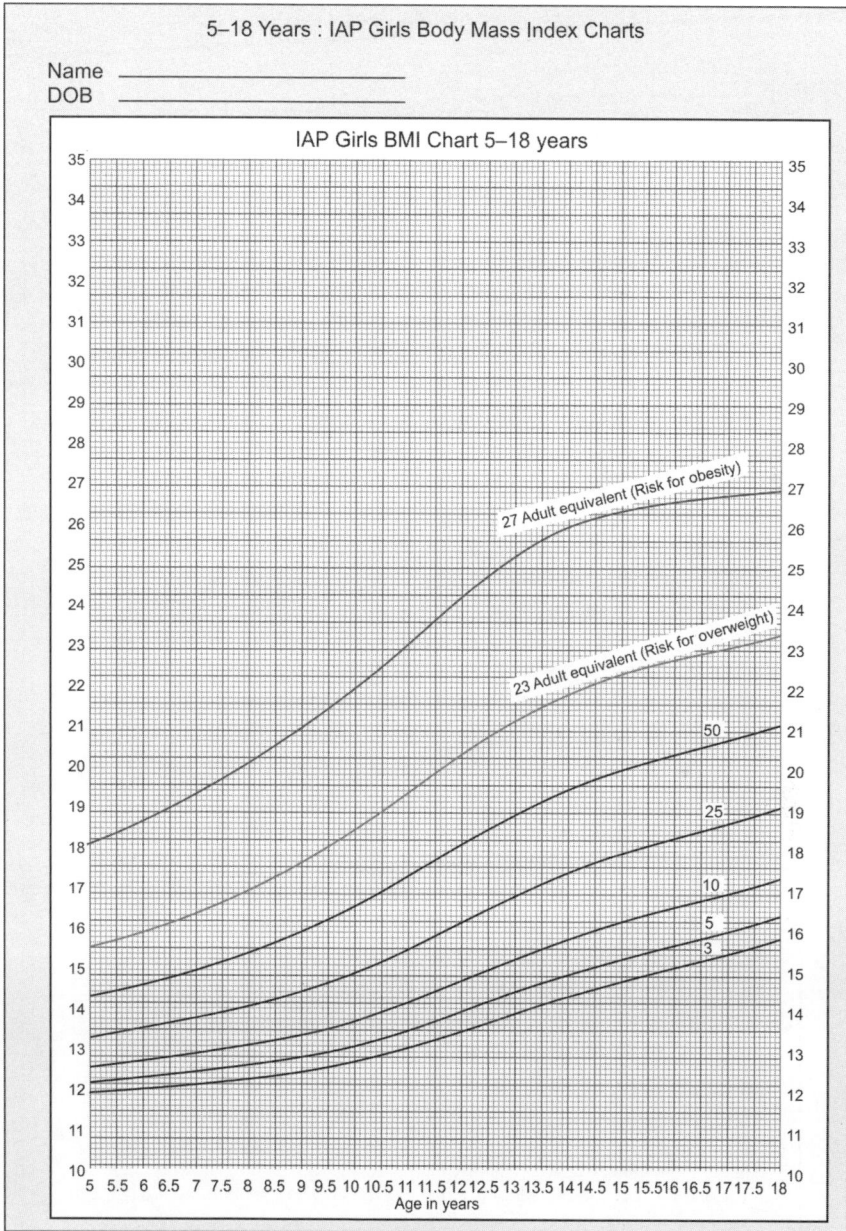

Fig. 3.11: BMI charts (girls) 5–18 years

Refer 3. IAP Growth Charts Committee. Khaldilkar V, Yadav S, et al. Indian Pediatrics. 2015;52:47-55

There are different classifications used by different workers to categorize children as normal or malnourished. For malnutrition, further classifications have been made to differentiate between varying degrees of malnutrition

5–18 Years : IAP Body Mass Index Charts

Name _____

DOB _____

IAP BMI Chart 5–18 years

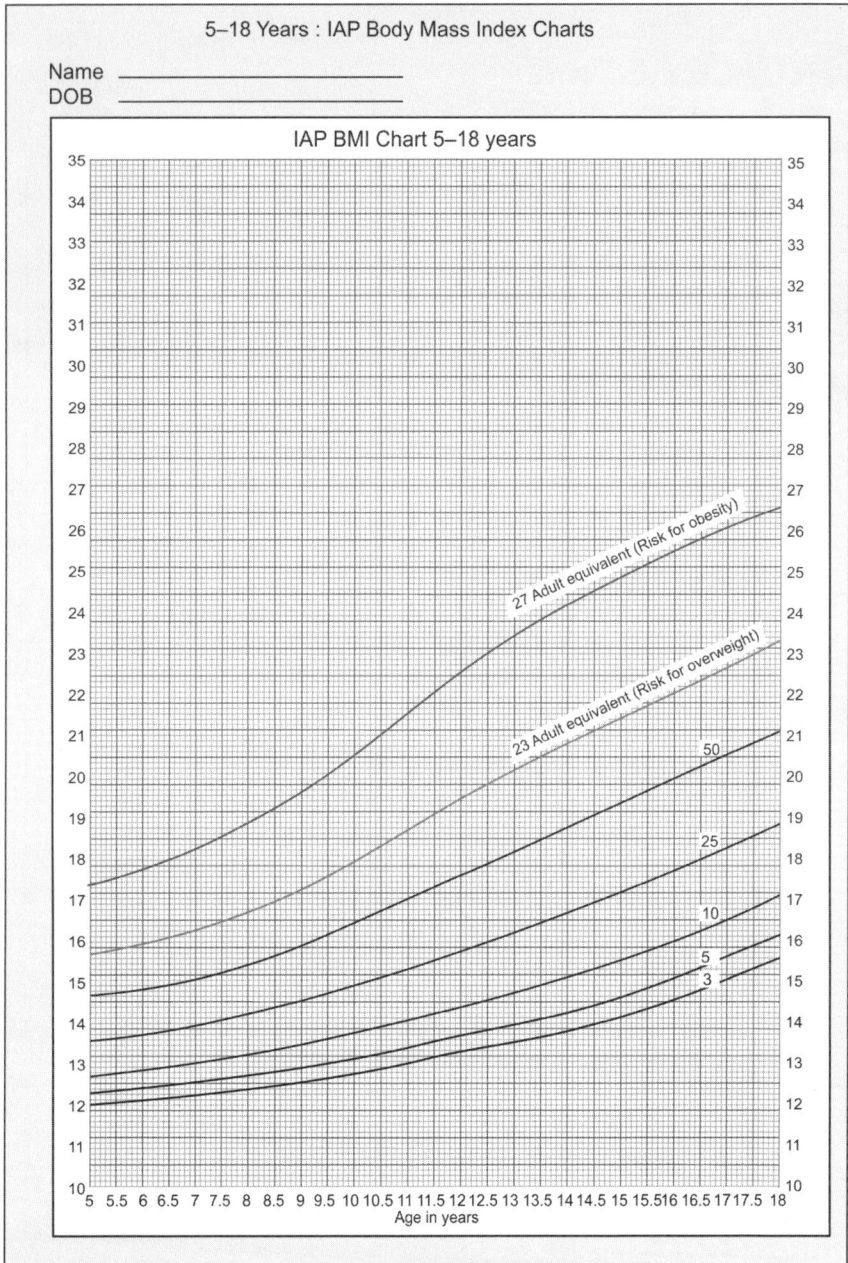

Fig 3.12: BMI charts (boys) 5–18 years
Refer 3. IAP Growth Charts Committee. Khaldikhar V, Yadav S, et al. Indian Pediatri.2015;52:47-55

from mild to severe. The most widely used are the Gomez classification and the Indian Academy of Pediatrics (IAP) classification.[7,8] as given in Table 3.2 and 3.3.

Table 3.2: The Gomez classification

% expected	Classification	Category of nutr. Status wt. for age
>90%	Normal	Normal
76–90	Mild malnutrition	1st degree malnutrition
61–75	Moderate malnutrition	2nd degree malnutrition
<60	Severe malnutrition	3rd degree malnutrition

Table 3.3: The IAP classification

% of expected weight (wt. for age)	Nutritional classification*
>80%	Normal
71–80	Grade 1
61–70	Grade 2
51–50	Grade 3 (severe malnutrition)
<50	Grade 4 (severe malnutrition)

*If coexisting edema of nutritional origin, the letter K is suffixed along with grade of malnutrition to denote kwashiorkor.

HEIGHT/LENGTH

In case of infants and children up to age 1–2 years, the length can be measured placing the child lying down using a horizontal measuring rod or an infantometer. The child is made to lie down flat on the back with the head just touching against the fixed end with a vertical board. The legs are stretched with the knees pressed together and the other mobile end (foot end) is made to touch the heels with feet at right angles. This procedure requires at least two people to take the measurements. The accuracy is usually up to 0.5 cm. It may be worth mentioning here that height for any age may not always be a correct indicator of the nutritional status of a growing child. But it does definitely give an idea of any past or chronic malnutrition. Height is largely genetically predisposed also; therefore such factors may reflect possible variations in any age group.

WEIGHT FOR HEIGHT

Weight for height is age independent. This criterion may not give a true picture of nutrition of a child since height measured at a given time may not always co-relate to the weight for height standard. In case a child has the desired weight for height but his linear growth is inadequate, it would be wrong to term this child as normal, even though his actual growth is inadequate. Therefore, height for age also needs to be accounted for along with weight for height. This criteria had been proposed by Seoane and Lytham (Table 3.4).[9] This criteria has been found to be better than other criteria as reviewed by Sastry and Vijayraghvan.[10]

Table 3.4: Seoane and Lytham classification

Nutritional status	Height for age (cm)	Weight for age (kg)	Weight for height (cm)
Normal	Normal	Normal	Normal
Past chronic malnutrition	Low	Low	Normal
Current short-duration malnutrition	Normal	Low	Low
Current long-duration malnutrition	Low	Low	Low

MID ARM CIRCUMFERENCE (MAC)

This measurement is made on a nondominant arm, midway between the acromial and olecranon processes, with the arm hanging relaxed. Measurements are done using a simple flexible measuring tape, gently without applying any pressure. This reading should be taken to the nearest 0.1 cm. MAC corelates well with weight for height. The cut off points used to determine malnutrition using this criterion are as follows:

Normal   —   14.00 cm
Mild/Acute malnutrition   —   12.4–14 cm
Severe malnutrition   —   <12.5 cm

HEAD CIRCUMFERENCE

This is also referred as occipitofrontal circumference (OFC) which is measured using a flexible measuring tape being firmly placed over the most prominent region of the occipital and frontal crests. The measurement is taken accurately to the nearest 0.1 cm. However, this parameter is of value for children up to about 2 years only, since by this age the increase in head circumference is usually complete.

CHEST CIRCUMFERENCE

This measurement is also done using a flexible tape and is taken at the level of the nipple, with the child sitting, midway between inspiration and expiration. In infancy, the OFC is more than the chest circumference, but by one year of age, both are almost equal, after which the chest circumference takes over the head circumference. In malnourished children, this ratio of OFC to chest continues to be >1, i.e. OFC continuing to be more than chest circumference.

TRICEPS SKINFOLD (TSF)

This is done using a Harpenden skinfold caliper and is calculated to the nearest millimeter. This measurement is made on the back of the nondominant arm mid way between the acrmial and the olecranon process, with the arm hanging relaxed

MID ARM-MUSCLE CIRCUMFERENCE

This is derived by using the MAC and the TSF using the following equation:
MAMC (cm) = MAC (cm) – TSF (mm) x 0.314

MID PARENTAL HEIGHT (MPH)

This criterion is not usually used as a routine. However, where the child is presented with growth retardation or short stature, this formula proves to be a helpful tool. The estimate for boys and girls is done as follows:

$$\text{Boys} = \frac{\text{Father's height} = \text{Mother's height} + 13}{2}$$

$$\text{Girls} = \frac{\text{Father's height} = \text{Mother's height} - 13}{2}$$

The values obtained for all the above measurements are compared to percentiles based on the child's age and sex as given in the growth charts. Values of less than 5% are indicative of significant malnutrition where as above 95th percentile denote over nutrition or obesity.

Apart from all the above parameters used to assess nutritional status, there are certain criteria made use of for quick bedside evaluation of the child's status. This formula is referred to as the Weech's formula or the NCHS criteria. In this formula, the expected weight is based on the assumption that *birth weight doubles by 5 months and triples by 1 year (10 kg) and quadruples by 2 years (12 kg). Thereafter, add 2 kg per year for children up to 6 years of age, and beyond that add 3 kg per year till puberty. Similarly, for height also, assuming birth length to be 50 cm, it becomes 75 cm at 1 year and 87.5 cm by 2 years. Birth length doubles by 4 years, after which 6 cm per year is added on till puberty. Birth length triples by 12 years.*

For head circumference, at birth it is considered 35 cm. It increases to 40 cm by 3 months, 45 cm by 9 months, 47 cm by 1 year, 49 cm by 2 years and 50 cm, by 3 years. The approximate increase is 2.0 cm per month in the first 3 months, 1 cm per month in the next 3 months and 0.5 cm per month in the next 6 months.[6] These bedside calculations are summarized in Table 3.5.

Table 3.6 shows formulae for calculating average weight, height and head circumference in children from birth to 12 years.[4]

ROAD TO HEALTH CHARTS

The commonly used growth charts that are used in most child health centers and wellness clinics and ICDS programs are given in Fig. 3.13. These colored charts are popularly termed as Road to Health Chart. The health worker plots the actual weight and height on them on each visit. The curve so formed

Age (years)	Weight (kg)	Height (cm)	Head circumference (cm)
Birth	3	50	33–35
3/12	5	60	39–40
6/12	7	66	42–44
9/12	9	71	44–45
1	10	75	45–47
2	12	87	47–49
3	14	94	49–50
4	16	100	50–51
5	18	106	50–52
6	20	112	51–52
7	23	118	
8	26	124	
9	29	130	
10	32	136	
11	35	142	
12	38	150	

Table 3.5: Bedside calculation for weight*, height**, head circumferences

*Add 2 kg/year in 1=6 years of age and add 3 kg/year thereafter till puberty
**Add 6 cm/year after 2 years of age till puberty

depicts the status of nutrition in that child. If the curve is within the green zone in the colored chart, if indicates normal nutrition. If the curve falls along the lower 'red zone' it will indicate severe malnutrition. Similarly, if the curve is along the 'blue or yellow zones, they will be considered as mild to moderately malnourished.[4]

DIETARY ASSESSMENT

After assessing the anthropometry, the next step to evaluate the nutritional status is to do the dietary assessment. This can be done in two ways. One is the qualitative intake and the other is the quantitative aspect. Qualitative assessment is done mainly to get information on the type of food consumed in a particular population or section of population with regard to their social or cultural background and food practices. These methods are more relevant in institutions or group of population for survey studies. The other being the quantitative evaluation which deals with the actual amounts of different foods consumed in terms of cooked and raw amounts and subsequently, the nutrients derived from these foods. These intakes are then assessed in terms of their adequacy vis a vis the RDA for any particular group of population. It is this aspect of the dietary evaluation which is relevant in the present context.

Table 3.6: Formula for average weight, height and head circumference in children (children birth to 12 years)

Weight	kg
Birth	3
3–12 months	$\dfrac{\text{Age (month)} + 9}{2}$
1–6 years	$\text{Age (year)} \times 2 + 8$
7–12 years	$\dfrac{\text{Age (year)} \times + 7 - 5}{2}$
Height	**cm**
Birth	50
3 months	60
6 months	66
1 year	75
2–12 years	$\text{Age (year)} \times 6 + 77$
Head circumference	**cm**
Birth	35
Infant	$\dfrac{\text{Length (cm)}}{2} + 9.5 \pm 2.5$
3 months	40
6 months	43
1 year	47
2 years	49
3 years	50
4 years	50.4
5 years	50.8

In order to know whether the child's intake in terms of macro- and micronutrients is adequate or not, a detailed dietary history needs to be elicited from the mother. In our country, the mother is the best source of providing the information, since she is the only one who is actually cooking and feeding the child. The two commonly used criteria used for assessing the dietary history are as follows:

24-hour Dietary Recall Method

Food Frequency Method

Recall method: The mother is asked to recall the diet consumed by the child over the past 24 hours in detail. She is asked to recount all the ingredients or

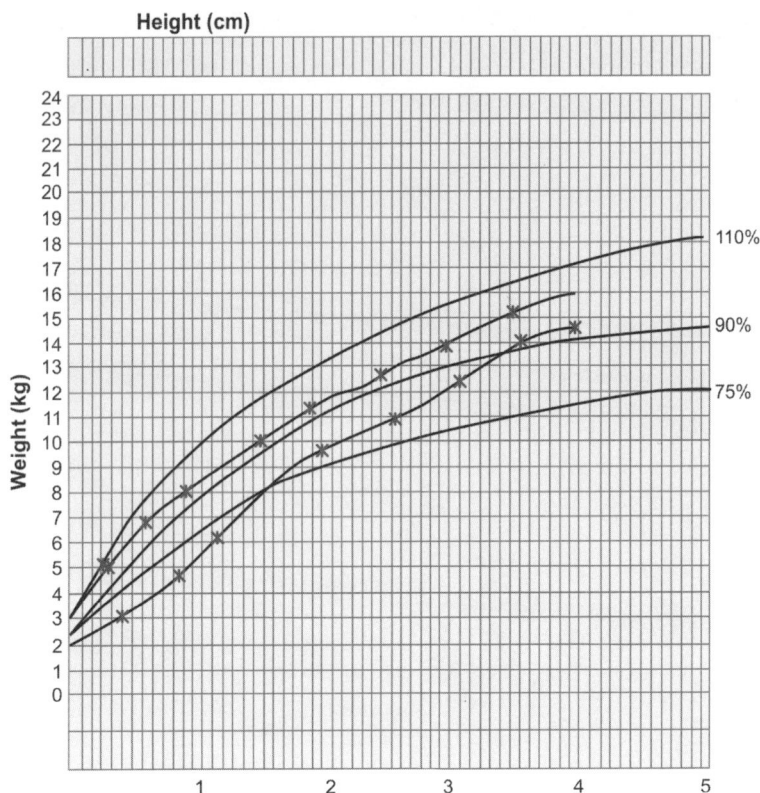

Fig. 3.13: Road to health chart[4]

foods that the child has consumed in terms of quantitative household measures which are standardized like spoons, cups, glasses or 'katoris'. For instance, a standard glass tumbler generally of 200 mL, or a tea cup is equated to 150 mL or a teaspoon is of 5 mL. In case of cooked food like a roti of 25, 30 or 35 g small, medium or large size generally is equivalent to raw weight of flour amounting to 25, 30 or 35 g respectively. Table 3.7 represents some of the foods used daily, their portion size and their calories/protein content.[11]

The raw weights then elicited from the cooked portions, the nutritive value of various macro- and micronutrients can be calculated using the standard ICMR reference tables.[11]

We can also make use of the Food Exchange Table 3.8,[11] to calculate the nutrients, mainly the macronutrients. By this method, portion size of the main food groups are so fixed so that one exchange equates to 100 calories. The amount of food consumed can be assessed in terms of number of exchanges and the approximate calories derived from those foods can be calculated; e.g one medium roti which is equivalent to about 30 g is of around 100 calories. Similarly, one medium katori of cooked dal equates to about 30 g which again equates to roughly 100 calories. The portion content of the different food exchanges can also be fixed for easy reference using Table 3.9.[11]

Table 3.7: Nutritive values of common household measures of cooked foods

Foods	Measure (cooked)	Volume/ amt. (raw)	Energy	Protein g	Fat g	Carbohydrate g
Buffalo milk	1 glass	250 g	292.5	10.75	16.25	12.5
Cow milk	1 glass	250 g	167.5	8	10.25	11
Paneer	1 cube	25 g	66	4.6	5.2	0.3
Skimmed milk	1 cup	250	72.5	6.25	0.25	11.5
Paneer (buffalo)	1 cube	25 g	73	3.35	5.2	0.3
Curd	1 cup	100 g	60	3	4	3
Roti (small)	1	25 g	85.25	3	0.42	17.35
Roti (big)	1	30 g	102.3	3.63	0.41	20.82
Dal (wash)	1 katori	30 g	105	17.7	0.74	6.87
Dal (whole)	1 katori	30 g	105.5	15.5	1.47	7.55
Vegetable	1	100 g	23	1.3	0.2	4
Leafy veg		100 g	42.8	4.2	0.92	4.52
Root veg		100 g	57.71	1.1	0.2	13
Banana	1 medium	100 g	11.6	1.2	0.3	27.2
Apple	1 medium	100 g	59	0.2	0.5	13.4
Citrus fruit	1 medium	100 g	46	0.8	0.4	9.78
Egg	1	50 g	86	6.6	6.6	-
Chicken	-	100 g	109	26.0	0.6	-
Fish	-	100 g	104	18	1.9	3.65
Mutton (with bone)	-	100 g	118	21.4	3.6	-
Veg oil	1 tsp	5 mL	45		5	
Butter	1 tsp	10 g	73		8	
Cream	1 tsp	5 g	10		1.0	
Sugar	1 tsp	5 g	20			5
Honey	1 tsp	5 mL	16			4
Brown bread	1 slice	15 g	36.6	1.32	0.21	7.35
White bread	1 slice	15 g	36.75	1.17	0.11	7.79
Biscuit (Marie)	2 no.		56		1	
Biscuit (Good day)	2 no.		100		6	

Table 3.8: Food exchange Table I

Cereal exchange (100 calories)	Meat exchange (80 calories)	Milk exchange (100 calories)
Chapati = 1 (flour—30 g) Bread = 2 slices Rice = 25 g (raw) = 65 g (cooked) (2/3 cooked katories) Country porridge = 20 g Oatmeal porridge = 20 g Dall = 85 g (cooked)	Egg = one Fish = 90 g Chicken = 100 g Meat = 50 g C. Cheese = 20 g Curd (g) = 150 g Dall = 30 g (1 katori cooked)	Cow's milk = 1 cup (150 cc) Tone milk = 1 cup (150 cc) Buffalo's milk dd-dd ½ cup Skimmed milk = 3½ cups Curd = 3½ cups (200 g) Butter milk = 600 cc

Fruit exchange (50 calories in each portion)

Items	Qty.	Weight	Items	Qty.	Weight
Apple big = small =	½ 1	80 g	Orange	1 medium	100 g
Mausami	1 medium	125 g	Lemon	2 medium	100 g
Papaya	¼	150 g	Per	1 medium	100 g
Arhu	2 medium	100 g	Alucha	4–5	100 g
Kharbuja	¼ slice	300 g	Amrud	1	80 g
Lichi	2–3	80 g	Jamun	6–7	80 g
Loquate	5–6	120 g			

Source: NIN.

This method may not be 100% accurate, but will suffice for bedside calculation of a child's intake and thereby assess his/her nutritional status. It can give us an idea whether the child's intake in terms of the macro- or micro-nutrients are adequate or not. These estimates can be corelated with their clinical, anthropometry or biochemical parameters, thereby giving a fair idea of the nutritional status of the child. For more accurate estimates required in surveys over a larger population, the same recall method is used but with more details. Besides eliciting the quantitative and qualitative intake, the volume of total cooked food is recorded too. Using the standardized measures, the distribution of the food by all family members is also recorded. The nutritive values are calculated from the raw weight of food stuffs using the formula:

$$\text{Individual intake (volume)} = \frac{\text{Individual intake (volume)}}{\text{Total cooked quantity (volume)}} \times \text{raw amount}$$

Ideally, this method of 24-hour recall should be done on three consecutive days and the mean of the three days can give a fair idea of the actual diet intake. Care should be taken to avoid feasting and fasting days in order to have a true picture. The advantage of this method is that it is useful in quick recapitulation of one's habitual diet and also gives an idea of extreme variations that might occur.

Food frequency method: In this method, the frequency of different foods consumed over a given period (daily, weekly, fortnightly, monthly or rarely)

Foods	Exchange	kcals	Protien g	Cholestrol g	Fats g	Ca mg	Fe g	Fiber g
Table 3.9: Food exchange table II								
Cereals	1 (30 g)	100	3.5	20	–	48	4.9	1.9
	(25 g)	80	3.0	17	–	45	4.0	1.5
Pulses	1 (25 g)	80	5.0	15	–	75	3.8	1.5
	(30 g)	100	7.0	20		80	4.0	2.0
Vegetables								
Group A	100 g	16	1.0	3.0	–	25	0.5	1.0
Group B	100 g	36	2.0	7.0	–	28	0.75	1.5
Fruits	100 g	40–50	–	10–15	–	15	0.5	1.4
Milk	1 (250 mL)	165	8.0	11	8.0	300	0.5	–
Meat/egg		80	6.0	–	6.0	60	2.1	
Egg	40 g							–
Chicken	40 g (1 med.)							
Fish	40 g							
Cheese	30 g							
Paneer	35 g							
Liver (sheep)	35–40 g							
Fats/oils	1 tsp (5 mL)							
Oil/ghee	2 tsp (10 g)	45	–	–	5.0	–	–	–
Cream	1 tsp (5 g)	40						
Butter								
Dry fruit	6 Pcs (8–10 g)	45			5			

Source: NIN

is recorded and this information can be corelated with the 24-hour recall information, to give a more accurate picture of the child's intake. For this a questionnaire is prepared enlisting all foods that are possibly consumed at different frequencies and intervals and intakes recorded (Table 3.10). Wherever required, the total cooked volume of food and its distribution among the number of family members is recorded from which the intake of an individual is derived. For foodstuffs like fats, where it is difficult to quantify individually, a better way is to record the total consumption of all types of oil, ghee etc. on monthly basis among a fixed number of family members. The individual intake can be calculated by dividing the total fat consumed (lts.) per month by number of members and the figure so derived, divided by 30 would give the amount consumed by one member per day.

This method has the advantage of providing information where evidence is required of an association of a child's existing nutritional status with diet in general rather than any specific nutrient.

Questionnaire method: This method involves recording the diet history but without an interviewer being involved. Here the questionnaire is distributed or posted to the respondents who in turn fill them up and return or post it back to the interviewer. But this method is not applicable for assessing the nutritional status of children in a hospital setting or in the out patient clinic.

Table 3.10: Food consumption frequency questionnaire

Foods\	Amt. g/mL	Daily	3–4/wk	1-2/wk	2-3/mth	1/mth	Rarely
Cereals:							
Wheat flour							
Rice							
Suji							
Bread							
Other							
Pulses							
Green loafy vegetables							
Other Vegetables							
Root Vegetables							
Fruit							
Milk							
Curd/Paneer							
Eggs							
Chicken/Meat							
Oil/Ghee/ Butter							
Sugar							
Sweets savory							
Chips							
Cold d							
Biscuits							
Cake/Pastry							
Ice Cream							
Noodles							
Pizza/Burger							
Fried snacks							

Moreover, this method also requires the respondent, the mother in this case, to be literate enough to be able to comprehend and fill up the form correctly and independently. However, it can be used to collect data on large scale samples in short periods with limited resources.

Biochemicalmethod: Besides anthropometry and dietary history, biochemical parameters are also used to corelate with the available information and the given clinical picture. Blood and urine samples are the most commonly used specimens used to determine the level of the required nutrients. These parameters can depict deficiency or any abnormality in absorption or utilization of any particular nutrient which can further be corelated clinically; e.g. hemogram showing levels of Hb can demonstrate prescence or absence of anemia which most often is related to iron deficiency in the diet. Serum lipid profile can give an idea of the levels of total cholesterol, HDL, triglycerides, etc. denoting hypercholesterolemia which can be corelated with dietary intake of fats.

Age	Serum albumin (g/100 mL)		
	Deficit (high risk)	Low (medium risk)	Acceptable (low risk)
0–11 months	-	<2.5	<2.5
1–5 years	<2.8	<3.0	>3.0
6–12 years	2.8	2.8–3.4	>3.5

Table 3.11: Serum albumin levels in children with PEM[12]

Serum albumin levels are commonly used to assess protein-energy malnutrition. Serum albumin and transferrin levels reflect long-term changes in the nutritional status, serum retinol binding protein and thyroxine binding prealbumin show more rapid changes. These values are mostly of use to monitor protein status during convalescence. Table 3.11 presents guidelines to interpret serum albumin in protein-energy malnutrition in children.[12]

CLINICAL ASSESSMENT

Clinical signs to assess nutritional status have been used but are always corelated with biochemical or anthropometric status also. These signs can manifest as marginal changes which may be short term. However, independently this assessment is not considered a very useful tool. The various organs by which we can assess nutritional status clinically are the eyes, skin, oral cavity, dental history and the skeletal system. Presence of Bitot spots in the eyes can be related to vitamin A deficiency, or pallor of the under side of the eyelids can be corelated to iron deficiency anemia. Koilonychia (spoon shaped nails) are also indicative of anemia. Cracks at the corners of the mouth are suggestive of thiamine deficiency or loss of papilla on the tongue can help identify deficiency of vitamin B_2 or riboflavin. Similarly, bleeding or inflamed gums may suggest deficiency of vitamin C, presenting as scurvy. On examining a child, appearance of bow legs or beading of ribs may indicate rickets, deficiency of vitamin D.

Overall appearance of a child showing wasting with or without edema can immediately be associated with protein-energy malnutrition. Flag sign of the hair showing color change can also be associated with protein deficiency in the form of kwashiorkor. Edema of the feet in certain hepatic disorders is also a sign of protein depletion.

REFERENCES

1. World Health Organization, Measuring change in nutritional status, Geneva, WHO, 1983.
2. Center for Disease Control and Prevention, National Center for Health Statistics, CDC Growth charts: United States, http://www.cdc.gov/growth charts/May 30,2000.
3. Indian Academy of Pediatrics (IAP) Growth Charts Committee. Khaldikhar V, Yadav S, Agarwal KK, Tamboli S, Banerjee M, et al. Revised IAP Growth Charts

for height, weight and BMI for 5-18 years old children. Ind Pediatr. 2015;52:47-55 (PubMed).

4. Elizabeth KE. Normal growth in children. In: Nutrition and Child development, 3rd Ed. Hyderabad: Paras Publishers; 2004.

5. Cole TJ, Green PJ. Smoothing reference centile curves: The LMS method and penalized likelihood. Stat Med. 1992;11:1305-19 (PubMed).

6. Cole TJ, Lobster T. Extended International (IOTF) body mass index cut off for thinness, overweight and obesity. Pediatr Obes. 2012;7:284-94 (PubMed).

7. Ramos GF, Galvan R, et al. Mortality in second and third degree malnutrition. J Trop Pediatr. 1956;2:77-83.

8. Nutrition Sub committee of the Indian Academy of Pediatrics, Report. Ind Pediatr. 1971;17:98-104.

9. Seoane N, Lytham MC. Nutritional anthropometry in the identification of malnutrition childhood. J Trop Pediatr. 1971;17:98-104.

10. Sastry JG, Vijayaraghvan K. Use of anthropometry in grading malnutrition in children. Ind J med Res. 1973;61:1225-32.

11. Gopaln C, Rama Sastri BV, Balasubramnian SC. Nutritive Value of Indian Foods, National Institute of Nutrition, Indian Council of Medical Research, Hyderabad, 2002.

12. Sauberlich HE, Dowdy RP, Skala JH. Laboratory tests for the assessment of nutritional status. CRC Critical Reviews in Clinical Laboratory Sciences. 1973;4:215-340.

Feeding of Infants (0–6 Months)

INTRODUCTION

The first consideration that comes to mind when we talk of feeding infants is the newborn child, and feeding a newborn obviously takes us to the most natural God given gift to the mother, that of breast milk. As soon as the child is born, nature prepares both, the mother and the baby to make the best of this natural gift. Soon after birth the mother starts secreting milk and it requires an effort on the part of the baby to suck, so that secretion is further enhanced. In our country from generations this gift of nature is well accepted and justified because the thought of feeding her child comes naturally to the mother and she is mentally geared to do so. The baby also responds spontaneously to the mother's love and the natural instinct of suckling is smoothly initiated. But, unfortunately, in our own country over the years this spontaneous practice of making the best of 'Nature's Gift' is slowly eroding with the result that both mother and child face a lot of problems. Therefore, to bring our attention to this problem and help the mother revert to the dying practice of utilizing nature's gift, WHO has dedicated one week (1–7th August) every year as 'Breastfeeding Week'.

To begin with we shall first discuss why breastfeeding is important and the various factors associated with failure to feed or 'nurse'.

ADVANTAGES OF BREASTFEEDING

The main advantages of breastfeeding are as follows:
- It is **a complete food** by itself for the baby till 6 months of life in all respects. The proportion of all macro- and micronutrients are such that it is tailor made for the newborn. It is rich in fats, especially the essential fatty acids and the protein quality is just right for the baby. It is unique that it is rich in lipase an enzyme which is poor in other sources of milk
- It has water content which is adequate to meet the total requirement of the baby in the driest of summers. There is **no need to feed water as long as the baby is exclusively breast fed**. Offering water to a baby on breast feeds

Table 4.1: Nutritive values of various types of milk

Nutrients	Human milk	Cow's milk	Buffalo's milk	Goat's milk
Calories (kcal)	65	67	117	72
Proteins (g)	1.1	3.2	4.3	3.3
Fat (g)	3.4	4.1	6.5	4.5
Carbohydrates (g)	7.4	4.4	5.0	4.6
Calcium (mg)	28	120	210	170
Phosphorous (mg)	11	90	130	120
Sodium (mg)	-	73	19	11
Potassium (mg)	-	140	90	110
Iron (mg)	-	0.2	0.2	0.3
Vitamin A (µg)	41	53	48	55
Thiamine (mg)	0.02	0.05	0.04	0.05
Riboflavin (mg)	0.02	0.19	0.10	0.04
Niacin (mg)	-	0.1	0.1	0.3
Folic acid (µg)	-	8.5	5.6	1.3
Vitamin B12 (µg)	0.02	0.14	0.14	0.05
Vitamin C (mg)	3	2	1	1

Source: 2, Goplan C, Rama Shastri BV, Balasubramanian SC, NIN, ICMR, 2012

can actually cause a reverse effect of reducing the mother's milk output by suppressing her prolactin concentration in the plasma. This fact has been well demonstrated by studies from Brazil by WHO.[1] It was shown that introduction of water or tea even if continuing breast feeds were twice as likely to stop breastfeeding before 3 months compared to those who were fed exclusively for 6 months

- It **is rich in antibodies** in the form of immunoglobulins and leucocytes, which help the baby fight against any infections. A bacterium called *lactobacillus bifidus* present in breast milk prevents the baby from possible infections. The breast milk protein consists of whey protein (80%) in the form of lactalbumin, and easily digestible too, thus making it superior to cow's milk.[1] Table 4.1 gives a comparison between various types of milk[2]
- The **Ca:P ratio is ideal** in breast milk as compared to other milk source.
- Though low in iron, the bioavailability is high due to **presence of lactoferrin** which prevents the baby from being anemic
- Breast milk is **available at just the right temperature for the baby** avoiding the need to cool or heat it as required appropriate for consumption
- The **mother is free to move around anywhere with the baby** without the hassle of organizing to carry formula milk or in premixed form or reheating it or carrying sterilized bottles along with

- **It is very economical** as it saves the family from spending on expensive formula available in the market
- It **is sterile with minimum chances of contamination**. The enzyme lactoferrin is bacteriostatic thereby inhibiting *E. coli* by rendering iron unavailable to it. An exclusively breast fed infant is about 14 times less likely to die from diarrhea, nearly 4 times less likely to die from respiratory diseases and almost 3 times less likely to die from other infections than a non breast fed infant[3]
- Breast milk ensures stability by **emotional bonding of mother and child**. It also gives a feeling of security to the child
- It ensures certain maternal benefits also by **decreasing postpartum bleeding**
- It burns off extra fat deposited during pregnancy besides possibly **decreasing the risk of ovarian cancers in mothers at a later stage**
- Exclusive breast feeding up to 6 months also **helps spacing between two**
- **pregnancies**. As per WHO/UNICEF estimates, contraceptive prevalence would have to increase by 11% in order to compensate for 25% decline in breastfeeding[4]
- Contrary to the general myth among young mothers of the present generation, breast feeding **helps her to lose the extra weight** she had gained during the course of her pregnancy and **helps regain her figure.**

COLOSTRUM

This is the first viscous yellowish milk which is secreted soon after delivery. Unfortunately, most often this 'early' secretion is discarded by most mothers in certain communities, with the explanation that it is toxic for the baby. On the contrary colostrums is the richest source of proteins and immunoglobulins and the fat-soluble vitamins like A and E. It is rich in secretory IgA, which prevents the baby from any gastrointestinal infections. However, it is lower in fats and carbohydrates as compared to mature milk. This secretion may not be secreted in large volume and lasts for only about 2–3 days, but is very crucial for the baby as it helps in stimulation of mature milk by 2–10 days after birth. It also helps in stimulating peristalsis and acts as a lubricating protective effect on the mother's nipples.

The Indian Academy of Pediatrics (IAP) has spelt out the guidelines for Indian infants, termed as 'Infant and young child feeding practices' (IYCF).[5] The goal of these guidelines is:

1. To ensure normal growth and development from 0 to 2 years of age.
2. To formulate, endorse, adopt and disseminate guidelines related to infant and young child feeding from the Indian perspective.

These guidelines are used for

- Feeding of infants from 0 to 6 months of age
- Feeding of infants from 6 to 12 months of age
- Feeding of young child from 1 to 2 years of age.

As per WHO guidelines and also endorsed by IAP, exclusive breastfeeding should be done for the first six months of life. No other liquid including water should be offered except for drops or syrups like vitamins, mineral supplements or medicines. Some important points of the guidelines include:

- Breastfeeding to be initiated within 1 hour after birth for all normal delivery or born by cesarean section
- Colostrum not to be discarded, but be fed for the first 2 days as long as it is secreted. No other prelacteals to be introduced
- Exclusive breastfeeding to be practiced for first six months
- No other food or liquid be given to an infant below six months, unless medically indicated
- Baby to be fed on demand at day and night. This is called demand feeding, unrestricted feeding or baby-led feeding
- An average Indian mother produces about 600 mL of milk in the first six months, which is adequate to meet the baby's requirements
- Mother's working outside maybe supported by either allowing extended maternity leave or alternatively arrange for "Hirakani's rooms" (arrange rooms for facilitate mothers to feed the babies at work place—based on a legend of a woman called Hirakani who jumped from a hill top to feed her baby)
- Mothers to be encouraged to breast feed even during illness unless medically contraindicated
- Artificial feeding, bottle feeding or any advertizing of infant milk substitutes to be discouraged
- In event of discontinuation of breastfeeding due to some reason, 'relactation' should be attempted at the earliest and assisted by a health care worker.

Positioning of Breastfeeding

Breastfeeding can be done in a way most suitable to the mother as well as the baby. Positioning the baby to enable him/her access and suckle at the breast comfortably is very important for successful feeding. A new mother needs the support of the elders or trained professionals to teach them how to do so correctly. Although it can be done in lying or sitting position, the best suitable is for the mother to be seated on the bed or chair, and her forearm should be able to hold the baby's head close to the elbow, at about 45 degrees angle as shown in Fig. 4.1.

The baby should be helped to 'latch on' to the breast in the correct position, with the baby's chin close to the breast rather than only at the nipple (Fig. 4.2A).

Preparing for Breastfeeding

The mother should prepare for the breast feeding process during the antenatal period itself. The nipples should be checked and in case of retracted or involuted nipples, medical help can solve the issue by easy maneuvering as shown in Fig. 4.2B.

All antenatal health workers involved, should also counsel mothers during the pre natal visits, regarding the importance of exclusive breastfeeding for the first six months and desist from any formula feeds.

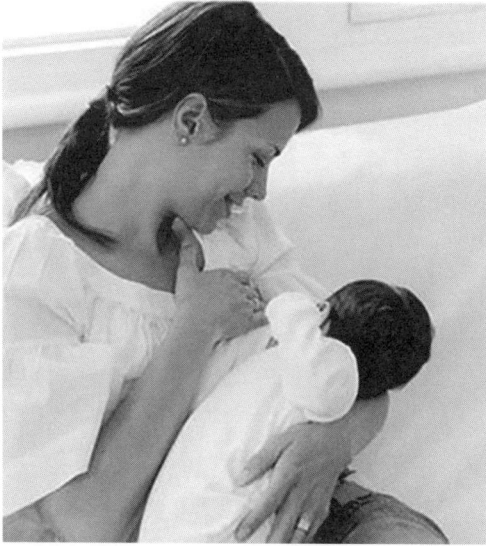

Fig. 4.1: Positioning of baby while breastfeeding

It is equally important that the mother take care of her own diet which should be well balanced with all required nutrients. This can be achieved by inclusion of fruits and vegetables, milk and milk products, legumes, nuts and whole grain cereals.

FACTORS CAUSING LACTATIONAL FAILURE

As mentioned earlier, breastfeeding is such a natural phenomenon which should be a spontaneous function, but still we find the incidence of successful breastfeeding practice gradually declining. There can be a number of factors leading to lactation failure. We shall discuss in detail and see what steps can be taken to prevent this problem.

- **Initiation of breastfeeding:** Breastfeeding should be initiated within half to one hour after delivery in the case of normal delivery and at least 4–6 hours after a cesarean section delivery. At birth, the baby is completely ready and alert to begin sucking. In an ideal environment, the onus lies on the part of the family members or the immediate care givers present around to put the baby to the mother's breast so that the sucking reflex is initiated. It should be impressed upon the mother that the initiation of lactation is influenced greatly by the sucking reflex and if she on her part fails to make an effort at that time, lactation failure is bound to set in. Mature milk starts from the third to fourth day and the volume increases gradually from about 100 mL on the second day, rapidly increasing to 500 mL by the second week and going onto about 700–800 mL by 5–6 months. The mechanism involved is that sucking stimulates the production of prolactin (milk production) and

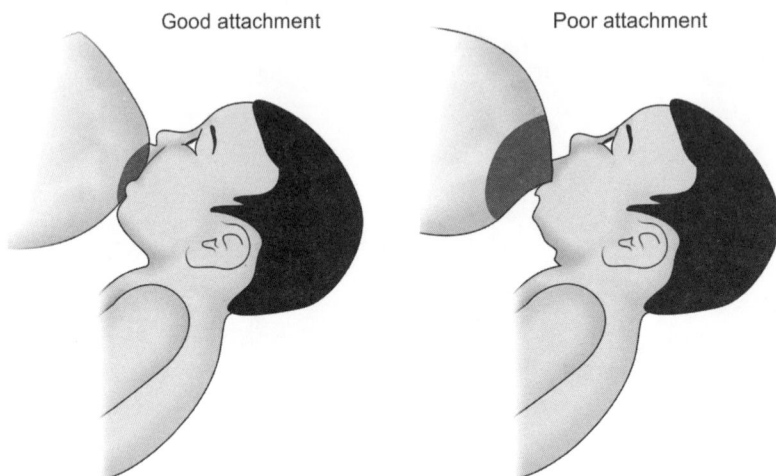

Fig. 4.2A: Correct and incorrect attachment to the breast

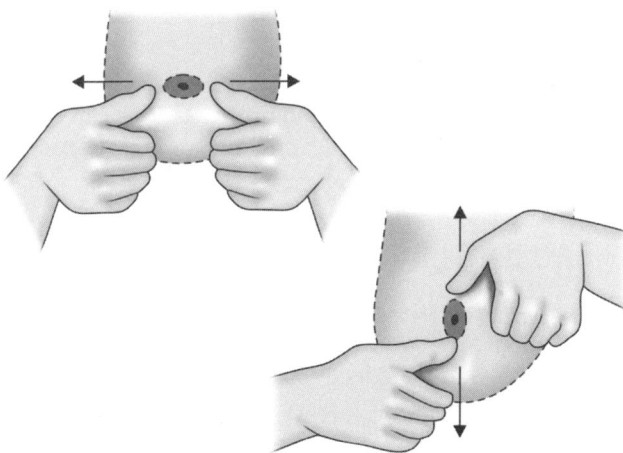

Fig. 4.2B: Way to maneuver inverted nipples

oxytocin (milk ejection) so that lactation is maintained. Oxytocin reflex is also known as the 'let down reflex' due to its role in 'letting down' milk production (Fig. 4.3)

- **Role of prelacteals:** In most communities it is customary for elders in the family to offer pre lacteals to the new born. These can be indifferent forms in different communities like, honey, 'janam ghutti' goat's milk or 'saunf' water etc. This practice is not healthy due to the risk of any infections being passed on to the baby. Honey which is commonly offered as the first food in many communities can actually be responsible for passing any fungal infections. 'Janam ghutti' is usually given as pacifier and considered good

Brain
1. Hypophysis at base of brain
Hormones are released
from here into blood
and thus, sent to breast

1.

2. Prolactin reflex
Increases milk production
(hormone, prolactin)

2.

3. Let-down reflex
Pushes milk towards the
nipple (hormone, oxytocin)

3.

4.

4. Sucking reflex
Sends impulses to hypophysis
by the vagus nerve

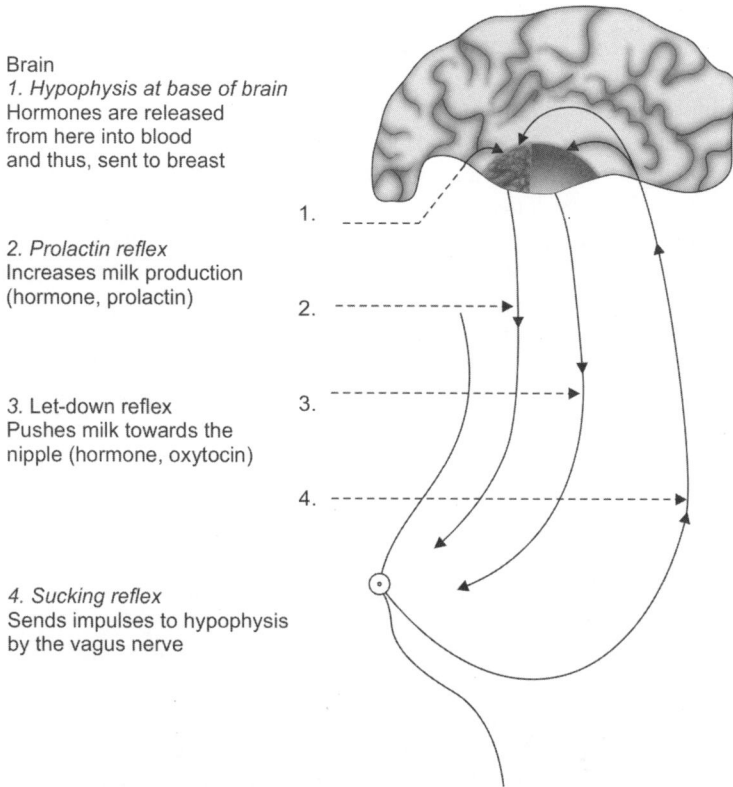

Fig. 4.3: Diagram of physiology of lactation

for digestion. Bloating of abdomen due to aerophagia is very common due to which the baby cries. Mothers then resort to such practices which can indirectly harm the baby's system. Even plain water, either as such or boiled with saunf etc. is not required. Such practices can adversely affect the sucking reflex which in turn suppresses milk output. There can be a risk of aspiration also into the air passages or lungs and secondly highly prone to infections if proper hygiene is not maintained. Therefore, the baby should be put on the mother's breast within half an hour of birth to stimulate the let down reflex by inducing the oxytocin

- **Family support:** The role of the female family elders is very crucial in influencing good or poor lactation. If the mother, mother in law or any one closely associated with caring for the new mother encourages her to feed by re-enforcing its importance, the mother is bound to follow their advice and be 'mentally geared' to feed her baby. On the other hand, if these same people give their own remarks about the baby not 'getting satiated by the mother's milk or that her 'milk is not adequate', or that the mother is 'too weak to feed', the mother is psychologically discouraged and begins to lose confidence in her own ability to satisfy her baby with her own feed. The lack of confidence is enough to inhibit the 'let down' reflex and gradually the milk production also dwindles. Added to this, is the fact that because of this reason, the mother herself or the family members begin to offer formula milk or cow's milk in their attempt to be over concerned. It may be noted that the milk production is inversely proportionate to the 'artificial' or 'top milk' fed to the baby, i.e. the more the baby is fed by the bottle; the lesser will become the breast milk output. Therefore, a 'positive attitude' needs to be instilled in the mother and the caregivers to maintain successful breastfeeding. Artificial feeds include water also which should not be offered before 6 months due to the fact that the water content in breast milk is adequate enough for the baby's requirement as mentioned earlier. It is noteworthy to point out here that just supplementing water also along with breast milk is enough to suppress the 'let down' reflex and lead to diminished milk output. Besides these factors, it is important that the mother be totally stress free, with no anxiety of any sort and comfortable since the let down reflex is greatly influenced by these factors

- **Lack of privacy/rooming in:** We live in a society and hence, social interaction is an integral nature of all humans. As per our traditions and social obligations, when a newborn arrives, there is a row of visitors making a bee line to bless the mother and the child. Or, at other times, in families with limited space, the mother does not get a chance to be on her own or have any privacy to be able to nurse the child in peace. This can often lead to distraction of her focus from the baby which itself can be a causative factor in lactation failure. Moreover, the mother is seen feeding her baby amidst other members of the family where there is some discussion going on or her attention is focused on the television or she may be attending any visitors too. This distraction from the baby can reduce the let down reflex further leading to decreased lactation. Therefore, it is very important that some 'rooming in' be allowed to the mother and the child so that she can focus completely on her baby. This allows 'one to one' contact eye contact with the child and may be some verbal communication between the two which helps 'bonding' between the mother and child

- **Early introduction of top feeds:** Ideally breastfeeding should be done 'exclusively' for 6 months as recommended by WHO.[6] But at times mothers in their zeal to feed their babies adequately end up 'overfeeding' them by resorting to artificial feeds. They feel that breast feeds are not adequate or he remains 'hungry', or is not growing adequately. As a result they initiate top feeds in the form of formula, milk substitutes and even semi solids much before 4–6 months. This results in decreased output of breast milk by mothers and again to make up for this deficit, they further add more solids. This vicious cycle ultimately results in further decreased output and lactation failure. On the contrary, if the mother continues to breastfeed at frequent intervals, the milk output is maintained and may normalize eventually. Approximately 700–800 mL milk is secreted per day in a healthy normal lactating women and this is sufficient till 5–6 months

- **Mother's employment:** In our grandmother's age, lactation failure was unheard of as mothers mostly were housewives and their total energy and commitment was focused on the family and their needs. In the process with the arrival of the newborn, the attention of the mother is totally focused on her baby and its care. Nursing comes naturally to her without which she can continue without ever having the fear of discontinuing it. But in the present scenario, where majority of the mothers are working, there is a latent fear in their minds that sooner or later they will have to leave the baby at the hands of her mother in law, or the care taker or in the crèche. In such a condition she will have to resort to artificial feeding. So, in order to allow the baby to' acclimatize' to the top feeds, the mother tends to introduce these much earlier. As a result, her own feeds gradually decrease and the baby is deprived of the several benefits of her own feeds. This is particularly true of working mothers who have maternity leave and unable to continue nursing their child once they go back to their jobs. Therefore, the fear that the baby may accept the bottle later on, drives her to initiate the child to this technique, so that it is easier for the caregiver or baby sitter to feed the child. This in a way also is enough to overcome her own guilt complex of not being able to feed her child herself. Besides, it is easier for the caregiver to put the bottle to the baby's mouth rather than make an effort to feed him/her with a cup and spoon
- **Problems related to the breast:** A very common problem encountered my some mothers which can contribute to lactation failure is related to engorgement of breasts, mastitis or obstructed ducts or sore nipples. But it may be stressed here that these problems are rather a result of inadequate or improper feeding and the cure lies in more or proper feeding technique rather than discontinuing nursing.

Engorgement

This is a result of inadequate milk removal, poor ejection or failure to 'let down' or insufficient or in frequent nursing. Treatment comprises frequent nursing, warmth, massage or use of breast pumps.

Duct Obstruction

This can be due to tight-fitting clothes exerting local pressure which can be relieved by frequent nursing, moist heat and massage.

Mastitis

This problem is a result of prolonged engorgement or duct blockage if not tackled promptly. There can be development of abscess also, which may require antibiotic treatment. Management again involves counseling of proper nursing technique or removal of milk from blocked ducts. Analgesics can help mitigate the pain to the mother.

Sore Nipples

This is also due to improper feeding or holding the baby to the breast. When there is improper latching onto the breast, the baby is not able to suck adequately, at the same time hurting the mother's nipples leading to cracks and soreness. Correct positioning of the baby to the mother's breast and the mother's own posture while feeding can help avoid this problem. As seen from Figure 4.2, the baby is 'latched on' in the right position when the baby's chin is close to the breast, rather than only at the nipple. More of the alveola is visible above the baby's mouth, unlike in the wrong position post of the alveolar area is visible and the baby's mouth is not wide open. In the right position, the mouth is wide open. Moreover, if not attached properly, breastfeeding becomes painful for the mother unlike in the right attachment where the baby sucks deeply with slow, regular movements of the tongue. Feeding should not be discontinued due to this problem since correct positioning and 'latching on' to the breast will gradually heal the affected area. In a good attachment, the baby's chin is close to the breast while in the improper latching, the chin is away from the breasts. More of the areola is visible above the baby's mouth than below it and the mouth is wide open with lower lip turned outwards. Nursing is not painful for the mother and the baby sucks slowly. In the wrong attachment, mouth is not wide open and much of the areola is outside the baby's mouth. Breastfeeding is painful for the mother if the latching on is incorrect.

Certain basic precautions if taken heed of can help avoid problems related to soreness of the nipples or blocked ducts, etc.

- Frequent expression of milk both manually or by use of breast pump can stimulate the 'let down' reflex and help in adequate lactation
- Frequent short feeding, e.g. every 2 hourly for 5–10 minutes after the 'let down'. The mother can offer from one side first and after feeding for about 5–8 minutes, the child is satisfied, she can feed from the other side the next time she feeds. This will ensure uniform flow from both breasts. With increase in its requirement with age, it might become necessary to feed from both sides
- Proper 'latching on' of the infant to the breast
- After the baby is satisfied, the mother should try to dislodge the baby from the breast gently by inserting her finger into the corner of the infant's mouth
- The nipple should be washed only with plain water without using soap or any disinfectant solution
- The nipple should be allowed to dry before covering. In case of severe pain or soreness, the mother can express manually rather than allowing the baby to suck, to avoid further pain
- If soreness is very severe and painful, it would be wise to stop nursing at that nipple and express manually from the other side for 24–48 hours
- A mild analgesic can help reduce pain to some extent
- **Expressed breast milk (EBM):** In event of unavoidable circumstances for the mother to go out for work, she can still feed her own milk, by expressing

it manually or using a pump which are easily available (Figs 4.4A and B). This can be left at home with the caretakers who can feed the baby with a spoon. This expressed breast milk (EBM) should be collected in a stainless steel container or cup and refrigerate it if required to be kept for more than 7–8 hours. The refrigerated EBM can safely be utilized for up to 12 hours. At the time of feeding this milk can be brought out and kept at room temperature till suitable for feeding, or the milk container can be placed in another container of warm water to bring it to room temperature faster. Use of glass or plastic bottles or cups for EBM should be avoided as the white corpuscles in the milk tend to stick to the glass making them unavailable to the baby. EBM can be expressed every 3 hours in a boiled and cooled utensil and can be stored at room temperature for 8 hours or 12 hours in a refrigerator or also can be frozen for months. Heating EBM directly on gas or microwave should be avoided

- **Feeding twin babies:** In case there are twins, the mother can be helped to feed both the babies together, one on each breast in a double football hold or double clutch position (Fig. 4.5A) and cradle hold position (Fig. 4.5B). The mother has to judge how well which of the babies is able to latch on and accordingly adopt the suitable position. Each baby can also be offered

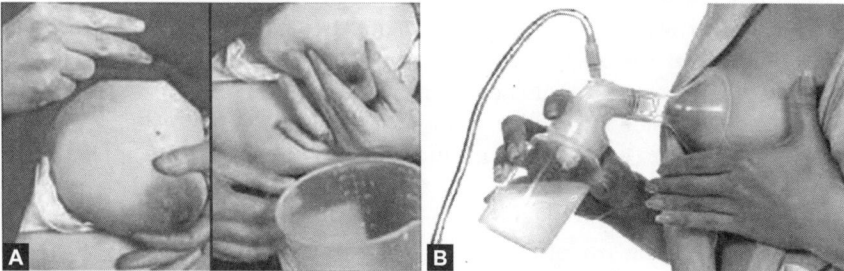

Figs 4.4A and B: (A) Manual expression of EBM; (B) EBM using pump

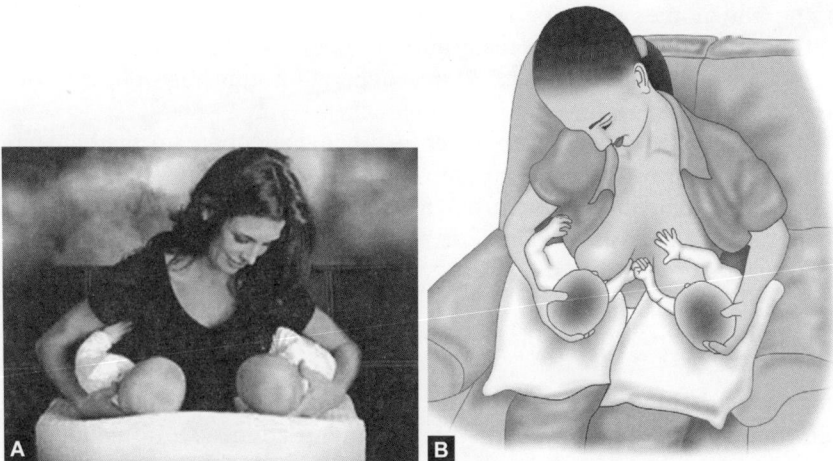

Figs 4.5A and B: (A) Football-hold position; (B) Cradle-hold position

one breast at one feed and then switch them on the other breast alternately. A pump to express the milk also will be helpful to maintain a record of the amount of feed each one of them has had. Each baby may have a different style of feeding, so the mother has to learn by experience which mode of feeding would be most suitable to each one of her babies. The services of a lactation expert may be helpful to mothers in such situations.

Considering the above points, the key to successful exclusive breastfeeding may be summarized as below:

a. Encourage her to relax.
b. Encourage confidence in her to be able to feed optimally.
c. Encourage 'rooming in' by providing reasonable space and privacy.
d. Encourage her to maintain optimum nutrition without food fads.
e. Encourage her to have adequate fluids.
f. Encourage her to 'bond' with the baby by allowing her to handle him/her personally, thereby building a sense of security in the baby also.

FREQUENCY AND DURATION OF EXCLUSIVE BREASTFEEDING

The baby is the best judge in self regulating its timing of feeding. There should not be any fixed schedule of feeding. Demand feeding is the norm advised. Each baby differs from the other in getting satisfied and may have varying stomach capacities. Some may be satisfied earlier but may demand more frequently. Others may continue to be quiet for longer periods, but at a time may feed well from both breasts. Generally 5–8 minutes on each breast is sufficient to satisfy the baby and give a feeling of fullness. A 'crying' baby generally is taken as a signal of a 'hungry baby' by the mother and feeding him generally satisfies him. But crying may not always indicate hunger. At times a wet baby might cry too or he may be ill or experiencing some sort of discomfort in any form. 'Teething' can also be painful or irritable for a child and he may express that by crying. The mother with experience learns to assess the need of her baby and will know whether the child is really hungry or not. Usually babies themselves set their own schedule of about 3–4 hours depending upon how optimally they are able to suck at one given time.

The mother can be assured of her feed being adequate for the baby, by maintaining a record of his weight gain and the frequency of urination. If there is an upward trend in weight gain and if the baby passes urine about 5–6 times per day, she can rest assured that her milk is adequate for the baby and need not resort to formula feeds.

ARTIFICIAL/FORMULA FEEDING

Mothers with the fear of their babies being left underfed, generally resort to formula feeds right from early infancy. In our country, formula feeding is generally discouraged due to the high risk of infections, and bottle contamination. There is also risk of over dilution leading to failure to thrive. Under exceptional conditions where either the mother has expired or the baby is adopted from unknown parents, or there are twins and the mother is not able to breast feed adequately, formula feed may be resorted to. Ideally cow's milk or the regular dairy milk can be used in undiluted form. The common myth that whole undiluted milk can not be tolerated by the infant should be dispelled off by proper counseling. Even it is whole buffalo milk, the excess cream formed after keeping for a few hours may be skimmed off in the early few weeks only, gradually shifting to whole milk. The main draw back of dairy milk or the locally available milk is that it is devoid of iron and therefore, iron supplementation may have to be given to prevent anemia setting in. Multivitamin drops too can be given along with. To counter the effect of higher sodium content and osmotic level in dairy milk, it is a good idea to feed plain water two to three times a day. Formula fed infants may not require iron or water supplements, since most commercial milk substitutes are all well fortified. The only drawback of formula milk, if used by the lower socioeconomic group, is that the dilution may be in excess of the instructions provided on the packaging, thereby leading to inadequate weight gain and if the water used for reconstituting is not sterile or hygienic, there can be added risk of gastrointestinal infections. In situations where the mother has to join back to work before 6 months, it would be a wise decision for her to express her milk (expressed breast milk or EBM) and leave it behind with the caretaker to be used with the other milk substitute being used. This EBM should be given with a clean spoon and cup. It can be safely kept for 4–6 hours without being contaminated. Refrigerating the EBM can keep it for almost 24 hours. Heating it may curdle it so it can be given as such. At times wet nurse is available who can nurse the baby, thus providing the benefits of human milk to the baby.

ADVERSE AFFECTS OF BOTTLE FEEDING

Although bottle feeding is widely practiced and accepted in the western world, in the developing countries this practice should not be encouraged due to the associated risks of infections and contamination of the feeds. As mentioned earlier in this chapter, the introduction of the bottle in early infancy also can lead to nipple confusion and the maternal milk output begins to decrease prematurely. The various reasons to avoid the bottle in our country are as follows:

- There is increased risk of gastrointestinal infections due to inadequate maintenance of the bottle hygiene. Even the mothers belonging to lower socioeconomic status tend to introduce the bottle due to the ease with which it can be put in the baby's mouth and the effort and time spared for attending to their household chores
- The baby is confused between the bottle nipple and mother's nipple and finds it easier to latch on to the bottle than to the breast
- Introduction of the bottle in early infancy also suppresses the mother's own milk output, thus depriving the baby of the essential nutrients which can be provided by breast milk

- The baby gets addicted to the bottle and develops a dependency on it, probably seeking security. This addiction prevents him to wean on to the cereal based semi solids in the second half of the first year, gradually leading to getting anemic, as milk is a very poor source of iron
- Many children who are hooked on to the bottle continue to use it for prolonged duration and even prefer to take other sweetened beverages/drinks from the bottle only, thereby compromising on their appetite
- As the baby might tend to overfeed with the bottle, there can be a risk of these babies getting over weight also due to excessive milk intake, sometimes going up to 1–1.5 liters per day. The milk used also may be full cream, which can be a contributory factor for increased fat cells in the body from childhood itself. These fat cells once formed can not be reduced later in life and these children would continue to be 'chubby babies' growing ultimately into 'obese adults'.

On the other hand, there is another extreme spectrum of bottle fed babies—those with 'failure to thrive'. This happens in the lower socioeconomic group of mothers who tend to dilute the milk in order to stretch the limited available resources with them. This satisfies the baby for a short while but is deprived of the essential nutrients required for his optimum growth and development. Again, since it is easier and convenient for the mother to feed with the bottle (sparing her the precious time available for other household chores) and equally comforting for the baby to suck from the bottle, he will not accept any solid food offered to him. The cereal pulse based solid feed has to be chewed and this requires an effort on the part of both the mother and the child to feed, chew and swallow it. This makes it easier for both to give into the temptation of using the bottle for feeding mother and the child to feed, chew and swallow it.

BURPING AFTER FEEDING

This is a very important step to be followed each time the baby is fed. Along with ingesting milk, babies take in a lot of air also, and if it is not expelled, the baby will cry soon after he is allowed to lie down. This is due to the abdominal distension caused by aerophagia. To relieve this problem, it is advisable to allow the baby to burp after each feed, by holding him upright with his head on the mother's shoulder and gently patting on the back till the baby burps out extra air. It is advisable to make the baby lie on the right lateral side after feeding to prevent any aspiration or choking.

DURATION OF BREASTFEEDING

Exclusive breastfeeding should be done for 6 months as per WHO guidelines and continued along with cereal supplements till 2 years of age. However, most often it is observed that many mothers come with problems of the child not accepting any semi-solid food despite their best efforts. On further probing, it is found that mothers continue to exclusively breastfeed well beyond 6 months without encouraging much of semi solids with the result that the baby sort of gets addicted to the breast and refuses to accept anything else. Besides, prolonged breastfeeding gradually leads to anemia which in turn results in loss of appetite. Therefore, if the child is gradually weaned over to semi solids after 6 months, he gets acclimatized to a variety of foods and develops a taste for a variety of foods. But, yes breastfeeding should continue for as long as possible in addition to cereal supplements. In specific conditions, when the child is not accepting solids at all because of prolonged breastfeeding, the mother can be asked to stop breastfeeding, so that the child gets to accept solids.

BREASTFEEDING DURING ILLNESS

There are very few indications when the mother is advised against breastfeeding her child. By and large a mother should continue to breast feed her child even if she is ill like in viral infections, even tuberculosis, hepatitis or any other infectious diseases. In mastitis or breast abscess, the mother can express her milk and feed the child. In case of the mother suffering from tuberculosis, she should be under constant supervision of a clinician for appropriate treatment for her own self as well as monitoring of the baby too for transmission of infection. In conditions where mother may be HIV positive, it is generally advised to continue breastfeeding keeping in mind the overall advantages of it as compared to the risk of transmission. If the baby is also positive, then there is no benefit in discontinuing breastfeeding in any case, but even if the baby is not positive, breastfeeding should be continued to be encouraged, as it can prevent further likely recurrent infections. As per the recommendations of WHO, breastfeeding should be promoted in HIV positive mothers in view of its role in providing immunity against other HIV related complications in already infected infants.[6] Perinatal transmission of the disease is known to be around 30%. Moreover, in situations where there is lack of adequate support for children of such mothers it is considered justified for the mother to continue breastfeeding. The few conditions where the mother is advised against breastfeeding are when she is on certain drugs like in conditions of malignancy, thyroid or some psychotic problems. Drugs like laxatives also can affect the baby's gastrointestinal system temporarily.

In case of a child being ill also, except when indicated otherwise, like in situations where there may be risk of aspiration, etc,[7] there is no indication of withholding breast feeds. In fact, breastfeeding should be continued since the child may not accept solids easily; in which case at least breast feed can help tide over that brief period of low intake. In conditions of viral or diarrhoeal illness which are very common in infants, breastfeeding should be encouraged to prevent them from dehydration and negative energy balance. It should be explained to the mothers that passage of stool after every feed in an exclusively breast fed baby does not indicate diarrhea and no medication should be offered. Over treating such babies with antibiotics can actually lead to drug-induced diarrhea which can worsen the situation. It is a perfectly normal phenomenon for a breast fed baby to pass stool after every feed. Only after

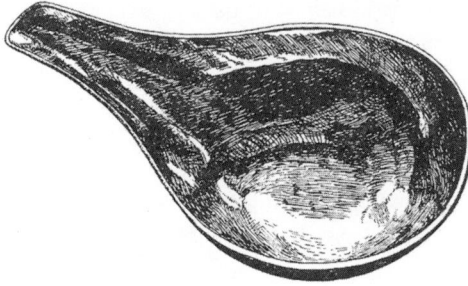

Fig. 4.6: Traditional feeding spoon (pallada)

solid feeds have been introduced, do the stools begin to be slightly formed and decrease in frequency.

A baby born with cleft palate might encounter some difficulty in breast feeding, if the palate is involved. In such conditions, he can be fed expressed breast milk by spoon and cup or if required there are specially designed spoons available termed 'pallada'[7] in local terminology (Fig. 4.6).

These have a long teat like design which can go easily into the baby's mouth for feeding milk. Care should be taken to avoid choking by maintaining an upright position of the baby while feeding.

SOME MYTHS AND FACTS RELATED TO BREASTFEEDING

1. **Myth:** Newborn babies should be given honey soon after birth
   Fact: Feeding of honey or any other prelacteal should be discouraged due to risk of infection.
2. **Myth:** Janam ghutti is good for baby's digestion or for a crying baby.
   Fact: No. It can work as an intoxicant and may make the baby's digestion sluggish.
3. **Myth:** Babies should be fed by the clock.
   Fact: Demand feeding is recommended. Each baby will have his/her own style of feeding and may not necessarily have a uniform amount each time. It can vary from time to time thus making him/her hungry accordingly.
4. **Myth:** Mother who delivers by cesarean section should avoid feeding the baby till a few days or hours.
   Fact: She should be encouraged to feed within 1–2 hours of the baby's birth.
5. **Myth:** Mothers with twins should resort to formula feeds, as her milk will not suffice for both.
   Fact: She can feed both of them simultaneously, alternating each one at each breast.
6. **Myth:** Babies can be fed with a feeding bottle at night.
   Fact: Feeding bottles should be avoided strictly as they can cause infections to the baby.
7. **Myth:** If baby is not gaining weight, it means the mother's milk is inadequate or unsuitable for her.

Fact: Failure to gain weight despite mother feeding the baby, could signify some underlying problem. So she must visit her pediatrician at the earliest to rule out any pathological/physiological factor. Reassurance rather than blaming the mother is very important in such situations, so that her lactation is not affected

8. **Myth:** A crying baby means he/she is hungry

   Fact: It could be a sign of any other problem bothering the baby like an ear infection, a blocked nose and unable to breathe properly or any gastrointestinal related issue. Reassuring the mother and a check up by a pediatrician is the best option to seek remedy.

9. **Myth:** Lactating mothers should be on a specific, restricted diet by avoiding 'cold', 'hot' or 'gassy' foods.

   Fact: She can consume a normal family pot diet without any restriction of any foods. However, high fat, high sugar and spicy foods may be taken with caution.

10. **Myth:** Lactating mothers should avoid drinking too much water as the abdomen gets distended.

    Fact: In fact she should be having water before and after each feed in small amounts, over the whole day to produce adequate milk.

11. **Myth:** Baby may not be satisfied by mother's milk.

    Fact: If a baby is playful and happy, it indicates her milk is adequate. A growth chart can be used to keep a track of the velocity of weight gain of the child. This will give an idea whether the baby is feeding adequately or not. Another way to assess the amount of breast milk is to express milk from both breasts, only once, and measure the amount collected. This amount when multiplied by the number of times the baby is fed in 24 hours, will give the total amount produced. This should work out to be about 600 mL, considering the baby is fed every 2 hours in 24 hours on an average.

BREASTFEEDING PROMOTION NETWORK OF INDIA (BPNI)

A national network has been formed for the cause of promotion of breastfeeding in our country known as the Breastfeeding Promotion Network of India (BPNI). A global agency exists for the same cause known as World Alliance for Breastfeeding Action. In 1992, UNICEF organized a global program of Baby Friendly Hospital Initiative (BFHI), which was adopted by India in 1993. Many hospitals today have been certified as 'BFHI' for which certain policies have been laid down:

* Hospitals need to have an official policy to protect, promote and support breastfeeding
* All staff involved in maternity and child care hospitals/centers are trained in skills of promoting breastfeeding
* To assist mothers in early initiation of breast feeding within half hour of birth for normal deliveries and within 4–6 hours of a cesarean section

- All mothers are taught the right technique of breastfeeding and to maintain lactation
- To ensure no food or drink or any other mill substitute other than breast milk be offered to the baby and are strictly prohibited in the hospital
- Mothers should be encouraged to breast feed on demand
- Any use of artificial teats, pacifiers, soothers and feeding bottles are strictly prohibited in the hospital
- Maximum follow-up support and assistance for exclusive breastfeeding up to 6 months be made available to all mothers.

The Infant Milk Substitute Act (IMS Act)

Around the same year in 1993, another act known as Infant Milk Substitute Act (IMS Act) was passed, relating to regulation, production, supply and distribution of all types of milk substitutes including feeing bottles and infant foods. The World Health adopted an international code for marketing of breast milk substitute way back in 1981. This code was subsequently adopted by the Government of India in 1993 and passed as an act (Central Act 41 of 1992). This act calls for strict prohibition of free samples of infant formula and other gifts, posters and advertisements and any financial inducements to health personnel. The Indian Academy of Pediatrics (IAP) has also adopted this code strictly.

Summary of Provision of the Code

- No direct promotion to the public by way of advertisement or distribution of discount coupons, free samples (Article 5.1 and 5.3)
- No promotion of products in health care facilities (Article 6.2 and 6.3)
- No free samples or gifts to mothers (Article 5.2 and 5.4)
- No contact with mothers by company sales personnel (Articles 5.5 and 6.4)
- No promotional samples or gifts to health workers (Article 7.3).

    Information provided by manufacturers and distributors regarding products should be restricted to scientific and factual matter and should not convey the belief that bottle feeding is equivalent or superior to breastfeeding.

NUTRITION IN LOW BIRTH WEIGHT BABIES

A baby is defined as low birth weight (LBW), when his birth weight is below that of a full-term baby which is generally about 2.5 kg. But in special abnormal conditions, be it either due to maternal factors or any other congenital abnormalities, a baby might be born much below the expected normal. Babies might be very low birth weight (VLBW) or low birth weight. If they are full-term babies with low birth weight, they are termed as small for gestational age (SGA). If they are appropriate for their gestation age, even if low weight, they are termed appropriate for gestational age (AGA) or they might be even large for gestational age (LGA), if they are more than expected for their gestational age. All full-term LBW are small for date but all preterm LBW babies may or may not be AGA or SGA.

LBW babies are commonly seen in most developing countries and it is estimated that approximately 70% of the LBW babies have intrauterine growth retardation (IUGR).

In India, about 30–40% of the babies are LBW who are mostly SGA.[8]

Extensive studies on Indian LBW babies have shown that by 4 years of age, one third of them were found to be in the normal range for weight and one fourth of them were found to be in the normal range for height and head circumference.[9] It has been observed that two third of the LBW babies achieve normal development, 20% tend to show mild to moderate impairments while 10–20% end up with cerebral palsy or mental retardation. As per estimates, 30% of all cerebral palsies occur in LBW babies.

The nutritional requirements of LBW babies have been laid down by the European Society for Pediatric Gastroenterology and Nutrition (ESPGAN) which is widely accepted, as given in Table 4.2.[9]

As observed from Table 4.2, the mean energy requirement of about 130 cal/kg/d can be adequately met with a fluid volume (breast milk) of about 150–200

Table 4.2: RDA for preterm infants	
Nutrients	*RDA*
Energy	130 cals/kg/d
Protein	1.5 g/kg/d
Fat	4.7 g/kg/d
Fluids	50–200 mL/kg/d
Vitamin A	1000 IU/d
Vitamin D	400 IU/d
Vitamin E	15 IU/d
Vitamin K	0.5–1 mg at birth
Vitamin C	10–60 mg/d
Folic acid	60–65 mcg/d
Calcium	100–200 mg/kg/d
Phosphorous	50–150 mg/kg/d
Iron	2–2.5 mg/kg/d
Zinc	1–2 mg/kg/d
Magnesium	6–20 mg/kg/d
Sodium	>1.3 mmol/kg/d
Potassium	3.5 mmol/kg/d
Multivitamin suppl.	Yes*

At following vitamin doses: A–300 mcg; D–20 mcg; E–5 mg; K–3 mg; B_1–50 mcg; B_2–200 mcg; B_6–100 mcg; C–20 mg; folic acid–60 mcg.

Table 4.3: Composition of term and preterm milk (PTM)/100 mL*

Nutrient	Term	PTM 1st wk.	PTM 2nd wk.	PTM 3rd wk.	PTM 4th wk.	PTM 5th wk.	PTM 6th wk
Energy (kcal)	67	64	67	67	67	67	67
Protein (g)	1.1	2.3	1.9	1.6	1.5	1.4	1.3
Sodium (mmol)	0.6	1.7	1.3	1.2	0.9	0.8	0.8
Calcium (mmol)	0.8	0.7	0.7	0.7	0.7	0.7	0.7
Phosphorous (mmol)	0.5	0.5	0.5	0.5	0.5	0.5	0.5

* The values given are for banked term and pre term milk[8]

mL/kg/d. Breast milk is considered quite safe during the first week of life. The preterm milk (PTM) is adequate in all nutrients as per the requirement of the baby, but this differs from the first week to the sixth week (Table 4.3).[10] It has a higher content of total nitrogen, protein, sodium, chloride, magnesium, iron, copper, zinc and IgA as compared to term milk. As seen from Table 4.1, the PTM has higher protein content (2.3%), initially, which comes down to 1.1g% in term milk. The energy content however, is almost the same throughout except for in the first PTM where it gets slightly lower. The pancreatic lipase in such babies is lower, therefore they are prone to fat malabsorption. It is also rich in carnitine which helps in transportation of long-chain polysaccharides across mitochondrial membrane for oxidation. Since the synthesis of carnitine is defective in preterm infants, breast milk can help tide over this defect. The lactose content of breast milk too is more soluble in preterms as compared to the formula milk, which might lead to osmotic diarrhea due to their high lactose content.

The preterm baby can be fed by expressing the breast milk (EBM), if the baby is too weak to suck adequately or is admitted in an ICU set up, where the mother may be separated for some time. However, efforts should always be made first to keep the mother and child close to each other as often as possible, which is being practiced widely now under the 'kangaroo mother care' program. In this program, emphasis is laid to keep the mother and child close to each other such that adequate nutrition, warmth and care are provided by the mother herself.

In situations where the baby is an adopted one or the mother has expired or not accessible for any reasons, formula milk may have to be resorted to. All the same, even cow's or dairy milk available locally can also be given but with a little modification for VLBW babies as they may not be able to digest whole cow's milk. The modification made is by diluting 2 parts of cow's milk with 1 part of water and adding 5 g of sugar per 100 mL. This brings the cow's milk close to the range of breast milk—67 cals, protein 2.2 g, fat 2.5 g and carbohydrate 8.2 g per 100 mL. But this modification is advisable only under supervision in the ICU, and should not be advocated after the baby is discharged, since the dilution may exceed the required concentration, besides doubtful source of water used.

ROUTE OF FEEDING

It is widely accepted that preterm babies thrive best when on mother's milk. But this may not always be possible with very low birth weight babies, as they may not be able to suck efficiently. Even if they do attempt, they will spend more energy rather than conserving whatever little possible. In such cases, EBM can be fed using spoon and cup. Initially, fluid and nutrient requirement may not be possible to meet by breastfeeding alone, in which case intermittent gavage feedings can be given. Aspirate levels should be checked to prevent risk of aspiration. Small frequent feeding 1–2 hourly can be given to begin with. Along with this, intermittent breastfeeding should be encouraged even when there is no secretion as this tends to induce early breastfeeding by boosting the sucking reflex. This phenomenon has been described as non nutritive sucking[11], and also known to enhance weight gain.[12,13] Bottle feeding should be avoided at any cost because of the reasons already cited earlier in this chapter.

REFERENCES

1. Elizabeth KE. Low Birth Weight (LBW) Babies, In: Nutrition and Child Development. 3rd Ed. Hyderabad, India: Paras Medical Publishers; pp.40–53.
2. Gopalan C, Rama Shastri BV, Balasubramanian SC. Nutritive values of Indian foods, National Institute of Nutrition, ICMR, Hyderabad, 2012.
3. Victoria CG, Smith P, Vaughan JP, et al. Evidence for protection by breastfeeding against infant deaths from infectious diseases in Brazil. Lancet. 1987:2:319-22.
4. WHO/UNICEF. Breastfeeding in the 1990's: Review and implications for a global strategy based on the technical meeting, Geneva, 25-28 June (1990).
5. Tiwari S, Nagar. Infant and Young Child Feeding Practice Guidelines. Ind Pediatr. 2010;47:995-1004.
6. Akre J. Health factors which may interfere with breast feeding. In: Infant Feeding: The Physiological Basis. Bull WHO. 1989;67(Suppl):41-54.
7. Gosh S. Infant Feeding, Food and Nutrition Board, Department of Women and Child development, Ministry of Human Resource Development, Government of India, 1993.
8. Mathur NB. Nutrition for LBW in the Third World. In: Nutrition in Children Developing Countries Concerns, HPS Sachdeva (Ed), Panna Choudhary, 1994.
9. Elizabeth KE, Feeding of infants and children. In: Nutrition and Child Development, 3rd Ed. Hyderabad, India: Paras Medical Publisher; 2002.pp.1–28.
10. Wharton BA. Nutrition and feeding of Preterm Infants. Oxford, Blackwell Scientific Publications; 1987.
11. Field T, Ignatoff E, Stringer S, et al. Non-nutritive sucking during tube feeding: Effects on preterm neonates in an intensive care unit. Pediatrics. 1982;70:381-4.
12. Brostrom K. Human milk and infant formula: Nutritional and immunological characteristics. In: Textbook of Pediatric Nutrition. Suskind RM (Ed). New York: Raven Press. 1981;pp41-64.
13. Bernbaum JC, Periera GR, Watkins JB, Peckham J. Non nutritive sucking during gavage feeding enhances growth and maturation in pre mature infants. Pediatrics. 1983;71:41-5.

Nutrition for Infants and Toddlers (6–24 Months)

"Man is what he eats"

—**Ludwig Feuerbach**

INTRODUCTION

The fact that exclusive breastfeeding should continue for till 6 months of life has been well established. Gopalan has emphasized the need for mothers from lower socioeconomic status to continue exclusive breastfeeding till at least 6 months since in poor communities, living under poor hygienic conditions, the theoretical benefits of early supplementation, if any, may be more than off set by diarrheal episodes, which are a major deterrent of infant growth and nutrition.[1] The same has been supported by Underwood and Horfrander in the recommendations made by Swedish Academy of Pediatrics, that no added calories are better than dirty calories.[2] However, the Academy has also stressed the fact that if for some reasons growth faltering is observed, appropriate measurements should be taken even earlier in the form of cereal supplementation. In any case, beyond 6 months exclusive breast feeding will not be able to sustain optimum growth of the infant thereby resulting in growth failure. The nutrient requirements of the child increase from birth to 12 months as shown in Table 5.1.[3] It is here that the transition of the child's diet takes place from exclusively milk based to cereal based which is popularly referred to as the weaning process.

WEANING OR COMPLEMENTARY FEEDING

Weaning initially had been referred to as getting 'accustomed to'. It has been later described by WHO/UNICEF as 'a systematic process of introduction of suitable milk in order to provide the needed nutrients to the baby.' Earlier on, the term 'weaning' was wrongly associated with the indication of stopping breast feeds once cereals were introduced which was not at all desirable, nor meant to be conveyed so. Therefore, the modified term, 'complementary feeding' was introduced and widely accepted to refer to the introduction of

Table 5.1: Nutritional needs of an infant (birth to 12 months)		
Nutrients	**Birth to 6 months (body weight—5.4 kg)**	**6–12 months (body weight—8.4 kg)**
Energy (kcals)	92 kcals/kg/body weight	80 kcals/kg/body weight
Protein (g)	1.16 g/kg/body weight	1.69 g/kg/body weight
Fat (visible) (g)		19
Calcium (mg)	500	500
Iron (mg)	46 µg/kg/body weight	5
Vitamin A (µg) Retinol (µg) B carotene (µg)	- - -	- 350 2800
Thiamine (mg)	0.2	0.3
Riboflavin (mg)	0.3	0.4
Niacin (µg)	710 µ/kg/body weight	650 µg/kg/body weight
Pyridoxine (mg)	0.1	0.4
Vitamin C (mg)	25	25
Folic acid (µg)	25	25
Vitamin B$_{12}$ (µg)	0.2	0.2
Vitamin D (IU)	200	200
Magnesium (mg)	30	45
Zinc (mg)	-	-

Source: NIN, ICMR, (2011).
Source: Dietary Guidelines for Indians—A Manual, National Institute of Nutrition, ICMR, Hyderabad, 2nd ed. 2011).

cereal based semi solids to a child's diet by 6 months of life in addition to continuation of breastfeeding.[4]

Complementary feeding should be well balanced (feed+food+diet) constituting 55–60% of energy from carbohydrates, 25–30% of energy from proteins and the rest 25–30% from fats. This can be achieved by including foods from various groups like cereals, pulses, vegetables, fruits, nuts, milk and milk products and fats and oils. Sugar or better still jaggery can also be used in moderate amounts for some of the preparations. As laid out by WHO,[4] principles of complementary foods should be:

- **Adequate in terms of quantity or volume**, implying to begin gradually at six months and steadily increase the volume; e.g. beginning with 1–2 tsps and building up to tablespoons and katoris as the baby grows older. Feeding inadequate amounts will also defy the goal and lead to growth failure
- It should be **dense in energy and other nutrients** in proportion to the baby's age, without increasing the volume too much. For this oil/butter or ghee can be made use of to make it energy dense. Feeds should be able to provide adequate vitamins and minerals like the B complex group, iron, magnesium, zinc, sodium and chloride. Some amount of fiber too should

be part of the diet which can be obtained easily by foods like green veggies, fruits and whole grain cereals
- **Breast feeding to be maintained** in between solid feeds
- Foods prepared should **be prepared hygienically** to avoid risk of infections
- **Consistency of feeds to be proportionate** to the age of the baby—not too thick so that the baby is unable to swallow with ease, nor too thin to compromise the nutrient density. It should be proportionate to the development of the baby as he/she is ready to munch, chew and swallow
- **Frequency of feeding should also be gradually increased with age**, beginning from 1–2 feeds per day at 6–8 months and going up to 3–4 per day by age 9–12 months and beyond
- **To follow responsive feeding**, meaning the caregiver should be responsive to the clues given by the baby by psychosocial stimulation, through age appropriate play and communication activities. Self feeding should be encouraged without bothering about spilling over on clothes and encouragement by praising the baby's efforts to feed him/her. Forced feeding, threats or anger should be avoided during feeding process
- **Bottle feeding to be discouraged** completely.

TIME OF COMPLEMENTARY FEEDING

The birth weight of the child nearly doubles by 5 months of age, thereby increasing the nutritional demands by about 600–700 calories. Since the breast milk can provide only about 400–500 calories by this time, the need for complementary food arises. Moreover, since the calcium and iron stores of breast milk also get depleted by 6 months of life, these have to be provided by additional supplements. It is known that by 4 months of age the baby is 'biologically ready' to 'accept' solids as the head control is achieved by now, the intestinal amylase matures, the gum hardening begins prior to teeth eruption and thus the baby is 'geared' to accept cereals and pulse-based foods. However, it should be kept in mind that 'too early' introduction of complementary feeding also at times can lead to intolerance of foods. Many allergies related to foods have been reported by early introduction of foods especially the protein-rich sources known as protein sensitization. Certain food allergies like the wheat allergy (coeliac disease) has been corelated to early introduction of these foods in some children. 'Too late' supplementation on the other hand can lead to growth faltering due to the inability of just breast milk or formula milk alone, to meet the increased demands. Anemia is another very common problem encountered among the 6–12 month old infants, as it is well known that milk alone is a very poor source of iron, be it from any source, and without adequate cereal/pulse supplementation the iron requirement cannot be met. Besides, the baby gets sort of 'addicted to the breast' and is unable to accept solids for a long time later. But of course, with a judicious approach, ideally breastfeeding should be continued for as long as possible (till about 2 years) along with complementary feeding of semi solids.

The feeding recommendations as given by the Integrated Management of Neonatal and Childhood Illness (F-IMNCI) as given in Table 5.2, gives a fair idea of the flow of complementary feeding schedule which should be borne in mind for children from birth to 2 years and older.[5]

The Weaning Bridge—Safety Net

The weaning period has been described by Jelliffe as bridge which acts as a safety net during the transition phase from that of exclusive breastfeeding to

Table 5.2: Feeding recommendations (0–24+ months) (IMNCI)

Up to 6 months	6–12 months	12–24 months	24 months and older
Breast feed as on demand, day and night, at least 8 times/24 hrs. No other fluids including water. Remember— • Continue breastfeeding if child is sick	Breast feed on demand Give at least 1 katori serving at a time of: • Mashed roti/bread mixed in thick dal with added ghee/oil or khichdi with added oil/ghee. Add cooked vegetables in the servings • Sevian/dalia/halwa/kheer prepared in milk or • Mashed boiled / fried potatoes • Offer banana/biscuit/chickoo/mango/papaya • 3 times/day if breast fed; 5 times/d if non breast fed Remember— • Keep the child in your lap and feed with your own hands • Wash your own and child's hands with soap and water every time before feeding	Breast feed on demand Offer food from the family pot. Give at least 1½ katori serving at a time of— • Mashed roti/bread mixed in dal with added ghee/oil or khichdi with added ghee/oil or • Mashed roti/rice/bread mixed in sweetened milk or • Sevian/dalia/halwa/kheer prepared in milk or • Offer papaya/banana/biscuit/chikoo/mango—5 times/day Remember— • Sit by the side of the child and help him to finish the serving • Wash your own and the child's hands with soap and water every time before feeding	Give family foods at 3 meals/d Twice/day in between nutritious food—banana/chikoo/papaya as snacks Remember— • Ensure that the child finishes the serving • Teach your child to wash hands with soap and water each time before feeding

Source: Facility Based Integrated Management of Neonatal and Childhood Illness (F-IMNCI, Chat Booklet: Published by Ministry of Health and Family Welfare, Govt. Of India, New Delhi in collaboration wit WHO and UMICEF, 2009).
Source: IMNCI, WHO/UNICEF, 2009.

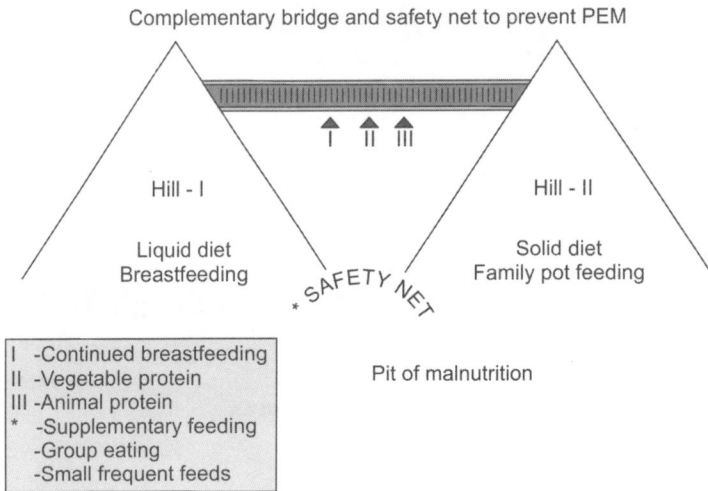

Fig. 5.1: Weaning bridge

the postweaning phase.[6] He has named this bridge as the 'three plank protein bridge' to prevent protein–energy malnutrition. This bridge prevents the child from falling into the pit of malnutrition, if not taken care of adequately (Fig. 5.1). The three plank bridge comprises:

1. Continued breastfeeding.
2. Vegetable protein.
3. Animal protein
   - Supplementary feeding
   - Group eating
   - Small frequent feeding.

CAUSES OF FAULTY WEANING PRACTICES

Despite best efforts of health personnel in educating the mothers to introduce complementary foods by 6 months, a large section of our population still fail to implement these practices due to various avoidable reasons as:

1. **Ignorance**: Mothers are ignorant of the significance of complementary feeding due to the belief that for small babies their own feed or top milk is sufficient and may even tend to over feed with just milk. This milk may be diluted again out of ignorance due to the belief that top milk is 'heavy' for the baby and may cause indigestion.
2. **Myths**: Then there is this concept of 'cold' or 'hot' or 'heavy' foods, which should or should not be given to the child due to its ill effects, e.g. banana is considered 'heavy' and producing 'phlegm' so should be avoided. In certain communities, cereals are considered 'heavy' for the liver to digest. Others consider absence of teeth eruption as indication for nonfeeding.
3. **Food not customized for the child**: There are families, where food is offered to the child as is cooked for the rest of the family with spices, etc. If the child

is offered such food to begin with, the irritation caused may deter him from accepting any cereal food later on for a long time.

4. **Lack of time**: Lack of time devoted to feed a child is another very common cause why children are unable to accept solids. They become so dependent, rather addicted to milk, either breast milk or formula, that they do not develop a taste for solids at all. It is easier for mothers too to feed them milk as it takes much less effort and time to feed milk, especially if fed by the bottle.

5. **Bottle addiction**: The introduction of the bottle for feeding is the main contributory factor for the child to get addicted to it and shun any cereals offered to him/her.

6. **Breast addiction**: In some cases it is also observed that because the baby is put to the breast each time he/she cries, the appetite is suppressed, due to feeling of 'satiety' and the child then refuses any solids offered subsequently. Therefore, the mother has to be reassured and referred to a pediatrician for help.

A WORD OF CAUTION

In the developing countries like ours, the supplementation process or in other words 'the weaning dilemma' can be fraught with some risks too if adequate precautions are not taken. If not done hygienically, recurrent diarrheal episodes can in fact put a great set back on the growth process, ultimately leading to failure to thrive.[6,7]

WHEN AND WHAT TO ADD

4–6 Months

In our country, introduction of new cereal foods in a child's diet is associated with many traditional, cultural and religious beliefs. These practices vary from state to state. In some parts of the country, like in the south, there is a ceremony called 'anna prassana', where the first cereal in the form of rice is introduced. Similar practices prevail in west Bengal also. The age at which these ceremonies are done, vary from 6 months to/or as late as 8–12 months. In such communities, respecting the sentiments of the elders, the parents can be educated regarding the risks involved in delayed supplementation. They can be given wheat and rice-based diets, mashed potatoes, vegetables, etc. Care should be taken to make use of locally available home-based foods and should be introduced one at a time. More variety can be added gradually. The various foods which can be offered are mashed rice with milk, suji, halwa, dalia, mashed banana, fruit juice, some vegetable oil or butter and mashed moong dal. All these foods should be in semi liquid or solid form for the babies to be able to swallow easily. These foods can be given 4–6 times a day. If a child refuses a particular food or develops any sort of reaction, the child need not be forced into it. May be after some days it can be tried again. Breast milk however, should be continued, but the frequency gradually decreased. A better option can be, to first offer the cereal supplement and then give breast feeds, because otherwise the child having been satiated by breast feeds, may refuse the supplement.

It has been shown that the minimum energy density of a supplement to meet the requirements of a child in a breast fed infant would be lesser than that of a non breast fed baby. A 4–6 month old breast fed baby would need a supplement of about 20–30 calories per 100 g to be fed 4–6 times a day and if given only twice a day would need a minimum of 60 cal/100 g. On the other hand, a non breast fed baby of the same age would require as much as 50–80 cal/100g to be fed 4–6 times a day. But, if fed only twice a day, they would need up to 160cal/100g. This is not very practical to implement as the stomach capacity of the child is not big enough to hold this amount. If given forcefully, it can result in vomiting/regurgitation and even refuse feeds.

6–9 Months

By this time, the child's requirements also increase with simultaneous weight gain. Breast milk also decreases both in quantity and quality and is unable to meet the total requirements. At this stage, since the child is already in to cereal foods, the quantity can be further increased. Foods like khichdi, 'churi' (parantha mashed with ghee and sugar/jaggery), panjiri, porridge, etc. can be given, increasing the amount to about 50 g. Vegetable soups are not a very good idea to feed children as being poor both in energy and proteins, it will only contribute to the volume of feeds without much nutrients except for small amounts of may be vitamins and minerals.

The top milk required to be given to the child at this stage should be preferably in a mixed cereal form rather than milk alone to enhance the nutrient density of the feeds. At this stage, since the child begins to sit up and teeth eruption begins, he may like to use his own hands to feed himself. Therefore, crisp pieces of bread, rusk or carrot slices, etc. can be given to him which he can nibble. This will also help soothe his gums which may feel irritable due to the teething process.

9–12 Months

Around this age, the aim should be to feed from the 'family pot', modified to the child's acceptability. More variety of foods can be introduced. A variety of seasonal fruits can be offered. In nonvegetarian families, eggs can be begun, but the yolk should be offered first and the white portion introduced later if there is no adverse reaction to the yolk part. The popular belief that raw egg mixed with milk (egg flip) is more nutritious is unfounded. On the contrary, it is not without health hazard. There is a risk of *Salmonella* borne infection which is quite common through eggs. Heating or cooking can destroy the bacteria and prevent any adverse affect. Secondly, since egg yolk which is rich in biotin, is made unavailable by the anti biotin factor called avidin. Avidin being heat labile is made unavailable thus, enhancing its absorption. Breastfeeding should be continued but the frequency may be decreased further gradually.

By one year of age the child's intake should be equal to half of the mother's intake and by two years it should be half of the father's intake.[8]

1–2 Years

A child having reached one year of age and through the second year would have more variety in his diet besides increased amounts of cereals and pulses and may be some amounts of added fat. The increased requirements can be met by following a 5 meal pattern. The feed and feeding schedule should coincide with the family's diet which is about 5 times a day. By this way the extra burden on the mother to prepare the feeds each time can be minimized and at the same time the child can learn to have meals along with the family members. Whole grain cereals, pulses, leafy vegetables and other seasonal vegetables and fruits should be included in some form. They will not only make the diet more palatable but also make it more energy dense. Home made cereal diets should be encouraged rather than tinned products. These diets prove to be cheaper, more nutritious and can be catered as per individual taste of the child. Vitamin and mineral supplements are not required if adequate cereal diets are started and continued subsequently.

The nutrient requirements of infants and older children are as shown in Tables 5.2 (a) and 5.2 (b),[3] and the amounts of food portions to be consumed, to meet these requirements can be seen in Table 5.3.[9]

The type of complementary feeds to be given for children can be summed up as follows (Table 5.4)[9]

- Energy dense—can be done by addition of fats
- Easy to digest and hypoallergenic
- Semi solid in consistency
- Low in bulk and viscosity
- Fresh and clean
- Home based and easily available
- Preferably culture/tradition based
- Should be free from spices
- Aim to feed from the family pot by 1 year of age
- Should be given in small frequent feeds
- Prepare separate feeds of measured volume.

SOME PRACTICAL ASPECTS OF COMPLEMENTARY FEEDING

- Maintenance of hygiene while handling food
- Should be of the right temperature-neither too hot nor too cold
- Child's individual likes and dislikes to be considered
- Avoid introduction of the feeding bottle

Table 5.2 (a): Recommended nutrient allowances for children (macronutrients and minerals)—ICMR 2010

Group	Particulars	Body weight (kg)	Net energy (kcal/d)	Protein (g/d)	Fat (g/d)	Calcium (mg/d)	Iron (mg/d)	Zinc (mg/d)	Magnesium (mg/d)
Infants	0–6 months	5.4	92 kcals/kg/d	1.16 g/kg/d	–	500	46 µg/kg/d	–	30
	6–12 months	8.4	80/kg/d	1.69 g/kg/d	19		05		45
Children	1–3 years	12.9	1060	16.7	27	600	09	5	50
	4–6 years	18.0	1350	20.1	25		13	7	70
	7–9 years	25.1	1690	29.5	30		16	8	100
Boys	10–12 years	34.3	2190	39.9	35	800	21	9	120
Girls	10–12 years	35.0	2010	40.4	35		27	9	160
Boys	13–15 years	47.6	2750	54.3	45	800	32	11	165
Girls	13–15 years	46.6	2330	51.9	40		27	11	210
Boys	16–17 years	55.4	3020	61.5	50	800	28	12	195
Girls	16–17 years	52.1	2440	55.5	35		26	12	235

Source: ICMR, 2010.

Table 5.2 (b): Recommended nutrient allowances for children (water soluble and fat soluble vitamins)—ICMR 2010

Group	Age (yrs)	Body Weight (kg)	Vitamin A (μg/d) β carotene	retinol	Vit. B1 (mg/d)	Vit. B₂ (mg/d)	Niacin (mg/d)	Vit. B₆ (mg/d)	Vit. C (mg/d)	Diet folate (μg/d)	Vit. B₁₂ (μg/d)
Infant	0–6 months	5.4	350	-	0.2	0.3	710 μg/d	0.1	25	25	0.2
	6–12 months	8.4	350	2800	0.3	0.4	650 μg/kg	0.4			
Children	1–3	12.9	400	3200	0.5	0.6	8	0.9		80	0.2–1.0
	4–6	18		3200	0.7	0.8	11			100	
	7–9	25.1	600	4800	0.8	1.0	13	1.6		120	
Boys	10–12	34.3			1.1	1.3	15	1.6	40	140	
Girls	10–12	35.0			1.0	1.2	13	1.6		140	
Boys	13–15	47.6	600	4800	1.4	1.6	16			150	
Girls	13–15	46.6			1.2	1.4	14	2.0			
Boys	16–17	55.4			1.5	1.8	17			200	
Girls	16–17	52.1			1.0	1.2	14				

Source: ICMR, 2010.

Table 5.3: Balance diet for infants, children and adolescents—ICMR 2011

Food groups	Infants 6–12 months	Years								
		1–3	4–6	7–9	10–12		13–16		16–18	
					Girls	Boys	Girls	Boys	Girls	Boys
Cereals and Millets (g)	15	60	120	180	300	240	320	420	330	450
Pulses (g)	7.5	30†	30†	60†	60	60† 60†	75†	60†	90†	60†
Milk (mL)	400	500*	500	500	500	500	500	500	500	
Roots and tubers	50	50	100	100	100	100	100	100	200	
Green leafy vegetables	25	50	50	100	100	100	100	100	100	
Other vegetables	25	50	100	100	100	200	200	200	200	
Fruits	100	100	100	100	100	100	100	100	100	
Sugar	10	15	20	20	30	30	25	20	25	30
Fat/Oils (visible)	20	20	25	30	35	35	40	45	35	50

*Amount indicates top milk. For breast-fed infant, 200 mL milk is needed
†30 g pulses may be exchanged with 50 g of egg/meat/chicken/fish

Table 5.4: Summary of type of complementary foods to be given to an infant (6–24 months)

Age (months)	Texture	Frequency	Average amount of each meal
6–8	Start with thick porridge; mashed foods	2–3 meals/d + frequent breastfeeding	Start with 2–3 tablespoonfuls
9–11	Finely chopped/mashed foods and foods which baby can pick	3–4 meals+ breastfeeding; based on appetite offer 1–2 snacks in between	½ of a 250 mL bowl or cup
12–23	Family foods, chopped or mashed if needed		

- Undue stress on juices/soups to be avoided—mashed fruits/vegetables is better options
- Foods should be fed by a spoon, placing it slightly towards the back of the tongue for the baby to accept it
- Introduction of tea to be avoided
- Feeds can be made calorie dense by adding oil/ghee and sugar, keeping the bulk low
- Include variety in daily menu, with simple flavors rather than highly spiced curries

- Encourage finger foods like salad or fruit slices cut in finger size portions for nibbling
- Encourage peer group eating to promote healthy eating habits
- Avoid highly refined, fried or other junk foods and snacks. These foods can lead to childhood obesity and other adult-onset chronic diseases
- Discourage offering/introducing cola or other sweetened beverages to these children as they can be addictive and the child may insist on having it more often. These beverages can suppress appetite and also lead to problems like gastritis, bone demineralization and metabolic syndrome later in life.

AMYLASE-RICH FACTOR

Amylase-rich factor (ARF) is actually germinated cereal flour, which is rich in alpha amylase that can reduce the dietary bulk of any viscous food. It acts as a catalyst by cleaving long carbohydrate chain into shorter dextrin thus, reducing the viscosity.

Given the small capacity of a child's stomach, large bolus quantities may not be tolerated by him. Therefore, it is essential that the feed should be in small aliquots (energy dense) and offered frequently as many as 6–8 times a day. Most of the supplement foods offered in our communities are very bulky and low in energy[10] and therefore, not very suitable for the infant in terms of meeting most of his requirements. Most mothers are more than satisfied if their child had just 1–2 small servings in the whole day. The rest of the feedings are generally made up of tea or diluted milk which is not desirable.

Method of Preparing ARF

About 100g of wheat is soaked overnight. The following morning excess water is drained and the moist grain is tied up in a muslin cloth and placed in a dark place from 24–48 hours by which time the grain will sprout. These grains are then sun dried for 5–6 hours and roasted slightly. The sprouts and the dry husk are removed by rubbing the grain by both hands. The dried grain is then ground to a powder and stored in air tight jars. About 2.5–5 g of powder can then be added in any gruel or porridge which alters its consistency. Besides, it has the added advantage of being cheap and easy to prepare at home.

ENRICHING COMPLEMENTARY FOODS

The simple home-based complementary foods can be further enriched by fermentation process some of which are already being used in our age old recipes. Typical examples are, curd, buttermilk, etc. where lactobacillus acts as a fermentation agent. Dosa, idli, dhokla are some of the other fermented recipes which can be incorporated as complementary foods in the first two years of a child's life.

Germination of foods like sprouts can increase the nutritive value of the pulse like vitamin B_1 and B_2 and vitamin E besides enhancing the protein digestibility.

Powdered almond may be added in the khichdi or porridge prepared for the baby. Similarly to increase the energy and protein content of the food without increasing the volume, milk powder (skim or otherwise) may be added in any suitable preparation.

PREPARATION AND STORAGE OF COMPLEMENTARY FOODS

Hygiene and proper storage of the complementary foods is very important. Proper hand washing with soap and water is desirable every time while handling food. The utensils, cups, spoons, etc. should be washed well and stored in a covered place away from exposure to dust. The cooking area should be maintained hygienic and dry.

FEEDING INFANT AND TODDLERS STUDY (FITS 2002)

A multicentric study on infants and toddlers conducted in 2002 in the USA revealed that a majority of the children were offered foods of low nutrient density. They constituted mainly high fat and high sugar foods like, sweetened beverages and cereals, margarine, cookies, processed meats, bakery products— all of them contributing nearly 90% of the total energy consumed. Such dietary trends place the toddlers at increased risk for inadequate intake of essential vitamins and minerals like iron and calcium.[10]

The FITS study brought out certain relevant guidelines[11] to be borne in mind to encourage healthy weaning process:

- Encourage pregnant women to consume a variety of foods including vegetables, fruits and whole grains
- This helps maximize fetal exposure (through transmission to amniotic fluid and human milk) besides mothers own nutrition
- Promote breast feeding to foster early infancy exposure to a variety of flavors
- Education of mothers/caregivers to recognize developmental milestones signaling approximate time to introduce complementary foods in appropriate orders
- Emphasis on need for repeated exposures (8–10) to novel foods and need for variety and diversity in their diet
- Emphasis on avoiding too high fats and sugary foods so as to promote preferences for more nutrient dense foods and beverages.

MYTHS AND FACTS RELATED TO COMPLEMENTARY FEEDING

1. **Myth:** Complementary foods can be started only after the teeth have erupted

Fact: Complementary foods can be offered from 6 months of life (even before dental eruption) in mashed or semi liquid form, as the mother's milk may not be adequate to meet the growing needs of the baby for optimum growth and development.

2. **Myth:** The food should be low residue or without fiber.

   Fact: Fiber-based foods in mashed, pureed or semi liquid form are essential in order to maintain bowl movement and prevent constipation which is a common problem with most 'all milk diet' fed children. However, care should be taken to avoid making the feed very bulky with fiber so that the other nutrients are not compromised and the baby can have maximum density in minimum volume.

3. **Myth:** Ready to cook commercial foods for babies are superior than home-cooked foods.

   Fact: In fact home prepared complementary foods are better as they are in a natural form and also feeding processed foods for a prolonged time can have other adverse health benefits for the baby in the long run. Moreover, processed foods have high amounts of sodium and other emulsifiers which are not healthy for prolonged use. These may be made use of in emergency situations or while travelling .

4. **Myth:** Banana, citrus fruit juices or rice, etc. are foods that may trigger cold or cough or phlegm and hence, avoided.

   Fact: This is not true. In fact these fruits provide immunity against allergies and also energy and fiber.

5. **Myth:** Dairy milk especially buffalo milk should be diluted for the baby as it is 'heavy' and indigestible for the baby.

   Fact: Infants up to 24 months need full fat milk for optimum development, especially the brain, and diluting the milk will compromise other nutrients too. Full cream milk also will take care of the vitamin A and D requirements of the child.

6. **Myth:** Eggs should not be given to babies in summers as they are 'hot'.

   Fact: Eggs can be offered to a child all through the year, but it should be gradually introduced into their diet. Begin with egg yolk first at about 9–10 months and once it is accepted and tolerated well, the whole of it can be given in boiled or any cooked form. Raw eggs should never be offered as it can lead to any gastrointestinal infections or intolearance.

7. **Myth:** Oil or ghee should not be added to the baby's food as they will not be able to digest it

   Fact: In fact oil/ghee should be used in maximum number feeds as it will increase the energy content of the food without increasing the bulk. It will also add to the flavor of the food and the child is more likely to accept it readily.

8. **Myth:** Pulses or dals offered to infants in complementary foods should be in the form of 'dal water' or diluted form.

   Fact: The dal offered to infants should be in the normal thick form as taken by the family. Giving dal water will be devoid of any nutrients, especially the proteins and the energy content.

9. **Myth:** Infants should be fed with vegetable soup rather than whole vegetables.

   Fact: Vegetable soup is not a recommended feed for a baby, since it will act as a filler, suppressing appetite for denser foods. The best way to make children have vegetables is by mixing them in their cereal preparation like dalia, upma or the dough used to make roti.

10. **Myth:** When babies are sick, they should not be fed or be given tea instead.

    Fact: On the contrary a sick child needs to be fed more frequently as he/she will not take adequate amounts at one time. Tea should be strongly discouraged as it can lead to loss of appetite, anemia and gastric irritation. 'Starving a fever' dictum should never be strictly discouraged.

SOME COMPLEMENTARY FOODS

Suji Kheer

Suji — 5 g
Oil — 5 mL
Sugar — 10 g
Milk — 200 mL.

Method: Heat oil in a pan, roast the suji slightly till light brown and add sugar and milk. Stir constantly and let it simmer till well done and the desired consistency reached.
Calories — 150/100 mL
Protein — 3.9 g.

Khichdi Feed

Rice — 6 g
Moong dal — 10 g
Oil — 10 mL
Water — to cook and make vol. to 200 mL
Salt — as per taste.

Method: Boil rice and moong dal along with oil or ghee in a saucepan and cook till well cooked and well blended. Then add water to make up the volume to 200 mL and boil till well blended into a semi liquid consistency. Serve without straining.
Calories — 80/100 mL
Protein — 1.75 g/100 mL.

Enriched Milk

Milk — 100 mL
Sugar — 10 g
Oil — 3 mL
Water — 100 mL.

Method: Mix oil and sugar in 100 mL water and add equal amount of water to make up the volume to 200 mL. Boil once and serve.
Calories — 80/100 mL
Protein — 1.75g/100 mL

Paushtik Ahar

Roasted wheat atta — 20 g
Roasted gram flour — 10 g
Skim milk powder — 5 g
Sugar — 15 g.

Method: Dry roast wheat atta and gram flour slightly, add coarsely ground sugar and mix the skim milk powder. Mix all the ingredients thoroughly. Serve as desired. If required, a teaspoonful of oil or ghee too may be added while roasting for improved flavor.
Calories — 182/50 g
Protein — 6.0 g/50 g.

Fruit Custard (175 g)

Milk — 150 mL
Custard powder — 1/2 tsp
Sugar — 25 g
Apple — 10 g
Banana — 10 g
Chikoo — 10 g.

Method: Dice all the fruits finely. Premix the custard powder in a little cold milk till all lumps are removed. Boil rest of the milk and add the custard milk mix gradually, while stirring constantly. Boil till the desired consistency attained.
Calories — 400
Proteins — 6.45 g.

OTHER COMMON HOUSEHOLD COMPLEMENTARY FOODS

Halwa, idli, upma, dosa, sago kheer, pancake made of gram flour or rawa, dhokla, sweets like rasgulla or gulab jamun, stuffed parantha, egg or cheese omellete with bread slice, besan barfi, pudding using jaggery, sweet rice using jaggery, vegetable cutlets or tikkis without much spices.

REFERENCES

1. Gopalan C. Appropriate supplementation of breast milk. NFI Bull. 1981;2:4-5.
2. Underwood B, Hofvander Y. Appropriate timing of complementary feeding of breast fed infants. Acta Scand. 1982;(Suppl)294:5-32.

3. ICMR, 2010, Nutrient requirements and recommended dietary allowances for Indians. A Report of the Expert Group of the Indian Council of Medical Research.
4. Brown KH. WHO/INICEF review on complementary feeding and suggestions for future research: WHO/UNICEF Guidelines on complementary feeding. Pediatrics. 2000;106:4.
5. Facility Based Integrated Management of Neonatal and Childhood Illness (F-IMNCI) Chart Booklet: Published by Ministry of health and family Welfare, Govt. of India, New Delhi in collaboration with WHO and UNICEF, 2009.
6. Jelliffe DB. Weaning and early childhood. In: Textbook of Nutrition ed, McLarren DS. Churchill Livingstone; 1991.
7. Rowland MG, Barrel RAE, Whitehead RC. The weanling dilemma: Bacterial contamination in traditional Gambian Foods. Lancet. 1978;1:136-8.
8. Sachdeva HPS, Choudhary P. Excluisve breast feeding for prevention of malnutrition and infection. In: Nutrition in Children, Developing Countries Concern, 7th edition. BI Publications Pvt. Ltd; 1994.pp.1-5.
9. Dietary Guidelines for Indians- A manual, National Institute of Nutrition, ICMR, Hyderabad, 2011.
10. Huffman SL, Martin LH. First Feedings. Optimal feedings of infants and toddlers. Nutr Res. 1994;14:127-59.
11. Zieqler P, Briefel R, Clusen N, Devaney B. Feeding of Infants and Toddlers study. J Am Diet Assoc. 2006;106(suppl 1):S12-27.

Nutrition for Older Children

"Tell me what you eat and I will tell you what you are"
—Anthelme Brillat Savarin (1825)

INTRODUCTION

A child having completed his second year of life will gradually begin to show many changes which are a part of his normal growth and development. His association with food assumes a varied spectrum, right from a language of communication to a show of emotions, to the extent of acceptance or rejection or selection of food.[1] But the fact remains that 'food' or more precisely 'good nutrition' continues to remain fundamental to the child's physical and mental growth and development.

Growth and development is a continuous process whereby each year builds upon the preceding one.[1] It is here that the role of building good food habits assumes significance. Good food habits can not be acquired overnight or for one particular period. They have to be built over the years and these years begin right from one's childhood. At this point, parents, health workers and to some extent teachers can play a crucial role to help the child.

Unlike in the past when a child used to enter school not before the age of five, today, due to changing times, a child is exposed to the outside world as early as 2.5–3 years. It is here that the process of food becoming a social event begins, when the packed tiffin which is sent with him (to the Nursery or pre-preparatory school or crèches), becomes a medium of another school activity. This participation inculcates certain habits, such as sharing, widening circles of human relationship and also becoming a sociocultural activity.

BUILDING GOOD FOOD HABITS

Certain considerations towards building good food habits should be:
1. Maintaining regular meal timings in a pleasant environment.
2. Offering small in between snacks of a nutritious variety.

3. Avoiding monotony in various meals. Change is usually welcome and will help develop new tastes.

4. Food items should be such that the child is able to handle himself without messing or difficulty. Where and when required, adult help would be appreciated.

5. Avoiding use to tinned products or instant ready to mix preparations. A child fed on such feeds will not accept the simpler home-based family diet later.

6. When ever possible, one meal of the day should be a 'family affair' where all the family members sit together and enjoy food rather than considering it as just another routine affair.

7. Undue anxiety over food should be avoided as it can rebound as a reaction of food becoming a weapon by the child to win his point.

DIET FOR THE PRESCHOOL CHILD (2–5 YEARS)

Growth and development although have a set pattern at various stages, need not necessarily be a uniform process for all children. Therefore, no two children should be assessed on a comparative basis but as an individual by himself. The velocity of growth tends to keep changing at various stages. During the second year of life there is a further deceleration of the growth rate. An average child gains 2.5 kg and 12 cm during this year. The decrease in appetite which had generally started by about 1 year extends well into the second year. This causes loss of some subcutanous tissue, which had reached its peak by about 10 months of life.[2] As a result the 'plump look' baby gradually begins to change to a lean and muscular child. According to Beal, healthy well-nourished girls reduced their milk intake as early as six months and returned to higher intakes at 2–3 years of age. Boys showed a reduction in their intake around nine months, but increased their intake by the end of two years. Pattern of appetite was seen to vary from child to child. In Beal's study, appetite of some children improved by five years or earlier, while other continued to eat poorly well into their school years.[3]

During the third to fifth year of life, weight and height gains are relatively steady. It is generally about 2 kg and about 6–8 cm gain in weight and height, respectively.[2] Besides, dentition begins to appear by about 2½–3 years resulting in changes in food habits and likes and dislikes of specific food items. A study conducted by the National Nutrition Survey in its first phase was directed towards areas of low income in ten states. This study revealed an alarming amount of malnutrition which included every type of deficiency seen in underdeveloped countries. However, cases of severe deficiency states like kwashiorkor, rickets and goiter were few, but still occurred. The incidence of failure to gain weight at a satisfactory rate was high among preschool children. Anemia was widely seen in this age group and dental decay was found to be practically universal.[4] This study was in total contrast to the others where nutritional status of most children in USA was good, due to the fact that the latter studies were limited to children from middle income groups where such problems are uncommon.[3,5] Beal and her associates, in a longitudinal study, confirmed that at a given age set up, the individual patterns of growth varied widely just as their intakes of nutrients varied.[3] More recent observations made in the pediatric out patient department of PGI, Chandigarh also revealed similar trends. The intakes and nutritional status of children 0–2 years were found to be proportionate to the socioeconomic and literacy levels of the mothers. The better the socioeconomic status and literacy level, more satisfactory was the food intakes and consequently nutritional status of the children.[6]

RECOMMENDED NUTRIENTS AND FOOD GROUPS

Considering the RDA for various nutrients [Chapter 5, Table 5.2 (a) and 5.2 (b)], and those for various food groups (Chapter 5, Table 5.3), it may be appreciated that it is not very difficult to provide the recommended foods. These are basically the common day-to-day food stuffs prepared by every household. The concept of extra milk or fruit requirement does not hold any weight, because as observed from the RDA, it is the common cereal-pulse-vegetable combinations commonly prepared at home, that requires emphasis rather than milk, fruit or eggs, meat, etc. Even small helpings of vegetables can be adequate to meet the requirements. Moreover making use of Mother Nature's gift to man-'seasonal crop' can best serve the purpose. Carrots and most green leafy vegetables available in abundance during the winter season can fulfill our daily needs of vitamin A, iron and calcium, in fact, also store for the lean period. Similarly the practice of consuming jaggery or 'gur' in winters and also ground nuts can provide adequate iron and proteins to us. In fact, whenever available these should be consumed throughout the year. Fruits though not essential, if made use of seasons gift can also prove easily accessible. Mangoes in summers are in abundance which can take care of the vitamin A requirements and perhaps even in building the store. Similarly amla and guava—the cheaper fruits are in fact precious enough in terms of their high vitamin C content. This way a judicious selection of foods available and formation of healthy good habits can easily provide the required nutrients for any individual for any given day. It is not necessary to be able to spend more' to 'provide more'. Rather overspending also leads to 'over nutrition' or wrong nutrition, which, if unbalanced can prove detrimental to the health of the children. Some easy to prepare low cost nutritious recipes as given in the Annexure can be planned (Annexure).

DIET FOR THE SCHOOL CHILDREN (6–12 YEARS)

Growth rate of children between 6 and 12 years of age continues to remain steady more or less ending in a pre-adolescent growth spurt by about 10 years in girls and 12 years in boys. The average weight gain during these years is about 3–3.5 kg per year and about 6 cm in height correspondingly.[2] This period of life is full of vigor and activity with increased physical output. Appetite of these children also tends to show an increase and correspondingly they tend to show good gain in weight and height. Normally, the fat in the subcutanous tissue which had decreased between ages 1 and 6 years in both sexes begins to redeposit as early as 8 years in girls and 10 years in boys with normal nutrition. They again tend to become chubby and look full and rounder just before the increased velocity of growth at pre-adolescent stage of 12 years.[2] During this period, girls and boys become conscious of their growth spurt and other changer of physical development. It is quite common to see uneven distribution of fat in them which during adolescence tends to spread out uniformly.

During these years, environmental stress and strains are not uncommon and most often children fall prey to all kinds to infections, some minor like viral, etc. to the more severe forms like tuberculosis or recurrent diarrheas. In such conditions, appetite is the first to suffer and their intakes decrease drastically, added to the lost in appetite are various fancies of children for particular goods which may not necessarily be nutritious. These result in failure to gain weight, and complaints of easy fatigueability, decreased alertness in school and irritability are some commonly associated problems.

WHAT ARE FOOD FADS

Besides poor appetite consequent to injections, certain other factors are a major contributor to the poor or faulty dietary patterns among children. Old blind beliefs and wrong food fads of 'hot', 'cold', 'light' and 'heavy' foods are most commonly seen among the Indian population including the so called educated class. Restriction of specific foods not suitable during a specific illness or being a cause of certain diseases adds to the problem of poor intake or faulty food habits; e.g. restricting banana during an episode of cold and coughs or it causes phlegm, or curd during fever due to its' cold' effect, of rice causing joint aches and cold; fats, jaggery and ground nuts are considered hot and heavy and hence, avoided during summers. Treating most diarrhoeas and fevers with tea spiced with certain herbal leaves is another very common practice which can adversely affect the child's appetite besides compromising on their nutrition. On the contrary, banana being a good source of calories and potassium can provide enough nutrition during any illness. Rice-based simple soft foods can equally be good with some added fat to increase the calories besides making it palatable in an otherwise anorexic condition. Jaggery and ground nuts commonly blamed for being hot and difficult to digest are on the contrary very good sources of vitamin A, and iron and proteins and calories, respectively. These should be consumed not only during winters but throughout the years whenever available. Sweets made from jaggery and addition of 1–2 tsps of ground nut powder can make an excellent source of calories, protein, vitamin A and iron.

HOW TO MEET THE REQUIREMENTS (RIGHT SELECTION)

As observed from the RDA (Chapter 5, Table 5.3) with increase in age, the stress is more upon cereals and pulses, the other groups like milk, fats and sugars remain more or less consistent. This requires a proper selection of foods. This means a child aged 7–10 years should be having approximately 10–12 chappatis or its equivalent in terms of rice, dalia, bread, etc. Pulses also should form an essential part of a meal, because the requirement of 60–70 g can only be met, if had as at least one serving (approx. 1 medium katori, i.e. 100 g cooked) twice a day. The same may otherwise be incorporated in the form of mixed flour as 'missi roti' bread sandwhiches, 'khichri' or even mixed dalia.

In between small feedings or snacks in the form of besan pura or pan cakes of corn flour or bread pakoras with paneer on potato stuffings can be excellent cereal/pulse-based nutritious combinations. Besan ladoos or groundnut and jaggery-based sweets can also serve as good in between snacks to meet the day's requirements. Milk, however remains the same as in the early years (approx 200–300 mL). Seasonal fruits and vegetables in moderate amounts can easily meet the requirements of most vitamins and minerals besides providing adequate fiber. Here in lies the importance of proper selection of foods and building good food habits. As mentioned earlier in this article, good food habits can only be built over the years. A child may be having adequate or even extra calories but through milk-based sweets, chocolates or any such junk foods available readily in attractive displays. The media exposure to tempting eatables sold in attractive packets, e.g. of potato wafers or instant noodles or cream soups are a major contributory factor for inculcating wrong selection and food habits. All these items may be providing enough calories but without the much needed proteins, vitamins and minerals.

It becomes very essential therefore that some adult supervision for the right selection of foods is made so that a balance is maintained between the requirements and the likes and dislikes of the child.

Annexure

Low-cost Nutritious Recipes

Nutritious Laddoo

Wheat flour	½ cup
Besan	½ cup
Oil	½ cup
Jaggery powder	1 cup
Til	2–3 tsp.

1. Roast the til without oil.
2. Fry the wheat flour and besan in the oil till golden brown.
3. Mix jaggery powder to the above mixture along with til and form into laddoos.

Carrot/Pumpkin Barfi

Pumpkin/Carrot	250 g/4–5
Jaggery/Sugar	50 g

Oil   1 tsp
Coconut gratings   If available
  1. Peel the carrots and grate finely.
  2. Prepare sugar syrup till slightly thick.
  3. Add coconut gratings and cook till the mixture leaves the side of the pan.
  4. Pour the mixture into a greased plate and cut into squares on cooling.

Besan Barfi

Wheat flour   100 g
Besan   100 g
Groundnut powder   200 g
Oil   7–8 tsp
Til   50 g
Ground jaggery/sugar   200 g
  1. Roast ground nuts and after peeling grind into coarse powder.
  2. Roast til without oil till reddish brown.
  3. Roast both flours separately first and then together in oil.
  4. Mix til, ground nut powder and jaggery powder or sugar and store in a jar on cooling.

Soyabean Pulao

Soyabean   50 g
Rice   100 g
Onions   25 g (1)
Carrot   ½–1
Peas   2–3 tsp
Cabbage/Cauliflower   100 g
Tomatoes   2
Spinach   1–2 leaves
Oil   5–6 tsp
Salt/Spices   To taste
  1. Soak soyabeans overnight. Remove spin the morning and boil or pressure cook for 10 minutes.
  2. Clean and soak rice for 10–15 minutes.
  3. Peel and slice vegetables into moderate size pieces.
  4. Heat oil in a vessel pressure pan. Fry sliced onions and other vegetables slightly.
  5. Add the soaked rice with 1 tsp. salt and let boil or pressure cook till done.
  6. Serve with curd.

Moong dal/Black channa'chaat'

Moon dal/Black channa   25 g
Roasted groundnut powder   2 tsp
Tomato   ½
Patato   1 (boiled)

Roasted channa dal	2 tsp
Oil	1–2 tsp
Salt	To taste.

1. Soak the pulse overnight.
2. Next day remove from water and tie in wet muslin cloth and leave for 12–24 hours till sprouts appear.
3. Pressure cook or boil the sprouted pulse for 5 minutes to soften it.
4. Fry the vegetables lightly and add boiled potatoes later.
5. Add the steamed pulse along with salt and spices.
6. Serve with lime, coriander leaves and chaat masala.

Missi Roti

Wheat flour	15 g
Gram flour (based	15 g
spinach/fenugreek leaves)	3–4
Onion	½
Oil	1½ tsp
Salt	To taste

1. Chop spinach/fenugreek leaves finely after washing.
2. Knead the flour with chopped leaves and onion adding salt to taste.
3. Make small balls and roll out to make medium-size paranthas.
4. Fry on both sides with oil and serve hot.

Poha

Chidwa (rice flakes)	25 g
Groundnuts	10 g
Onion	½
Roasted gram dal	10 g
Potato	¼–½
Carrot (sliced)	½
Salt	To taste
Oil	2–3 tsp

1. Wash the chidwa and keep aside.
2. Slice potatoes, carrots and onions finely.
3. Heat oil and fry the above vegetables.
4. Add groundnuts and roasted dal to the above and fry till brownish.
5. Now add the wet chidwa along with some salt and turmeric powder and mix all the ingredients well.
6. If desired, add finely chopped coriander leaves and green chilli. Mix again and serve.

Upma

Suji	½ cup
Groundnuts	10 g
Carrots sliced	½

Potato sliced	½
Tomato	1
Onion sliced	1
Salt	To taste
Mustard seeds	¼ tsp
Oil	3–4 tsp
Water	1½ cup

1. Fry suji in oil till brown and keep aside.
2. In a karahi, heat oil and fry mustard seeds till they sprout. Then add the vegetables and groundnuts.
3. Add to the above thrice the amount of water as suji and boil adding salt.
4. Once the mixture boils well add the fried suji gradually, stirring simultaneously till the whole mixture forms into a smooth 'halwa' like consistency.
5. Serve with any chutney, pickle or sauce.

Coconut Groundnut Chikki

Coconut powder	50 g
Roasted groundnut	50 g
Sugar powder	50 g

Method:
1. Roast the groundnuts.
2. Remove husk with hands and grind coarsely.
3. Make sugar syrup by mixing sugar and water in a pan. Add 2 tsp milk in the syrup and filter it to make it clear of residue.
4. Mix all the dry ingredients and spread evenly on a greased plate.
5. Keep it to cool for 5–6 hours and cut into square pieces and store.

Fruit Smoothie

Papaya	50 g
Grapes	50 g
Strawberries/Apples	50 g
Dates	2 No.
Skimmed milk powder	3 tsp
Milk	150 mL
Sugar	3 tsp
Almond/Walnut powder	2 tsp

Method:
1. Take all the above fresh fruits and blend well.
2. Boil milk in a pan, let cool and add skim milk, sugar and powder and dates.
3. Serve chilled.

REFERENCES

1. Beal VA. "Dietary Intake of Individuals followed through and childhood. Am J. Pub Health. 1961;51(8):1107-71.
2. Behr-man RE, Kliegman RM, Jenson HB. Growth and Development. In: Nelson Textbook of Pediatrics Part I, 16th Ed. Harcourt Publishers International Co. 2000. pp 23-65.
3. Gopalan C, Rama Sastri BV, Balasubraminiam SC. Nutritive Value of Indian Foods, National Institute of Nutrition, ICMR, Hyderabad, 2010.
4. Madhu Sharma, Thapa BR. Impact of Socio-economic and literacy level on nutritional status of children (un-published).
5. Morgan AF Ed: Nutritional status, USA. Bull.769, California Agricultural Experiment station, Barkley, 1959.
6. Robinson CH. Nutrition for Children and Teenagers, In: Normal and Therapeutic Nutrition, 14th Ed. Oxford &IBH Publishing CO.;1972. pp 321-36.

Nutrition for the Adolescent

"We are indeed much more than what we eat, but what we eat can nevertheless help us to be much more than what we are"

—Adelle Davis

INTRODUCTION

Adolescence is the period of transition from childhood to adult and any transitional phase involves some stress and strain. An adolescent sometimes finds himself in a peculiar circumstance of adjustment to a new environment and may experience the pain of setting in to the groove of the big world. It is also a period of rapid growth and maturity, both physiologically and psychologically.

In the past few years, the adolescent group has become a focus of great interest for physicians, nutritionists, social worker and psychologists, due to the realization that this is the group that required a lot of support and right guidance in term of physical growth, sexual maturation, optimum nutrition and sound mental help.

About 35% of adult weight and 11–18% of adult height is acquired during the adolescent age. Nutrition plays a key role to support this rapid growth and development. More than 80% of the adolescent population lives in the developed countries where growth in number and proportion of children and adolescents has far exceeded in any other age group.

According to studies from National Institute of Nutrition figures,[1] the population projections for India indicate that the number of adolescents will increase from 200 million in 1996 to 215.3 million in 2016.

Adolescence has also been referred to as a window of opportunity to prepare for a healthy productive and reproductive life, and prevent the onset of nutrition-related chronic diseases in adult life. At the same time this is the last chance to address adolescent-specific nutrition issues and possibly, also correction of some nutritional problems originating in the past.

This is the period when they get conscious of their looks, figure and personality. Eating behavior during this period is greatly influenced by school pressures, peer pressures, media influence and parental support.

Anemia and chronic undernutrition, are the two major problems encountered during this phase. This picture of malnutrition is mainly the result of exposure to media and easy access to junk foods through more available money on hand. It would not be an overstatement, as endorsed by authors that undernutrition in the early teens is directly linked to lifestyle-related diseases of adulthood like diabetes, hypertension and cardiovascular disease.[2]

These lifestyle and eating behaviors, along with psychosocial factors are particularly important threats to adequate nutrition. Therefore, this period of adolescence can be considered a timely period to shape and consolidate healthy eating and lifestyle behaviors, thereby preventing or postponing the onset of nutrition-related chronic diseases in adulthood.

Certain nutrition issues are adolescent specific and need to be targeted with specific strategies and approaches. These include the following:

- Increased nutritional needs
- Growth assessment
- Adolescent eating patterns and lifestyle
- Nutrition related to early pregnancy.

INCREASED NUTRITIONAL NEEDS

The period of adolescence has also been termed as the period of 'youth'. This is that time of life which begins at puberty. For girls, puberty typically occurs between 12 and 13 years of age, while for boys it occurs between ages 14 and 15 years, and the velocity or spurt of growth is the fastest during this period.

Energy

As per ICMR estimates, energy requirement for children 1–10 years is lower than the value derived from food intake data, but thereafter for adolescents, it is higher.[3] The energy requirement of children and adolescents were estimated on children from 75% industrialized and developing countries. It is emphasized by experts that the values derived for adolescents are based on the assumption that they are physically active and in fact by this phase their activity has increased further as compared to younger age group.[4]

As seen from Table 7.1, the caloric needs of boys from pre-adolescent (10–12 years) begin from around 2200 calories, increases to almost 3020 by the time they are 18 years. Similarly for girls, the range begins from approximately 2000 calories at about 10–12 years and increases to about 2440 calories. This is a significant increase from childhood phase. The peak increase for both, boys and girls is around 16 years. The recommendation for distribution of these calories from carbohydrates, fats and proteins is 55–60%, less than 10% saturated fats and about 30%, respectively. Various studies from Indian group indicate a poor nutritional status of adolescents, especially in terms of energy intakes.

Table 7.1: Recommended nutrient allowances for adolescents

Age group (years)	Sex	Wt. (kg)	Calories/ day	Protein g/d	Fat mg/d	Calcium mg/d	Iron mg/d
10–12	Boys	34.3	2190	39.9	35	800	21
	Girls	35.0	2010	40.4	35	800	27
13–15	Boys	47.6	2750	54.3	45	800	32
	Girls	46.6	2330	51.9	40	800	27
16–17	Boys	55.4	3020	61.5	50	800	28
	Girls	52.1	2440	55.5	35	800	26

Source: ICMR, 2010.

Although, there is no data available for optimum level of physical activity, it is recommended that children should involve in moderately intense physical activity at least for one hour per day.[4]

This activity may be split in bouts of 10–20 minutes, even if it is not done in one stretch. The moderately intense physical activity inculcates activities that have body displacement and physical effort, which can be achieved through individual activities like walking, running or cycling or team sports and games. The physical activity level (PAL), (which is the ratio of energy expenditure for 24 hours and the basal metabolic rate (BMR) over 24 hours), is taken into consideration while computing the energy requirements for the various age groups as shown in Tables 7.2 and 7.3 for boys and girls, respectively. The PAL values are based on activity level, sedentary and vigorous activity.[4]

Proteins

Adequate intake of proteins is also very important for growth and maintenance of muscle mass. At adolescent age beginning from age 11 years boys and girls have different growth patterns and so their protein deposition rates too will differ. The safe values for protein derived from an Indian balanced diet are as given in Table 7.4.[4]

The safe requirements are more systematically derived values than the earlier values which were based on body weight increases and their protein component. Therefore these values can be adopted for Indian children. In terms of good quality proteins, safe intakes for Indian children have been proposed by FAO/WHO/UNU, and the values corrected for Indian cereal –pulse-milk based balanced diet for all age groups including adolescents as given in Table 7.4. The requirement for girls gradually increases from 40 g at age 11–12 to 56 g by age 17–18 years but steadily increases by 14–15 years to 57.7 g and peaking at 62.2 g by 17–18 years.

Table 7.2: Energy requirements and PAL of Indian boys at different activity levels

Age (years)	Weight (kg)	Sedentary[1]			Vigorous activity[2]		
		Total energy req[3]. (kcal/d)	Total energy req.† (kcal/kg/d)	Pal	Total energy req.[3] (kcal/d)	Total energy req.[3] (kcal/kg/d)	Pal
11–12	30.8	1700	55	1.5	2550	75	2.0
12–13	38.0	2020	55	1.5	2680	70	2.0
13–14	43.3	2160	50	1.5	3010	70	2.1
14–15	48.0	2280	50	1.5	3180	65	2.1
15–16	51.5	2530	50	1.6	3310	65	2.1
16–17	54.3	2600	50	1.6	3400	65	2.1
17–18	56.5	2660	45	1.6	3490	60	2.1

Source: ICMR 2010.
[1] Sedentary activities—A child not engaged in organized sport/games and went to school by motorized means
[2] Vigorous activity—Walking/cycling long distances daily in high intensity/energy demanding chores or games for several hours, or intensively practicing sports for several hours a day and several hours in a week
[3] Rounded off to the nearest 10 kcal/day
† Rounded off to the nearest 5 kcal/kg/day

Table 7.3: Energy requirements and PAL of Indian girls at different activity levels

Age (years)	Weight (kg)	Sedentary[1]			Vigorous activity[2]		
		Total energy requirement (kcals/d)[3]	Total energy requirement (kcal/kg/d)†	Pal	Total energy requirement (kcal/d)[3]	Total energy requirement (kcal/kg/d)[3]	Pal
11–12	34.8	1770	50	1.5	2350	65	2.0
12–13	39.0	1840	50	1.5	2450	65	2.0
13–14	43.4	1930	45	1.5	2570	60	2.0
14–15	47.1	2000	45	1.5	2660	55	2.0
15–16	49.4	2040	40	1.5	2720	55	2.0
16–17	51.3	2040	40	1.5	2730	55	2.0
17–18	52.8	2040	40	1.5	2860	55	2.1

Source: ICMR, 2010.
[1] Sedentary activity—Child who does not engage in organized sport/games and goes to school by motorized means
[2] Vigorous activity—Walking/cycling long distances everyday, engaging in high intensity/energy demanding chores or games for several hours, or intensively practicing sports for several hours a day and several days in a week
[3] Round off to the nearest 10 kcals/d
† Rounded off to the nearest 5 kcals/kg/d

Table 7.4: Protein requirement and dietary allowances for adolescent boys and girls

Adolescents (years)	Boys			Girls		
	Require[1][2] (g/kg/d)	Body Wt. (kg)	Total daily Requirement (g/d)	Requirement[1][2] (g/kg/d)	Body Wt. (kg)	Total Requirement (g/d)
10–11	1.18	30.8	36.3	1.18	31.2	36.8
11–12	1.16	34.1	39.6	1.15	34.8	40.0
12–13	1.15	38.0	43.7	1.14	39.0	44.5
13–14	1.15	43.3	49.8	1.13	43.4	49.0
14–15	1.14	48.0	54.7	1.12	47.1	52.8
15–16	1.13	51.5	58.2	1.09	49.4	53.8
16–17	1.12	54.3	60.8	1.07	51.3	54.9
17–18	1.10	56.5	62.2	1.06	52.8	56.0

Source: ICMR 2010.
[1] In terms of mixed Indian vegetarian diet protein
[2] Requirements for each age band taken as the protein requirement for the lower age limit at that age band

For communities like Punjab, Haryana and even Delhi, children belonging to the upper middle class and higher strata of life, these requirements may not be very difficult to achieve, given the consumption of milk and milk products and nonvegetarian foods which are pre-dominant in their dietary habits. However, in fast growing culture of media friendly youth, involved in a string of fashion competition, the fear of gaining extra kilos and preserving the ideal figure, may deter them from adequate and right type of dietary habits. In such scenarios, the protein intake may be compromised due to faulty eating behavior and over indulgence in empty calorie dense foods and beverages.

Fats

For all children right from 2 years to 17 years, it is recommended that the total fat intake should not be less than 25% to avoid compromising on their growth and development. As observed from Table 2.1 (chapter 2), the RDA for fats is around 35–40 g between ages 10–15 for both boys and girls, except for boys in the age range of 13–15 years where the allowance is slightly higher (45 g per day. But boys between ages 16–17 again require about 50 g of visible fat, after which the requirement again drops to that as that for adults (25–30 g). Considering the fact that less than 10% of total energy requirement is from saturated fats, this amount is adequate to meet the recommended allowances. The invisible fat in other dietary sources like milk, cereal, pulses and nonvegetarian foods, besides, nuts and oilseeds which go to make up a day's meal, should not exceed 15–20 g to comply with recommendation of less then 10% of energy from saturated fats.

	Table 7.5: Recommendations on types of visible fat
1.	Use correct combination/blend of two or more vegetable oils (1:1)## Oil containing LA +oil containing both LA and ALA* Groundnut/Sesame[1]/Rice bran[2]/Cottonseed + Mustard/Rapeseed** Groundnut/Sesame[1]/Ricebran[2]/Cottonseed + Canola Groundnut/Sesame/[1]/Rice bran[2]/Cottonseed + Soyabean Palmolein[3] + Soyabean Safflower/Sunflower + Palm Oil/Palmolein[3] +Mustard/Rapeseed** Oil containing high LA + oll containing moderate or low LA*** Sunflower/Safflower + Palmolein[3]/ Palm oil[3]/Olive Safflower/Sunflower + Palmolein[3]/Palm oil[3]/Ricebran[2]/Cottonseed
2.	Limit use of butter/ghee†
3.	Avoid use of PHVO as medium for cooking/frying
4.	Replacements for PHVO Frying : Oils which have higher thermal stability—palm oil, palmolein, sesame, ricebran, cottonseed—single/blends (home/commercial) Bakery fat, shortening, Indian sweets, etc.—Food applications which require solid fats: Coconut oil/palm kernel oil/palm oil/palmoloein/palm stearin and /their solid fractions and/their blends.

Source: ICMR, 2010.
All vegetable oils contain tocopherols and plant steroids
[1] seasame lignans, [2] oryzanols + tocotrienols,[3] †vitamins A and D
Furnish greater variety of nonglyceride components
*Approximately 30–40% PUFAs with >3% ALA
** Combinations with Rapeseed/mustard reduce erucic acid levels
*** Approximately 40–50% LA and <0.5% ALA, recommended only when intake of ALA from other foods/conventional foods is increased and adequate amount of fish is consumed

An important point to keep in mind about fat recommendations, besides the amounts or quantity of fat, the quality of visible fat is also very important to be considered while using fats in the diets of children, adolescents and adults. Tables 7.5 highlights the quality of fats recommended and how to achieve them in diet planning.

Calcium

The skeleton account for at least 99% of body stores of calcium and the gains in skeletal weight is most rapid during adolescent growth. About 45% of the adult skeletal mass is formed during adolescent growth. The largest gains are made in early adolescence between 10–14 years in girls and 12–16 years in boys. During peak adolescent growth, calcium retention is on an average about 200 g/d in girls and 300 g/d in boys. The efficiency of calcium absorption is only about 30%. Therefore, it is important that to reduce the risk of osteoporosis in later adult life, adequate calcium is provided in the diets of adolescents. The dietary requirements have therefore been revised to 800 g per day for this age group of children as seen in Table 7.1. Activities like cycling, gymnastics skating, dancing and supervised weight training for at least 30–60 minutes a day, three to four times a week can help build bone mass and density. In the well-to-do middle class houses where milk consumption is an essential component of a day's meal, especially in the North Indian community, deficiency is not very common. Of course, as mentioned earlier, with today's youth focused on more weight management, deficiency of calcium can pose a major risk.

Iron

Iron deficiency anemia is very common in adolescence, in view of their increased blood volume and muscle mass during growth and development. The increased lean body mass (LBM) composed mainly of muscle is more important in adolescent boys than in girls. In the preadolescent period, LBM is about the same for both sexes. With the onset of adolescence, boys undergo a very rapid accumulation of LBM for each additional kilogram of body weight gained during growth ending up with a final LBM maximum value, double that of girls. In girls increased body mass and onset of menarche also account for increased requirements. It has been observed widely among the youth, that their meal pattern is such that adequate tissue replacement cannot be met with. Good iron sources are, iron whole grains, pulses, green leafy vegetables, jaggery and nonvegetarian foods like egg yolk, organ meats like liver. Iron from nonvegetarian sources like lean meats and fish (known as hem iron) is better absorbed than iron from nonhem iron. But even in nonvegetarian families, these foods do not form a regular feature in majority of them. Therefore, left with the vegetarian sources, the adolescent of today's generation is quite averse to include whole cereals or leafy vegetables in their diet. Most of the refined or processed foods available at the supermarket, which they mainly rely on, are all devoid of iron which can be a significant contributory factor for anemia. Nutritional anemia itself is a major national nutritional problem and can be responsible for a host of eating and behavioral problems like anorexia, irritability and lethargy. Iron supplements can be given to those who tend to be anemic.

Recommendations for various nutrients in terms of the daily dietary intake for all age groups are as given in Chapter 5, Table 5.3.

Growth Assessment

Anthropometry is the one most important criterion to monitor growth assessment. The report of the WHO expert committee for anthropometric methods and reference data[5] includes specific recommendations for appropriate use of anthropometry in all age groups including adolescents, for screening or program response evaluation at the individual or population level. Reference data tables are provided, as well as calculations to convert weight and heights into BMI values. Anthropometric data may help identify stunting underweight, overweight and obesity. Stunting or short height for age may reflect maturation in the past irrespective of the current problem. The assessment of obesity and adiposity level is more difficult in adolescents than in adults due to rapid changes in body composition. The velocity of growth values at different stages of life, is greater during the first five years of life, then slows down, and again reaches its peak during the adolescent years. During puberty, boys gain about 20–38 cm in height, while girls about 16–25 cm. Similarly weight gain is about 20 kg in boys and 16 kg in girls by the time of puberty.

Growth pattern of adolescent Indian boys and girls (10–19 years) as per the National Nutrition Monitoring Bureau (NNMB) data is shown in Figs 7.1 and 7.2.[6]

The WHO recommended standard reference growth charts is the NCHS standard, validated in 1963–1975 and updated in 2000 on more than 20,000 well nourished healthy US population from birth to 18 years. The 50th centile of the normal distribution curve is the median and is considered as standard value or 100% of the expected. The International Obesity Task Force (IOTF) has defined BMI >18.5 as normal; >25 corresponding to 90th centile as overweight and >30 corresponding to 97th centile as obesity. Studies on Indian children[7] have reported that 79% of the poor rural girls from Rajasthan below 13 years have a BMI below 18.5, which is otherwise considered as normal. Therefore, it was suggested that values <15 be indicative of underweight or chronic energy deficit (CED) and <13 as severely underweight. The upper cut off of 22 for overweight and 25 for obesity in young adolescents during the growth period seems appropriate and in accordance with IOTF standards.

In view of the current trend of nutrition transition taking over in India, and consequently the growth pattern of children, Indian Academy of Pediatrics (IAP) has computed new growth and BMI charts for children from 5–18 years [Refer also BMI charts (Figs 3.11 and 3.12) for Indian boys and girls, Chapter 3].

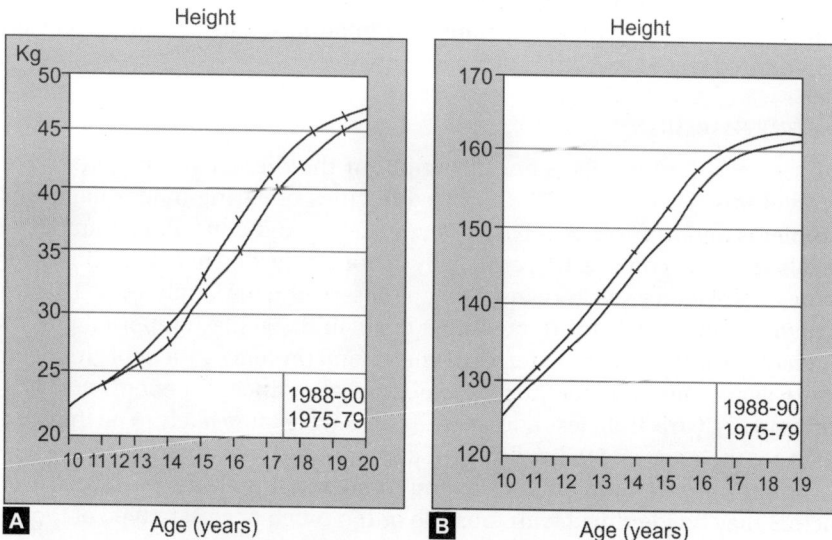

Figs 7.1A and B: Growth pattern of adolescent boys
Source: NNMB, NIN, Hyderabad 1975–1990.

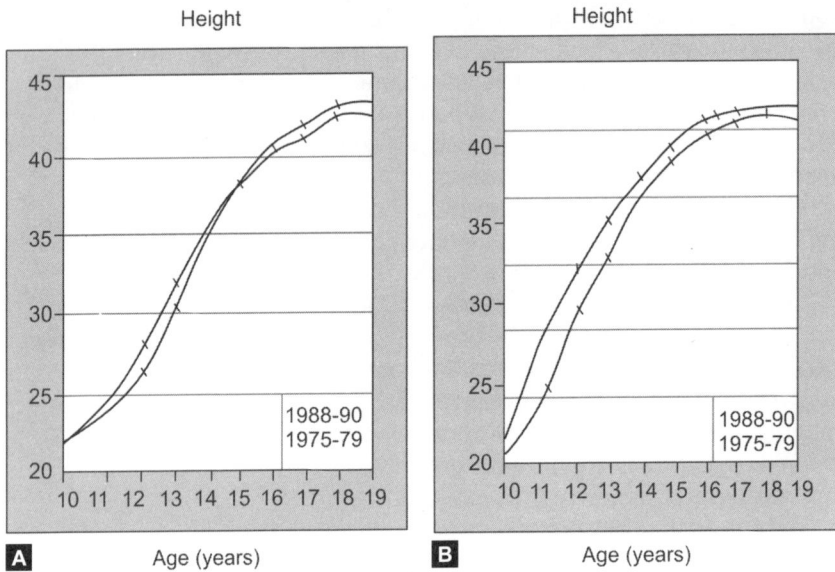

Figs 7.2A and B: Growth pattern of adolescent girls
Source: NNMB, NIN, Hyderabad 1975–1990.

In addition to weight, height and BMI, upper segment to lower segment ratio is also considered. An upper segment to lower segment ratio of 0.9–1.0 is expected among adolescents and in adults it is 1.1. Higher U/L segment ratio is characteristic of short limb dwarfism and bone disorders like rickets. BMI measurements of adolescents are recommended wherever and whenever feasible, irrespective of the type of nutrition problems to be expected. Whether too high or too low, inappropriate BMI in adolescents should trigger an appropriate response from health care providers.

Dietary Assessment

Diet assessment involves enquiring about the dietary intake pattern of individuals. This is intended to provide clues of eating inadequacies or problems and to serve as a basis for counseling and education. Number of meals and their composition especially in nonstaple food items, are powerful indicators of food security or insecurity as observed at the family level.[8] Dietary enquiries when conducted by Ahmed et al.[9] in Bangladesh reported grossly inadequate intakes, both in terms of energy and proteins, in school girls aged 10–16 years. Only 8% met the recommended allowances for energy and 17% for proteins. Girls from less educated families were more likely to be thin and short for their age and to have diets of poorer nutritional quality.

Inappropriate food choices owing to personal preferences or cultural factors may be identified with too little or too much of certain type of foods. Finally, the enquiry may reveal a risk of eating disorders, and for this, questions on body image and dieting are in order.

Adolescent Eating Pattern and Lifestyles

Dietary habits that affect food preferences are generally developed in childhood and particularly during the adolescent years.[10] The patterns of eating vary widely among the youth and are influenced by various social, economic, physiological and psychological factors.[11]

Adolescents today have a greater freedom to break away from the family dietary patterns and eat with their peers. This involves eating any type of food accessible easily in plenty. Such observations have been made by many workers.[12]

Irregular meal timings can also be one of the contributory factors to unhealthy food habits. A study on well-to-do boys and girls in Delhi revealed that the dietary intake in terms of energy and protein was less as compared to RDA in both sexes. The calorie deficit was 27% in case of girls and 25% in case of boys,[13] Observations from a study on adolescents from Chandigarh, revealed that the calorie distribution from macronutrients was highly skewed.[14] In the diets of these adolescents, the carbohydrates contributed about 50–64% of the total calorie, but that contributed by proteins was only around 11% against a desired level of 15%. On the other hand, as high as 29% of the calories came from fats against the RDA of 20–25%.

Factors Affecting Adolescent Eating Pattern

Changing Lifestyle

As the child moves on to his teens from the school phase, he undergoes a sea of change in his environment. He becomes more conscious of his looks and appearances. The same holds true for the girls also. They are highly susceptible to peer pressure with regard to their eating patterns. They become 'choosy' for selective foods, irrespective of whether it is nutritionally healthy or not. As a school child he carries tiffin along with him to be had during the break time. Certain schools too are particular regarding the type of food/snacks children bring to school. Others are day boarding schools where lunch is a social activity, supervised by house teachers. But as soon as they finish school and enter college life, the tiffin boxes disappear and they rely on college canteens for eating. They are very susceptible to peer influenced eating styles. Cold drinks, sweetened beverages, pizzas, samosas, burgers, noodles, etc. are a routine affair and replace meals. Besides, they enter into the big world to make a niche for themselves. The new culture of tuitions competing with their meal timings prevents them to devote adequate time to spend on eating. Meal schedules are disturbed and they tend to resort to whatever is available at hand to satiate them. Moreover, most of these foods available 'at hand' are highly bizarre, with nutritional content of little significance. On the contrary, they are high sugar, high fat based which gives them instant gratification, and consequently missing out on home-based balanced meal.

In addition, there is an increased culture of dining out, even among the middle class families. Any occasion which calls for celebration in the family, is focused around food. The only difference is that in the good old days, food was organized at home under the supervision of the elders, while today, it is much easier and convenient to hire caterers or even organize in big restaurants. Here again, the menu is vast and highly energy dense thanks to the liberal fat and carbohydrate contents of such recipes. Adolescents tend to get hooked on to these types of foods and develop a taste for them, as a result of which they begin to dislike home-based food.

Increased Consumption of Junk Foods

They tend to rely heavily on junk foods like potato chips or fries, burgers, pizzas, etc. Cold drinks like colas, aerated sweetened beverages and bakery products are consumed while on the move. Most of the foods may not feel very 'heavy', but being energy dense due to their high fat content, they are devoid of important minerals like calcium and iron, which make the adolescent highly 'at risk' for developing anemia and osteoporosis at a much younger age. The emergence of multinational fast food joints are patronized by a large number of adolescents and youngsters.[15] A study from Ludhiana on teenager's eating behavior observed that fast foods were mostly consumed in between regular meals, some of the favorites being samosa, bread pakora, potato chips, noodles, pastry, patties and cola drinks.[16]

Missing Meals

It has been reported that the number of meals missed or eaten away from home increases from early adolescence to late adolescence, reflecting their growing independence and more time spent away from home.[17] The meals omitted are generally compensated by snacks and other fast foods. The general trend is that the meal missed maximum is the breakfast, followed by lunch. Very often mothers seem to be satiated if their teenager has a glassful of milk in the name of breakfast. This is because due to the pressure of competition and matching up to the expectations of their parents/teachers, they do not have adequate time to partake a wholesome cereal-based breakfast. Lunch is often skipped due to the long working hours and again lack of time to be home for a good lunch. In the bargain they end up snacking on whatever is conveniently available. Observations made on the dietary pattern of adolescents in Chandigarh revealed that the snacks/junk foods comprised about 25% of the day's calories while percent calories from breakfast was 19% and lunch and dinner combined comprised 41% of the day's intake.[15] A study from Spain, showed that high-energy breakfasts were associated with higher intakes of minerals and vitamins, lower serum cholesterol levels and improved biochemical indices of nutritional status.[18]

Prolonged Television Viewing

Adolescents are easy prey to the television culture and this practice has led to an increased percentage of couch potatoes. It has been reported that television viewing is commonly associated with eating habits of teenagers amongst both under nourished and obese groups. In a study from Indore, 44% of underweight and 53% of the obese children associated television viewing along with meal timings.[19]

Nibbling

This is another very common habit, rather a time pass activity among most adolescent groups. It was found to occur in almost 54–70% of the children irrespective of normal or overweight children.[20] This incidence of nibbling could be also attributed to the fact that they feel hungry or 'munchy' more often, as most of them cannot or do not adhere to a regular three meal pattern with two in between snacks time. This makes them more vulnerable to lay their hands on whatever tit bits are available around. Secondly, most adolescents who 'are' concerned about their overweight status, resort to this practice, by skipping a whole meal to reduce calories and end up munching here and there to satisfy their hunger. They do this under the false concept that these foods tend to be 'light', where as actually they are energy dense (either high fat or sugar). They ultimately end up ingesting more calories than they would have done by a regular meal which would be balanced in all nutrients. Many authors have made similar observations from time to time at different periods.[21,22]

Meal Timings

An ideal meal pattern for a child or adolescent age group is a three-meal pattern with two inbetween snacks. These include breakfast, lunch and dinner. This pattern helps to meet the increasing energy and other nutrient requirements of these children. But in practice this concept has literally disappeared from the schedule of our youth. As mentioned earlier in this chapter, breakfast mostly is skipped (if at all they do so, it comprises nothing more than a glass of milk per force). Lunch timings may not be fixed due to their varied schedule or due to 'snacking' during the inbetween period. The last meal, dinner, may be a heavy one, if they are hungry or again it may be skipped, if in the name of dinner or supper, some snacks are consumed at some fast food joint along with their peers. As high as 41–44% of children do not follow any fixed meal pattern.[20]

Adolescent-related Nutritional Disorders

Obesity

Obesity is emerging as a very common nutritional related disorder and if timely intervention is not done, it can lead to serious chronic disorders in adulthood. The changing lifestyle of the present generation as discussed earlier, is the main contributory factor. Lack of physical activity and other outdoor games along with faulty eating habits takes a toll on their health. The major long-term health problems associated with adolescent obesity are its persistence in adult life and its association with cardiovascular disease risk in later life. Based on the Harvard Growth Study males who were overweight at age 13–18 years were found to be at increased risk of mortality five to six decades later compared to subjects who were lean during adolescence.[23]

In general, longitudinal studies suggest that obesity tracks into adulthood, particularly if it is present in adolescence.[24] It is well established that the amount of body fat and its distribution affects metabolic disease risk. In a cross-sectional study of Bogalusa, anthropometric measures of adiposity were found to be related to lipid and insulin concentrations, even before adulthood.[25] It is estimated that half of cardiovascular disease mortality is nutrition related, and 33–50% of type 2 diabetes cases. (WHO 1990).

Hypertension is another high-risk disease among obese adolescents. Other nutrition-related chronic diseases, such as cardiovascular diseases, diabetes mellitus Type II, and cancer may only appear in adult life, but are associated with dietary and lifestyle risk factors at adolescence, most of which are in association with obesity.

Stunting and Malnutrition

Stunting is commonly observed among adolescents in undernourished populations. Short stature in adolescents is usually caused by infection and inadequate dietary intake during the preschool years. Fetal mal formation may also be a contributory factor. In India, by and large the girls are found to be worse off than boys. This gender difference can perhaps be explained by the deeply rooted sociocultural and economic practices that discriminate against females of all ages. Various studies have shown that most of the growth deficit in adolescents occurred during the first 3 years of life. The positive effects of energy and protein supplementation during the first 3 years of life indeed persisted at adolescence: Height, weight and fat-free mass were still higher in the supplemented than nonsupplemented individuals.[26] The consequences of stunting and malnutrition are delay in maturation especially in girls, reduction of work capacity and ultimately high-risk pregnancy.

Iron Defiency Anemia

Anemia may either be the cause of malnutrition among young adolescents, or malnutrition itself may be the cause of anemia. Prevalence of anemia is estimated to be about 27% in developing countries while only 6% in industrialized countries. According to the ICRW/USAID studies[27] anemia in adolescents was quite high in Nepal (42%) and in India (55%). The prevalence was as high in boys as in girls. The high prevalence of anemia itself can also be a cause for stunting due to failure to achieve their full growth potential. The consequences of anemia can also affect the outcome of pregnancy, especially if it is a teenage pregnancy. Besides it can also result in high risk of low birth weight, prematurity, still births and maternal mortality.

Calcium Deficiency

It is well known that calcium requirements for skeletal development are greater during adolescent period, since maximum bone mass is acquired during adolescence. The amount of calcium reserves made during this period determines the risk of osteoporosis in adulthood. Deficiency of calcium also increases the risk of bone fractures even among adolescent period if atleast 60% of the RDA is not met with. Calcium deficiency during adolescence has also been corelated with postmenopausal bone loss. Regular consumption of dairy products during this period is associated with lower levels of postmenopausal bone loss.

Nutrition-related Dental Decay

According to WHO, in developing countries, dental health may deteriorate rapidly as a consequence of dietary changes. Sucrose or the common table sugar is the main carcinogenic factor since it is generally in a form which sticks to the teeth. Starch or complex carbohydrates are not harmful, therefore diets high in starch but low in sugar have a very-low caries producing potential. Also, partly hydrolyzed starch as found in highly processed foods and snacks items which are literally consumed by youngsters can be carcinogenic. Risk of tooth decay can increase with increased consumption of snack foods, processed or tinned products and other high-sugar foods. Therefore, early malnutrition and dietary changes associated with adolescent lifestyles and socioeconomic development may lead to increasing prevalence of dental decay in adolescents and adults.

Diet and Violence—A New Dimension

'We are what we eat' Our Vedas have long since dwelt at length on the effect of various types of foods we eat and how they can be responsible for the overall personality and behavioral temperament of an individual. The concept of 'cold' or 'hot' foods is deeply buried in the Indian psyche and any changes related to our physical, psychological and even sexual behavior have been attributed to the type of dietary lifestyle of an individual. According to the ancient science, food has been categorized as 'satvic' or 'tamasic', meaning either producing soothing and healthy effects or having a negative influence like aggression, violence, etc. Though not scientifically proven, there might be some basis for this concept.

Today, we can see this impact of dietary pattern on the personality and behavior of our young generation. Violence among children and adolescents is fast leading to a magnitude of epidemic. This trend has led many research workers to look into the depth of the etiology of this new problem, that of malnutrition as a cause of 'child violence'. This phenomenon is steadily spreading across the globe—the developed and the developing countries. Reports of kids killing their own peers over petty issues are increasingly being heard and seen. It is time now that this problem is tackled efficiently with the right approach. Several workers now have established this link between malnutrition and child violence. Malnutrition can involve either excess or deficiency of certain important nutrients during the growth of the child.

High-calorie (Junk) Malnutrition

The link between high-calorie malnutrition and crime and senseless violence has been well documented.[28] High-calorie malnutrition is defined as calorie excess with nutrient deficiencies, resulting in inadequate ability to utilize these calories efficiently. The possible hypothesis attributed is, the incomplete oxidation of some of the byproducts which are toxic and might interfere with the acid–based balance of the body. Most of these high calories are contributed by a high consumption of junk foods. It was seen that these high-calorie foods comprised too much sugar, refined foods and stimulants. Children thriving on such foods were the ones with violent behaviors and were found to be hyperactive. It is believed that hyperactivity and restlessness lead to impatience and a desire for instant gratification. These unfulfilled desires lead to frustration and anger, which may lead to violent behavior.

High-calorie malnutrition can create 'irritable brainstem' since this tissue, (brain) demands highly efficient oxidative metabolism. This 'irritable brainstem' can 'turn up the volume' of the response and in the worst scenario create temporary insanity and take over the complete behavior of the individual. Triggering factors for such behaviors can be as trivial as being refused an expensive car or watch or being rebuked for not concentrating enough on one's studies.

Vitamin and Mineral Deficiencies

Besides excess calories, lack of certain vitamin deficiencies can also trigger violent behavior. Deficiency of vitamin B1 (thiamine) is reported to result in irritability and poorly controlled behavior due to failure of cholinergenic behavior. Supplements of thiamine in the diets of such children for several months resulted in complacency of behavior, which initially were very aggressive and difficult. Other factors like medications (hormone therapy) can contribute to the mood swings and behavioral changes in women. Deficiency of vitamin B12 is also known to trigger violent behavior.[29] The role of other nutrients like iron, cobalt, zinc and iodine are also known to influence behavioral changes in children. A deficiency of iron, for instance is well known to impair mental performance.

Some foods commonly known to contribute to child violence are as follows:

- *Sugar and white flour:* These contribute to empty carbohydrates, leading to high-calorie malnutrition by providing calories without vitamins and other supporting nutrients, to assimilate these calories
- *Sugar drinks:* High in phosphoric acid which causes calcium depletion. They are also high in sugar contributing to 'high-calorie malnutrition'.

Caffeine in soft drinks is likely to stimulate the adrenal glands leading to nutrient deficiencies

- **Coffee and tea:** Besides caffeine, these contain tannin which inhibits absorption of vitamin B1
- **MSG:** Monosodium glutamate is an essential ingredient of all Chinese cuisine, is associated with violent behavior
- **Trans fatty acids:** These fats replace healthy animal fats that provide fat-soluble activators needed for mineral absorption
- **Liquid vegetable oils:** Being very high in omega 6 fatty acids, these inhibit the proper utilization of omega 3 fatty acids, which are vital for brain function.

Eating Disorders

Eating disorders in children are becoming a matter of concern besides posing a great challenge to the dieticians and the pediatricians. These may range from a state of starvation to that of excessive feeding, both of which can pose serious problems for an adolescent. These disorders can start as early as 9 years of age or before puberty. Girls are more commonly affected but it has been observed that 5% of all cases are males.[30] It is estimated that about 5–10% of postpubertal females are affected by these disorders. Girls are almost nine times more likely than boys to develop any sort of eating disorder. This has also been described as a 'wealthy persons' disease, implying that only families from the higher socioeconomic groups are susceptible.[31]

Anorexia nervosa, bulimia nervosa and binge eating disorders are complex, multidimensional disorders having psychological, medical, sociocultural and nutritional components.[30] These disorders are reported widely and alarming statistics support the need for serious interactive measures.

As per definition, diagnosis of eating disorders can be made when all features of the disorder are met.[32] These include:

- A fear of becoming fat and a drive to be thin
- An obsession with food, weight, calories and dieting
- The use and abuse of eating or not eating to cope with emotional discomfort, stressed life events and developmental challenges
- An increased incidence of depression, obesity, substance abuse and eating disorders in the families of sufferers
- A world view valuing external appearance over personal integrity
- **Anorexia nervosa:** Anorectics have an abnormal fear of gaining weight even if they appear very thin. They take pride in being thin and can go to the extent of remaining hungry and causing pain to themselves. They tend to regulate their intake by quantifying their food portions, rather than by depending upon their sensation for hunger. There are two types of anorectics:
    - Those who keep themselves emaciated through strict dieting and food restriction (dieters)

   – Those who are not able to lose the amount desired by dieting alone and hence, resort to self-induced vomiting and purging. (vomiters and purgers).

These children often feel they are not good enough when compared to peers and also other family members and have a distorted image of their ownselves. The clinical signs and symptoms of these patients include bradycardia, hypothermia, hypotension, constipation, insomnia, restlessness and depression. These features are known to revert upon refeeding and return to normal weight. Treatment of such patients involves:

- Nutritional Support
- Psychotherapy
- Family therapy.

For nutritional support, high-calorie diets in liquid or solid form as per the condition and acceptance of the patient is advised. Education regarding food, weight, body composition and normal growth and development is encouraged. Nutritional intervention to relieve the affects of starvation is accepted as an essential pre-requisite for desired results.

Specific principles for nutritional support include[33]

- A gradual weight gain is recommended since sudden weight gain can result in congestive heart failure, gastric dilation and malabsorption
- Meals should consist of adequate amounts of carbohydrates, fats and proteins, being nutritionally balanced. The food preferences need to be considered too
- Adequate dietary fiber from whole grain cereals is encouraged to avoid constipation
- Small frequent feedings may be encouraged to avoid a feeling of bloating
- Cold or room temperature foods can be advised to reduce satiety sensations
- If caffeine intake is in excess, it should be reduced.

Bulimia Nervosa

This disorder involves recurrent episodes of eating by rapidly consuming large amounts of food very fast. They seem to lose control on their eating behavior and may indulge in self-induced vomiting, purging by use of laxatives and diuretics, vigorous exercise to control weight and even strict dieting. Such disorders generally develop after a distressing life event like death of someone dear, some major set back or disappointment, even perceived personal failure or memories of childhood abuse. The frequency of this disorder can occur on an average of atleast 2 days a week for at least 6 months. Such patients tend to set unrealistic diet goals for themselves which may be quite rigid. They may lay undue stress on low fat foods like fruits, vegetables, non fat yoghurt, etc. Their focus is primarily to serve caloric restriction.

Treatment in this disorder involves counseling, education about food, weight, etc. Counseling is a very important mode of intervention in these patients which includes psychotherapy blended with nutritional issues.

Summary of Recommendations in Eating Disorders

- Establish patient goals for 'normal' eating. Set calorie level for weight maintenance to ideal weight control and reduced risk of increased hunger
- Ensuring at least three regular meals per day
- Small frequent meals may be helpful
- Food patterns can be maintained and eating patterns can be monitored
- Develop exercise guidelines that support moderation and are practiced
- Dispelling myths regarding diets, eliminating food rules
- Gradual negotiation with them to add foods from their preconceived forbidden list of meal pattern.

High-risk Groups of Adolescents

Adolescent Pregnancy

Pregnancy in adolescence adds more risks and complications for pregnant teens compared to any other age group. They have higher rates of low birth weight infants, especially among those younger than 15 years old. The nutritional status of the pregnant adolescent is influenced by both physiologic and environmental/social factors. Since the pregnant teen is still growing, there occurs a maternal and fetal competition for nutrients, thus indicating increased nutrient needs in addition to pregnancy. Besides, there is also a risk of low pregnancy weight and minimal nutrient stores at the time of conception. Other factors affecting the nutritional status are lack of adequate ante natal care, limited resources for a good healthy diet, poor eating habits and emotional stress.

Energy needs can vary greatly, depending on pubertal maturation and physical activity. The RDA of protein is 60 g, which is 14–16 g more than for a nonpregnant teenager. Adequate energy intake will spare the protein to be used for growth. An iron supplement is routinely prescribed, besides vitamin B6, C, folate and calcium.

Education and counseling are needed for the pregnant teen to accept the needed weight gain and avoid risks of possible complications.

Athletes

Adolescents involved in sports generally feel pressurized to maintain a certain weight or to perform at a certain level. In the bargain, some of them may be tempted to adopt unhealthy behaviors like crash dieting, taking supplements for muscle building, or to improve performance or eating unhealthy foods to fulfill their appetites.

Table 7.6: Recommended energy intakes for adolescent athletes

Age group (years)	Sports group	Suggested energy intake (per day)	
		Girls	Boys
12–15	All sports	2700 kcal (Diet A)	3200 kcal (Diet B)
15–18	All sports	3100 kcal (Diet A)	3500 kcal (Diet B)
>18	Skilled games	3100 kcal (Diet A)	3500 kcal (Diet B)
>18	Endurance events and team games	3500 kcal (Diet A)	4500 kcal (Diet D)
>18	Power games	4200 kcal (Diet C+ supplements*)	5200 kcal (Diet D+ supplements*)

*Supplements providing 600–700 kcal, as specified in the diet scale
Source: SAI and NIN.

Table 7.7: Diet scales for various sports groups

Food articles	Quantity			
	Diet A	Diet B	Diet C	Diet D
Wheat soya flour	120 g	180 g	210 g	310 g
Other cereals	200 g	260 g	300 g	400 g
Pulses	30 g	30 g	40 g	60 g
Green leafy vegetable	100 g	100 g	100 g	100 g
Other vegetables	200 g	200 g	200 g	200 g
Roots and tubers	100 g	100 g	100 g	100 g
Fruits	150 g	150 g	200 g	200 g
Milk	750 g	750 g	750 g	750 g
Soya oil	25 g	25 g	30 g	40 g
Butter	15 g	15 g	15 g	25 g
Sugar	30 g	30 g	30 g	30 g
Meat/Fish/Poultry	100 g	100 g	100 g	100 g
Eggs	Two (no.)	Two (no.)	Two (no.)	Two (no.)
Energy	2775 kcal	3195 kcal	3528 kcal	4459 kcal
Protein	114 g (16.4%)	146 g (18.3%)	161 g (18.3%)	206 g (18.5%)
Fats	92 g (29.8%)	92 g (25.9%)	97 g (25.0%)	112 g (22.6%)
Carbohydrates	373 g (53.8%)	445 g (55.8%)	500 g (56.7%)	656 g (58.5%)

Source: SAI and NIN.

There are certain guidelines to be followed to plan for a day's diet of an adolescent. These are based on their nutrient requirements, as recommended by Sports Authority of India training centers and National Institute of Nutrition,

Table 7.8: Supplements for power games

S. No.	Food article	Quantity
1.	Eggs	Two
2.	Milk	500 mL
3.	Meat	100 g
4.	Fruit	100 g

Energy: 660 kcal
Protein: 44 g
Fats: 25 g
Carbohydrates: 65 g

Source: SAI and NIN.

in 2002–03 during the training and competing phase. Ideally they should meet the daily calorie requirement as per the age and sex. Drastic changes in body weights should be avoided. A typical balanced diet for an athlete should comprise around 55% carbohydrates, 15% proteins and 35% fats. On an average an adolescent weighing around 50–70 kg may require about 3000–3600 calories per day, keeping in mind the sports activity that he/she may be involved.[3] The suggested energy intakes for different age groups are as given in Table 7.6.[3]

To meet these requirement, scales has been fixed for the various food groups as given in Table 7.7.[3] Additional supplements have been recommended for those involved in high intensity power games as given in Table 7.8.[3]

REFERENCES

1. Venkaiah K, Damayanthi K, Nayak MU, Vijayraghvan K. Diet and Nutritional Status of rural adolescents' in India. Nutrition News, National Institute of Nutrition, Hyderabad. 2003;24(4).
2. Rolland Cachera MF, Guillode DM, Batuileun Avons P, et al. Trekking the development of obesity from one month of age to adulthood. Ann Hum Biol. 1893;14:219-99.
3. Nutritive Requirements and Recommended dietary allowances for Indians. A report of the expert group of the Indian Council of Medical Research, ICMR, 2010.
4. Joint FAO/WHO/UNU: Human energy requirements. Report of a Joint FAO/WHO/UNU Expert Consultation, Rome, 17-24 Oct 2001. Rome, FAO/WHO/UNU, 2004.
5. Mercedes de Onis, Blossna M. The WHO Global database on child growth and malnutrition: methodology and applications. Int J Epidemiol. 2003;32:518-26.
6. National Nutrition Monitoring Bureau, National Institute of Nutrition, Indian Council of Medical Research, Hyderabad. 1975-1999.
7. Chaturvedi S, Kapil U, Gnaneskaran N, et al. Nutrient intake amongst adolescent girls belonging to poor socio economic group of rural area of Rajasthan. Indian Pediatr. 1996;33:197-201.
8. Ali M, Delisle HA. A participatory approach to assessing Malawi villagers' perception of their own food security. Ecol Food Nutr. 1999;38:101-2.

9. Ahmed F, Zareen M, Khan MR, et al. Dietary patterns, nutrient intake and growth of adolescent school girls in urban Bangladesh. Pub Health Nutr. 1998; 1:83-92.
10. Cusatis DC, Sharma BM. Influences on adolescent eating behavior. J Adolesc Health. 1996;18(1):27.
11. Rees JM. The overall impact of recently developed foods on dietary habits of adolescents. J Adolesc Health. 1992;22(1):14.
12. Bull NL, Barbet SA. Food habits of 14-25 years old living accommodation and social class as factors affecting the diet. Health Visitor. 1985;58:9-10.
13. Kapil U, Minocha S, Bhasin S. Dietary intake amongst 'well to do' adolescent boys and girls in Delhi. Indian Pediatr. 1993;30:1017.
14. Sharma M, Ray M. Nutritional status of children visiting the adolescent clinic in a tertiary care centre at Chandigarh, 2005 (unpublished).
15. Truswell AS, Hill ID. Food habits of adolescents. Nutr Rev. 1981;39(2):73.
16. Sadana B, Khanna M, Mann SK. Consumption pattern of fast food among teenagers. Applied Nutrition. 1997;22(1):14.
17. Guthrie HA. Nutrition from childhood through adulthood. In: Introductory Nutrition, 6th Ed. Times Mirror/Mosby; 1986.p 569.
18. Preziosi P, Galan P, Deheeger M, Yacoub N, Diewnowski A, Hercberg C. Breakfast type, daily nutrient intakes and vitamin and mineral status of French children adolescents and adults. J Am Coll Nutr. 1999;18(2):171.
19. Kanchanwala R, Husain MH. Food habits of adolescents in relation to their body weight status and impact of diet counseling. Applied Nutr. 2003;28(1 and 2): 33-9.
20. Bull NL. Studies of dietary habits, food consumption and nutrient intakes of adolescents and young adults. Wld Rev Nutr Diet. 1998;524-74.
21. Lawson M. Nutrition in childhood. Proceedings of a conference. London: Routledge. 1992.
22. Must A, Jacques PF, Dallal GE, et al. Long-term morbidity and mortality of over weight adolescents: a follow up of the Harvard Growth Study of 1992 -35. N Engl J Med. 1992;327:1350-5.
23. Serdula MK, Ivery D, Coates RJ, et al. Do obese children become obese adults? A review of literature. Prev. Med. 1993;22:167-77.
24. Freedman DS, Shear CL, Srinivasan SR, et al. Tracking of serum lipids and lipoproteins in children over an 8 year old period. The Bogalusa Heart Study. Prev Med. 1985;14:203-16.
25. Riveria JA, Martorell R, Ruel M, et al. Nutritional supplementation during the pre school years influences body size and composition of Guatemalan adolescents. J Nutr. 1985;125(Suppl 2):91-7.
26. Kurz KM, Johnson-Welch C. The nutrition and lives of adolescents in developing countries: Findings from the nutrition of adolescent girls research program. ICRW. 1994.
27. Lonsdale D. Crime and Violence: A hypothetical explanation of its relationship with high calorie malnutrition. J Adv Med Fall. 1994;7(3):171-80.
28. Dommisse JV. Subtle vitamin B12 deficiency in Psychiatry: A largely unnoticed but devastating relationship? Medical Hypothesis. 1991;34:131-40.
29. Levine M. How schools can combat eating disorders: Anorexia nervosa and bulimia. Washington DC. National Education Association; 1987.
30. Berg F. Afraid to eat. Children and teens in weight crisis. Hettinger D. Healthy Weight Publishing Network; 1997. p.69.

31. Garner D, Garfinkel P. Handbook of Psychotherapy for anorexia nervosa and bulimia nervosa. New York's Guilford Press; 1985.
32. Levine M. How schools can combat students eating disorders; Anorexia nervosa and bulimia. Washington DC: National Education Association; 1987.
33. Rock CC, Yager J. Nutrition and eating disorders: a primer for clinicians. Int J Eating Disorder. 1987;6:267-79.

Maternal Nutrition in Pregnancy and Lactation

INTRODUCTION

Maternal nutrition not only influences the health and well being of the mother but also has intermediate and long-term effects on the development and health of the infant.[1] The fact that maternal nutrition during the antenatal period directly influences the fetal outcome has well been recognized. When a precursory study into the link between nutrition and pregnancy was done in a series of women who consumed minimal amounts over the 8-week period, it was discovered that they had a higher mortality or disorder rate concerning their off spring than women who ate regularly since children born to well-fed mothers had less restriction within the womb.[2] Pregnancy and lactation are times of heightened vulnerability. The threat of malnutrition begins in the womb and continues through the life cycle. A mother who was malnourished as a fetus, young child or adolescent, is more likely to enter pregnancy stunted and malnourished. Her compromised nutritional status affects the health and nutrition of her own children. Growth faltering earlier in life leaves women permanently at risk of obstetric complications and delivering low-birth-weight babies.

PRECONCEPTION NUTRITION

It is estimated that a woman planning for a pregnancy be prepared even before the conceptual stage, which is known as the perinatal period. It requires a mother to be in good nutritional state prior to conception and that this state be maintained throughout pregnancy, labor and the period after birth. A mother well nourished before conception, will encounter fewer premature births and produce healthier babies.

The most important factor in prepregnancy nutrition is ensuring that the mother is healthy and without any major factors, which could worsen the chances of conception, like anorexia or bulimia, both of which can hinder conception. The minimum basal metabolic index (BMI) of 20.8 is a positive factor for preconception stage. Gaining weight restores fertility and a body fat content of at least 22% is necessary for a normal ovulatory function and menstruation.[3] On the other hand, the same is true for obese women with a BMI of more than 30, which is a direct result of decrementing amounts of insulin activity and sex hormones may reduce the viability of the ovum. If a woman planning to conceive needs to gain or lose weight, it is recommended to be done gradually. The ideal weight of a woman planning to conceive is thought to be optimal at BMI between 20 and 26. This together with good diet and nutrition before pregnancy, would also maximize the reserves of micronutrients which are required during pregnancy.[4]

Some nutrients are considered to be beneficial for the pregnancy state and it is recommended that the standard dosage of these is followed as per the RDA:

- Magnesium and zinc supplements for the binding of hormones at the receptor sites
- Folic acid supplement or dietary requirement of foods containing it for regular growth of the follicle
- Regular vitamin D supplement decreases the chances of deficiency in adolescence. It has an important role in reducing the incidence of rickets with pelvic malformations which can hamper normal delivery
- Vitamin B12 is known to reduce chances of infertility and ill health
- Omega 3 fatty acids help in prevention of premature delivery and low birth weight.[3] Good dietary sources are oily fish, flax seeds, walnuts and pumpkin seeds.

NUTRITION DURING PREGNANCY

- The postconception stage and the weeks following it are the most vulnerable, being the period when fetal development occurs within the womb. The energy needed for the organ and system development is derived from those present in the mother's circulation and around the lining of the womb. During the early stages, the placenta is not formed and hence, the transport of nutrients from the mother to the embryo is not possible. Therefore, it is important that the mother's diet is healthy comprising all the essential nutrients, so that the embryo is not deficient in these components. Diets should be rich in folic acid and iron to prevent neural tube defects.

Nutritional Recommendations during Pregnancy

Energy

- Energy requirements during pregnancy are variable due to the energy sparing adaptations which protect the mother or fetus from nutritional strains.[5] Energy supplements in pregnancy have been shown to have variable effects on birth outcome, with more obvious benefit in women who are nutritionally at risk during this stage. The National Institute of Nutrition (NIN), (ICMR) group has worked out the recommendations of various nutrients for the pregnant and lactating mothers. Based on the prepregnancy weight of 55 kg, 'the additional energy requirements' of an Indian woman as per the recommendations of NIN are as follows in Table 8.1.[6]

Table 8.1: Additional energy requirements of an Indian pregnant woman (based on prepregnancy weight of 55 kg as per the NIN recommendations[6])

	12 kg increase	10 kg increase
1st trimester	85 kcals	70 kcals
2nd trimester	+ 280 kcals	+ 230 kcals
3rd trimester	+ 470 kcals	+ 390 kcals

Therefore, an average recommendation of 350 kcals/d through the second and third trimesters, as additional requirement during pregnancy (for an Indian woman of 55 kg body weight and pregnancy weight gain between 10 and 12 kg) may be made.

Proteins

Protein intakes to meet the average requirements of women during pregnancy, have been worked out by NIN by rounding off high-quality protein for 10 kg gestational weight gain. These are 1, 7 and 23 g/d in 1st, 2nd and 3rd trimesters, respectively.6 A balanced energy/protein supplement (protein <25% of energy) tends to influence pregnancy outcome favorably, while a very-high protein supply may also be harmful.[7] It is therefore recommended that protein supplements are not required to meet this additional requirement during pregnancy. To achieve high-quality protein content in an Indian diet, the foods can be varied, selecting foods with high protein content. For instance, pulses or legumes which have an individual protein efficiency ratio (PE) of 28% can be added as a cup of lentils or whole gram at meal time, or even between meals. Similarly a greater use of milk or milk-based products (with a PE ratio of 15%), or nonvegetarian foods like eggs (PE ratio of 30%) or flesh food can further increase protein intake. All these food groups also add high-quality protein to diet.[6]

Gestational Weight Gain

Fetal growth is reflected by gestational weight gain. A low weight gain is a risk indicator of intrauterine growth retardation and perinatal mortality. On the other hand a higher gain is a risk indicator for maternal diabetes, macrosomia, delivery problems, birth trauma and asphyxia. It is now well known that intrauterine growth retardation and macrosomia may program obesity and metabolic syndrome later in life. The recommended total weight gain ranges for pregnancy are highlighted in Table 8.2.[8]

Table 8.2: Weight gain recommended for pregnancy

Prepregnancy weight category	Recommended total gain (kg)
BMI <19.8	12.5–18.0
19.8–26	11.5–16.0
>26.0–29.0	7.0–11.5

Source: Institute of Medicine. Nutrition during pregnancy, 1990.

Essential Fatty Acids

Some data exists in support of supplementation of essential fatty acids (EFA) like fish oil during pregnancy showing improved birth weight,[9] but random controlled trials have failed to elicit any such corelation.[10]

MICRONUTRIENTS IN PREGNANCY

Vitamins

Fat-soluble Vitamins

Requirement of vitamin D increases twice the normal during pregnancy, therefore besides consuming rich dietary source of vitamin D, exposure to sunlight increased the vitamin production in the skin. An average well-nourished woman would be having adequate reserves of the vitamin to sustain through the pregnancy period. Therefore, the extra supplement of vitamin A may not be required. Good dietary sources include milk and milk products, green leafy vegetables, fruits like mangoes, papaya, vegetables like carrot, jaggery (source of β carotene, a precursor of vitamin A). Vitamin E requirement also increases during the last 8–10 weeks of pregnancy. The role of this vitamin is to prevent oxidation of the total fat reserves which are stored for providing for the growing fetus. Good sources of vitamin E are oily fish, flax seeds and green leafy vegetables.

Iron

As well known, iron requirements increase dramatically during pregnancy. The absorption of iron is directly proportionate to the level of iron stores in the body. When dietary iron stores are inadequate for the increased demands of iron, the maternal stores are depleted. By the first trimester, the iron stores are low or absent in women. However, during pregnancy, the iron status of the fetus is maintained near normal, even if depletion of iron stores and subsequently anemia occurs in the mother. Iron deficiency during pregnancy can produce anemia, fatigue and irritability in the mother and may impair growth of the fetus. Iron supplements should be taken with food to enhance iron absorption (meat, fish and fruits and vegetables rich in vitamin C).

Zinc

Low zinc intake during pregnancy increases the risk of delivering a low-birth-weight baby and may increase risk of birth defects.[11] Zinc requirements are about 50% higher during pregnancy.

Magnesium

Deficiency of magnesium can cause fatigue and muscle cramps and increase risk of premature birth and maternal hypertension. An intake of 400 mg/d is recommended. In a cross-sectional study, birth weight has been shown to be positively corelated to magnesium intakes in early pregnancy.[12]

Calcium

During pregnancy about 30–40 g of calcium are transferred to the fetus during pregnancy, most of it during the third trimester.[8] The absorption of maternal calcium increases rapidly during pregnancy. An intake of about 1000–1200 mg of calcium throughout pregnancy reduces bone loss, since during late pregnancy, the calcium must be withdrawn from maternal bone and transferred to the fetus. Keeping in view the importance of most micronutrients, the deficiency of any of these can have adverse effects during pregnancy, both for the mother and the baby as shown in Table 8.3.[13]

DIETARY AND ENVIRONMENTAL HAZARDS DURING PREGNANCY

Alcohol

Consumption of alcohol during pregnancy is potentially hazardous due to the devastating effects on the outcome, termed as fetal alcohol syndrome (FAS).[14] It is characterized by abnormal facial structure and impairment in growth and intellectual development. The mechanism involves the crossing over of alcohol and its metabolites through the placenta. The fetus does not have the

Table 8.3: Effects of micronutrient deficiencies during pregnancy

Nutrient	Effect on mother	Effect on fetus/placenta
Vitamin D	Reduced bone density, may increase risk of osteoporosis	Impaired skeletal and tooth development, hypoglycemia, rickets
Vitamin A	Anemia	Low birth weight, premature birth
Vitamin E		Birth defects, spontaneous abortion
Folate	Anemia	Low birth weight, birth defects, miscarriage
Thiamine		Infant beriberi (severe B12 deficiency producing heart failure)
Iodine	Hypothyroidism	Severely impaired mental and motor development
Calcium	Increased risk of hypertension and eclampsia, decreased bone density may increase risk of osteoporosis	Impaired skeletal and tooth development, rickets
Magnesium	Increased risk of hypertension and eclampsia	Premature birth
Zinc		Birth defects, premature birth and low birth weight
Iron	Anemia	Low birth weight, premature birth, increased infant mortality

Source: Keen CL, et al. (Eds). Maternal nutrition and pregnancy outcome. Ann NY Acad Sci. 1993;678.

enzymes to breakdown these toxic products including alcohol, which remain in the fetal circulation over prolonged period, thus exposing the fetus to high concentrations of alcohol for a long duration.

Caffeine

In pregnancy, the metabolism of caffeine is known to slow down, taking 2–3 times longer to metabolize. Intake of >300 mg caffeine per day (equivalent to >3 cups of caffeine/d) can be devastating due to its causing impaired growth and development and increasing risk of miscarriage.[15] Caffeine tends to constrict the blood vessels in the placenta which can result in reducing the supply of oxygen and nutrients to fetus.[16] It is recommended that pregnant women should best avoid coffee, black tea, chocolates and colas.

Food Additives

Additives like nonsweeteners, i.e. saccharine, cyclamate and aspartame should be avoided by pregnant women due to the fact that these pass through the placenta and could be carcinogenic, especially when exposure begins in utero and continues through adult life.

Heavy Metals

Exposure of toxic metals like mercury, lead, cadmium and nickel can be harmful for the pregnant women, including the industrialized and agricultural chemicals due to their risk of being transported to fetus through the placenta. Even low levels of lead passing through the placenta increase the risk of premature birth, irreversibly impairing intellectual and motor development throughout childhood and lowering IQ.[13]

Hypervitaminosis A

Excess intake of vitamin A above the recommended levels during pregnancy (>25000 IU) has been linked to birth defects, including malformations of the skull, heart and the central nervous system.[17] It is interesting to note that deficiency of choline and vitamin E enhance the toxicity of high doses of vitamin A during pregnancy.

Tobacco

Children of mothers with history of smoking may have long-term impairments in physical growth and intellectual performance. The adverse effects are dose dependent and directly proportionate to the number of cigarettes smoked during pregnancy. The adverse effect is due to the reduced blood flow through the placenta and restricted oxygen and nutrient flow to the fetus.

Smoking can deplete maternal stores of zinc, vitamin C, vitamin B6, folate and vitamin B12.[17]

SPECIAL CONSIDERATIONS DURING PREGNANCY

Heartburn, Nausea, Constipation

A woman may encounter certain problems like heartburn, nausea and constipation during the entire period or specific periods of pregnancy. This is due to the changes in the hormonal levels during this period. The progesterone levels are raised which cause the muscle tone to relax and slow down the digestive process especially the peristalsis.[17] As a result there is a reflux of the gastric juices, at the lower esophagus, causing irritation and discomfort which is termed as heartburn. This can be minimized by eating smaller meals and avoiding taking meals immediately prior to physical activity or exercise. However, the relaxing of the muscle tone is otherwise beneficial as it helps to slow the transit time allowing increased nutrient absorption along with the gastrointestinal tract (GIT). The problem of reflux can also be alleviated by avoiding lying down immediately after meals (3–4 hours) and even when doing so to keep the head end elevated. Another common problem of nausea can be tackled by having small frequent meals and not with meals which can be of help too.[17] Nausea may also be controlled by supplemental vitamin B6 (25–75 mg/d) and magnesium (200–500 mg/d).[18]

Many women experience severe constipation and hemorrhoids during pregnancy which is due to increased water absorption from the stools which transits slowly along the GIT. Therefore, liberal fluids and high-fiber diet is recommended to ease the problem. Lots of fresh fruit and green vegetables and whole grain cereals can help the stool motility. Extra-vitamin C and regular moderate exercise can be helpful.

Hypoglycemia

Pregnant women are prone to develop hypoglycemia due to increased utilization of glucose by the fetus from the mother. This is particularly so at the early hours in the morning or if the woman has skipped a meal or is on a long fast. Skipping meals tend to produce more ketone bodies which can adversely affect the fetal development. Frequent small consumption of snacks and meals is recommended for these women to avoid hypoglycemic attacks.

Gestational Diabetes

About 5% of pregnant women may develop reduced ability to secrete insulin and control blood sugars resulting in gestational diabetes.[19] Hyperglycemia during pregnancy has an adverse effect on the fetus and the mother producing complications later on. Therefore, dietary modifications with moderate exercise can help maintain normoglycemia and thus, prevent complications. Supplemental zinc and chromium are known to enhance the action of insulin.[20]

Hypertension and Toxemia of Pregnancy

Extreme increase in the blood pressure during pregnancy can cause toxemia characterized by protein loss in the urine and fluid retention. This can prove fatal for both mother and the fetus.[21] These complications can be prevented by suitable dietary modifications. Too much restriction of salt can also increase the risk; therefore undue salt restriction should be avoided. Low calcium or zinc is known to increase the risk of toxemia. Calcium supplementation (2 g/d) during pregnancy can be beneficial. Supplemental B_6 (25–50 mg/d) may also be helpful in prevention and treatment of this disorder.[22]

LACTATION PERIOD

Nutritional Needs During Lactation

Breast milk is Mother Nature's unique gift bestowed upon the child through the mother. Milk production in the first 6 months of lactation averages about 750 mL/d, but women can vary in their output which can far exceed this volume being up to 2000 mL/d.

The composition of breast milk is unique due to the fact that it contains over 200 recognized components like:

All nutrients (energy, protein, essential fatty acids, vitamins and minerals) needed by the newborn for optimum growth and development.

- Enzymes to help the newborn digest and absorb nutrients
- Immune factors to protect the infant from infection
- Hormones and growth factors that influence infant growth.

All of the above components, though remain same in all mothers, the concentration of each of these are dependent upon her diet. Therefore, during the period of lactation it is very important that the diet of the mother for the first 6 months is optimum which can in turn optimize the breast milk formation. Breastfeeding mothers need significantly more energy, proteins and micronutrients during lactation to support milk formation. For an exclusively breastfeeding mother, who would produce an additional amount of milk for the first 6 months, would require 600 kcals, and for partially breastfeeding during 7–12 months, it would be 517 kcals or approximately 520 kcals.[6] The NIN (2010) recommendations have been computed by adopting the factorial requirement during lactation. This has been computed on the basis of secretion of 9.4 g/d of protein in milk during 0–6 months and 6.6 g during 6–24 months. Therefore, the additional mean and safe protein intake at different months of lactation have been rounded off to 19 g/d for safe allowance for a lactating woman during 1–6 months and 13 g from 6 to 12 months. As for pregnancy, protein requirements can be met from a balanced diet with a PE ratio between 12 and 13%.[6]

The requirements of most vitamins and minerals go up by 50–100% compared to the pregnancy period. The quality of the breast milk can be influenced by the quality of the food consumed while breastfeeding. The type of fat consumed during breastfeeding influences the fat content of the breast milk. Vegetarians produce more milk with greater amounts of fatty acids present in plant foods. This is important since essential fatty acids (omega 3 fatty acids and EPA and DHA) are essential for the development of the nervous system of the newborn.[23]

Vitamins like vitamin D are essential in the maternal diet since deficiency of this can lead to low levels in the infant too. Infants fed breast milk low in vitamin D may develop skeletal abnormalities and rickets.[24] There are other major minerals like calcium and magnesium which continue to be secreted in the milk despite low concentrations of the same in the maternal diet, draining from maternal reserves. Therefore, if maternal stores of calcium are continuously low, these can be totally depleted leading to osteoporosis later in their lifespan.[21] Calcium supplements along with vitamin D during lactation and during the weaning period are important to maintain calcium balance and maternal skeletal health.[25]

REFERENCES

1. Plagemann A. Perinatal programming and functional teratogenesis: impact of body weight regulation and obesity. Physiol Behav. 2005;86:661-8.
2. Rasmussen KM. The influence of maternal nutrition on lactation. Annual Review of Nutr. 1992;12:103-17.
3. Williamson CS. Nutrition in pregnancy. British Nutr Foundation. 2006;31:28-59.
4. Barasi EM. Human Nutrition-A health perspective, London: Arnold Publishing; 2003.
5. Prentice A, Goldberg GR. Energy adaptations in human pregnancy: limits and long term consequences. Am J Clin Nutr. 2000:S1226-S32.
6. ICMR, Nutrient Requirements and Recommended Dietary Allowances for Indians, A Report of the Expert Group of the Indian Council of Medical Research. 2010.
7. Otten JJ, Pitzi Hellwig J, Meyers LD (eds). Dietary Reference Intake (DRI) Washington, Institute of Medicine, National Academic Press. 2006.
8. Kramer MS, Kakuma R. Energy and protein intake in pregnancy. Cochrane Database Syst Rev. 2003;4.
9. Institute of Medicine (IOM). Nutrition during pregnancy: Report of the Committee on Nutrition during Pregnancy and lactation. Washington: National Academy Press; 1990.
10. De OnisM, Viller J, Gulmezoglu M. Nutritional interventions or prevent intrauterine growth retardation: evidence from randomised controlled trials. Eur J Clin Nutr. 1998;52:S83-93.
11. Ramakrishnan U, Manjerkar R, Rivera J, et al. Micronutrients and pregnancy outcome: a review of the literature. Nutr Res. 1999;19:103-59.
12. King JC. Determinants of maternal zinc status during pregnancy. Am J Clin Nutr. 2000;71:1334S.
13. Doyle W, Crafford MA, Wyan AH, et al. Maternal magnesium intake and pregnancy-outcome. Magnesium Res. 1989;20:205-10.

14. Keen CL, Bendich A, Calvin C. Willhite (Eds). Maternal nutrition and pregnancy outcome. Ann NY Acd Sci. 1993;678.
15. Beattie JO. Alcohol exposure and the fetus. Eur J Clin Nutr. 1992;46:S7.
16. Hinds TS. The effect of caffeine on pregnancy outcome variables. Nutr Rev. 1996;54:203.
17. Azais-Braesco V, Pascal G. Vitamin A in pregnancy: requirements and safety limits. Am J Clin Nutr. 2000;71:1325S.
18. Baron TH, Ramirez B, Richter JE. Gastrointestinal motility disorders during pregnancy. Ann Int Med. 1993;118:366.
19. Sahakian V, et al. Vitamin B6 is effective therapy for nausea and vomiting of pregnancy: A randomized controlled study. Obster Gynecol. 1991;78:33.
20. Jovanovic-Peterson L, Peterson LM. Vitamin and mineral deficiencies which may predispose to glucose intolerance of pregnancy. J Am Coll Nutr. 1996;15:14.
21. Ritchie LD, King JC. Dietary calcium and pregnancy induced hypertension: Is there a co-relation? Am J Clin Nutr. 2000;71:1371S.
22. Institute of Medicine. Nutrition during lactation. Washington DC: National Academy Press; 1991.
23. Crawford MA. The role of essential fatty acids in neural development: Implications for perinatal nutrition. Am J Clin Nutr. 1993;57:S703.
24. Greer FR, Marshall S. Bone mineral content, serum vitamin D supplements. J Pediatr. 1989;114:204.
25. Kalwarf HJ, et al. The effect of calcium supplementation on bone density during lactation and weaning. N Eng J Med. 1997;337:523.

Nutrition for the Athlete Child

It is well established that health and fitness of children is associated with the physical behaviors of parents,[1] thereby implying that family fitness should be encouraged. Physical involvement of children in their daily routine is well recognized by all sections of society, which is the reason why some time period is set aside for games and sports in most educational institutions. Inducting some form of activity for every child is considered very important in order to initiate lifetime habits of physical exercise.[2]

Taking part in recreational or competitive sports at a younger age helps developing skills, confidence, good health and fitness. Attitudes about physical activity and an active lifestyle are often formed in the first ten years of life.[3]

PHYSIOLOGICAL EFFECTS OF EXERCISE

Sports activity for a child has many physiological effects in children, especially cardiorespiratory, which is important for children and adolescents due to the following benefits:
- Improves strength and flexibility
- Conditions the cardiorespiratory system
- Increases endurance
- Develops power, agility and speed
- Aids in development of muscles
- Exercises neuromuscular skills
- Controls body fat percentage
- Provides mental well being.

It is recommended that at least 20 minutes of exercise be performed, which should involve large muscles, produce mild perspiration and ensure heart beat to be at 60-80% of maximum rate. Such an activity done at least 3-5 times a week can give the maximum benefits from cardiorespiratory workouts.[4,5]

Children preparing in sports activity should be assessed by physicians and health professionals to rule out any deleterious consequences of exercise activities undertaken by them. For participation and training in competitive sports by children, it is advisable to determine the match of maturation age with the sport, injury risk and general health status. This can be done prior to participation by a pediatrician or a physician trained in sports medicine.[6,7] Children preparing for sports activity also need to be imparted education on proper training, diet and injury prevention.[4]

NUTRITIONAL RECOMMENDATIONS

Good nutrition is crucial for appropriate growth, development and excellence in performing. Children participating in sports activities need to pay attention to their nutritional needs specific to their age and gender. The recommendations for such children are adequate supply of nutrients provided from a balanced, healthy diet as per the recommended dietary allowances (RDA). There is no indication that there are increased needs for any other nutrient beyond the RDA, although some teens may need more protein during periods of rapid growth.[8] In case of any individual deficiencies observed during the child's review, the specific nutrients can be supplemented and appropriate nutritional counseling session imparted. Arbitrary use of over-the-counter supplements however should be discouraged by the youth. Depending on the intensity of their activity and type of sport, the nutrient requirements may increase significantly which if not covered adequately can result in adverse effects of the growth and development of the children. Eating for sport activity should be an extension of healthy eating.

Principles of Healthy Diet for a Sports Child

The principles of a healthy diet for a child involved actively in sports should be:
- The child has a proper breakfast, comprising a cereal/bread, a drink like milk or fruit juice or a fruit
- The child has two main meals—lunch and dinner apart from the morning breakfast, with a mid morning and an evening snack. These could be dairy products, cereals or fruit
- The child has adequate fluids, preferably pure water or milk.

Pregame Meal

Before an event or a practice session, the diet of the child should be:
- High in carbohydrates for energy, maintaining normal glycemic levels. Complex carbohydrates like rice, pasta, suji, potatoes are good choices
- Moderate in protein (1–1.5 g/kg/d)
- Low in fat/fiber to reduce digestive stress
- Low in salt
- Preferred and familiar to the child's taste
- Should have taken about 3–4 hours before any intense physical activity (Table 9.1)[9] providing about 200–350 g of carbohydrates (4 g/kg). This helps improve performance efficiency

- Options of foods are low-fiber cereal, with milk, fruit, milk shake or milk with an apple
- The carbohydrate content of the food in the meal immediately preceding a meal should be reduced to avoid gastrointestinal distress
- Prehydration with 120–250 mL water or fluid helps to maximise absorption of fluid without urination. After exercise begins, the kidney slows down urine production to compensate for water loss.

Post Meal Diet/Refuelling

After an intense sports activity, the body needs to be 'refuelled' with the losses, preferably within 30 minutes of ending a sport activity. Delaying carbohydrate intake for too long after exercise reduces resynthesis of muscle glycogen. Resynthesis is most efficient when approximately 100 g of carbohydrates are consumed immediately or within 30 minutes of exercise.[10] The meal or snack should be a balance of carbohydrates and proteins depending upon the time of the day, whether it is meal time or a mid meal time of the day.

Energy

The base calorie requirement for the athlete is as per the recommended allowances. For the Indian athlete these recommendations are based on the guidelines recommended by Sports Authority of India and National Institute of Nutrition, as given in Table 9.1.[9]

To meet these requirements, scales have been fixed for the various food groups as given in Table 9.2.[9]

Any increase in the calories for an activity will depend on the child's age, sex, present weight, desired weight, particular sport and level of involvement. Achieving the desired weight and maintaining the same will be the indicators of adequate calories. Because of the variance in the age of sexual development for children and the connection of body fat composition to development, body fat measurement should not be used as a qualification of weight status or goal, as in adults.[8,11] Frequent monitoring is recommended if weight change is desired to prevent too rapid loss or gain, which otherwise can affect the performance. It is therefore advisable to make the weight changes prior to the sports season.[12]

Carbohydrates

The carbohydrate content of the child involved in an intense sport activity or one who might be involved for long duration of practice may be increased in the diet to provide extra energy. It is worth considering that carbohydrate feeding does not prevent fatigue, but only delays it. The carbohydrate should be of the complex types which are digested and absorbed easily. They are also important to improve the performance level of the young athlete. This nutrient can efficiently fuel the body before, during and after sports events or competition, but the timing of carbohydrate is important.[13] Carbohydrates consumed during endurance exercise lasting longer than 1 hour ensures the availability of sufficient amounts of energy during the later stages of exercise

Table 9.1: Recommended energy intakes for adolescent athletes

Age group (years)	Sports group	Suggested energy intake (per day)	
		Girls	Boys
12–15	All sports	2700 kcal (DIET A)	3200 kcal (DIET B)
15–18	All sports	3100 kcal (DIET A)	3500 kcal (DIET B)
>18	Skilled games	3100 kcal (DIET A)	3500 kcal (DIET B)
>18	Endurance events and team games	3500 kcal (DIET A)	4500 kcal (DIET D)
>18	Power games	4200 kcal (DIET C+ supplements*)	5200 kcal (DIET D+ supplements*)

*Supplements providing 600–700 kcal, as specified in the diet scale
Source: SAI and NIN.[9]

Table 9.2: Diet scales for various sports group

Food articles	Quantity			
	Diet A	Diet B	Diet C	Diet D
1. Wheat soya flour	120 g	180 g	210 g	310 g
2. Other cereals	200 g	260 g	300 g	400 g
3. Pulses	30 g	30 g	40 g	60 g
4. Green leafy vegetable	100 g	100 g	100 g	100 g
5. Other vegetables	200 g	200 g	200 g	200 g
6. Roots and tubers	100 g	100 g	100 g	100 g
7. Fruits	150 g	150 g	200 g	200 g
8. Milk	750 g	750 g	750 g	750 g
9. Soya oil	25 g	25 g	30 g	40 g
10. Butter	15 g	15 g	15 g	25 g
11. Sugar	30 g	30 g	30 g	30 g
12. Meat/Fish/Poultry	100 g	100 g	100 g	100 g
13. Eggs	Two nos.	Two (no.)	Two (no.)	Two (no.)
Energy	2775 kcal	3195 kcal	3528 kcal	4459 kcal
Protein	114 g (16.4%)	146 g (18.3%)	161 g (18.3%)	206 g (18.5%)
Fats	92 g (29.8%)	92 g (25.9%)	97 g (25.0%)	112 g (22.6%)
Carbohydrates	373 g (53.8%)	445 g (55.8%)	500 g (56.7%)	656 g (58.5%)

Source: SAI and NIN.[9]

and improves performance. The type of foods which can be consumed during the competitions and the timings when they can be best consumed are listed in Table 9.3.[14] Easily digested foods high in carbohydrate, but low in protein and fat should be had. Allowing time for partial digestion and absorption provides a final addition to muscle glycogen, additional blood sugar and also

Table 9.3: Eating during competition

3–4 hours before (600–700 cals)	2–3 hours before (300–400 cals)	1–3 hours before (100 cals)	2–3 hours after
Fruit/Vegetable juice	Fruit/Vegetable juice	Fruit/Vegetable juice	Bread, biscuits, muffins
Fresh fruit	Fresh fruit	Fresh fruit (low fiber, like plums, melons, peaches	Fruit yogurt
Bread, rusk	Bread, rusks, muffins	Sports drink	Large banana
Peanut butter, lean meat, low-fat cheese	No butter or cream cheese		Fruit juice
Low-fat yogurt			
Baked potato			
Cereal with low-fat milk			

Refer. 14

relatively complete emptying of the stomach. Some good sources of complex carbohydrates are whole grain cereals, brown bread, rice and liberal amounts of fruits and vegetables.

Proteins

Protein is required for muscle building, therefore adequate amounts should be provided in the diet though vey high amounts are not recommended. This can be achieved by a balanced diet as per the RDA. Consuming greater protein than required is not advisable, because by consuming more than that required, the carbohydrate status may be compromised, thereby affecting the ability to train and compete at peak levels. High protein intake may also result in diuresis and potential dehydration.[10] Studies have shown that the need for protein in exercise depends more on the energy intake, since proteins will be used as energy source if calories are insufficient.

Foods like dairy products, nuts and legumes, fish, poultry and soyabeans are good sources. It is worth keeping in mind that strong muscles come from regular training and exercise rather than excess of protein form the diet.

The traditional concept among athletes and body builders that they require high protein or amino acid supplements in the form of powders or pills is unfounded and should be discouraged. Large amounts of protein intake can cause dehydration, hypercalciuria, weight gain and stress on the kidney and liver. Moreover substituting amino acid supplements for food can also cause deficiencies of other micronutrients like iron, niacin and thiamine.

Fats

About 20–30% of the calories are provided by fats in a normal balanced diet for a young athlete. It is the most concentrated source of energy for fuel for light to moderate intensity exercise, besides providing the essential fatty acids. But severe fat restriction (<15% of energy) is also not advisable as it can limit performance by hindering intramuscular triglyceride storage, which is a significant source of energy at all intensities of exercise. Moderate to low-fat meal is recommended for the premeal diet as high fat intake can interfere with performance and also cause gastrointestinal discomfort.

Vitamins and Minerals

Besides the macronutrients mentioned above, vitamins and minerals too are essential for a healthy body with good stamina. Of particular concern for the young athlete is calcium for healthy and strong bones and iron for stamina and endurance. Lack of calcium can lead to weak bones prone to stress fractures. Calcium-rich foods are milk and milk products, while for iron, foods like meat, eggs, legumes especially soyabean and whole cereals are good sources. The iron from animal sources is the heme iron which is more easily and efficiently absorbed as compared to nonheme iron from vegetable sources like green leafy vegetables, cereals, legumes and dry fruits.

Fluids

An athlete child participating in a sport activity needs adequate hydration to prevent exhaustion and dehydration. Extra-fluids are needed to replace for losses through perspiration. Dehydration can lead to a feeling of overheating and exhaustion which can affect the child's performance level. The fluid needs include the amount required for normal hydration plus extra for training, participation and cool down activity.[12,15] Some common signs of dehydration should be explained to the athlete which are as follows:
* Thirst
* Dizziness
* Fatigue
* Nausea
* Headache
* Chills
* Muscle cramps.

If not treated promptly severe dehydration can be very serious. It is therefore recommended to drink adequate water before, during and after the events. The athlete should be taught to recognize signs and symptoms of dehydration so that he/she can act promptly and consume adequate fluids. The color of the urine is an early sign to look for. Dark, scanty urine indicates dehydration, while a good amount, pale yellow urine indicates adequate hydration.[15] A guide to the fluid schedule is given in Table 9.4.[14]

It should be explained to the young athlete that certain fluids should be avoided as they can cause gastric disturbances and affect performance. These are as follows:
* Carbonated drinks, regular fruit juice, fruit drinks, lemonade

Table 9.4: Fluid schedule before, during and after exercise

Time	Amount	Type of Beverage
4 hours or less before exercise	>250–500 mL (1–2 cups)	Water—best choice
2 hours or less before exercise	400–600 mL of fluid	Water—best choice
During exercise	Keep fluids with you when exercising; sip during work out—enough to replace losses through sweat (150–350 mL every 15–20 minutes advisable)	Water—best choice Sports drink—if exercising for >1 hour
Immediately after exercise	As per thirst if already had adequate during exercise (450–675 mL approx)	Water—best choice Other options—milk or chocolate milk,100% fruit juice, sports drink

Source: American Dietetics Association, Dieticians of Canada and the American College of Sports Medicine: Nutrition and athletic performance- Position Statement. J Am Diet Assoc. 2000;100:1543.

- Energy drinks containing lot of sugar or caffeine.

It is recommended that a child of about 10 years of age or younger should drink until he or she does not feel thirsty and then should drink an additional half cup of water. Older children and adolescents should follow the same guidelines, but they should consume an additional cup of fluid.[10] It is a good idea to allow children to allow children to leave the playing field periodically to drink. It may not be easy for children to get to drink adequate fluids in the form of water. Providing them a sport drink that will tempt them to drink and rehydrate is the key to prevent active children from becoming dehydrated.

Sports drink: These may be offered to a young athlete involved in active sports, but care must be taken that these should provide:
- Fluids to cool down the body and replace losses
- Carbohydrates for quick energy—40 g–80 g/L from sources like glucose, fructose, sucrose or maltodextrin
- Sodium and potassium lost in sweat—300–700 mg/L or at least 70 mg/250 mL
- Should be noncarbonated and free from fizz
- Should be free of amino acids, oxygen or herbal ingredients.

Exercise Recommendations in Specific Age Groups

Newborns—3 years

Unstructured safe play without special exercise equipment is good for the infant for healthy development.[16] Walkers and other baby equipment should be discouraged as they tend to hinder the muscle coordination of the child by restricting free movement.

Ages 3–8 years

Children tend to mimic parenteral activities, so the entire family should be involved in some physical activity so as to develop habit of participation by the children.[17] Activities in this age should be focused on participation and not on the aim of winning. However, it is important that children should not be imposed upon for an activity due to over zealousness of the parents.[13]

Ages 8–12 years

Children by this age should be encouraged to perform cardiorespiratory exercise which can continue into adulthood. Those interested in perusing serious sports involvement and/or competitions, their maturation level should be assessed by a health professional.[6,15,17]

There can be vast differences in the maturation level of children of the same age group, and it is obvious that an early matured child will excel in a sport due to his/her maturity associated skill and muscular level. Children should be explained the physiological changes that occur during puberty so that they can prevent unsafe practices aimed at changing body composition for sport participation or appearances.[17]

Ages 13–18 years

At this age eating habits of teens usually are erratic, unhealthy (mainly snacking and reliance on fast foods, etc.). It is important to impart normal healthy nutrition education through class rooms or incorporated into their lifestyle to build good dietary habits. Exercise for them should be a continuous activity all the year round, rather than concentrating only during the practice or training sessions.

Ergogenic Aids

Ergogenic aids are popularly used and recommended by trainers for increasing the performance level in competitions, and readily available over the couter but it must be kept in mind that these have not been tested in pediatric subjects and should be discouraged.

Most athletes are prompted to use ergogenic aids to boost performance by many coaches and trainers. Supplements like β hydroxyl-β-methylbutyrate and creatine are commonly prescribed and made available to athletes. However, there is no evidence to prove any extra-benefits of such products on the performance levels, even though such claims are made by various advertisements. The safety of long-term use of creatine too is not established either, even though there are no scientific reports of any deleterious side effects of these supplements. However, anecdotal claims of having had muscle cramps or dehydration problems have been reported.[10] Caffeine is another common ergogenic aid used by athletes but is not suitable for children because of its side effects. Moreover it is also considered as illegal in International competitive sports.[18]

REFERENCES

1. Ross JG, Gilbert GG. A summary of findings (The National Children and Youth Fitness Study). J Phys Educ Recreation Dance. 1995;56:1-48.
2. Healthy Children 2000, National Health Promotion and Disease Prevention. Objectives Related to Mother, Infants, Children, Adolescents and Youth. US Department of Health and Human Services, DHHS Publication No. HRSA-M-CH-91-2,1991.
3. Birrer RB, Levine R. Performance parameters in children and adolescent atheletes. Sports Med. 1987;4:211-27.
4. Sady SP. Cardiorespiratory exercise training in children. Clin Sports Med. 1986;5:493-514.
5. US Department of Health and Human Services. 1991:11-12. Physical activity and fitness risk reduction objective 1.4. In: Healthy Children 2000. US Department of Health and Human Services.
6. Emery HM. Considerations in child and adolescent athletes. Rheum Dis Clin North Am. 1996;22(3):499-513.
7. Goldberg B, Saraniti A, Witman P, et al. Preparticipation sports assessment: An objective evaluation. Pediatrics. 1980;66:736-45.
8. American Dietetic Association. Timely Statement of the American Dietetic Association: nutrition guidance for adolescent athletes in organized sports. J Am Diet Assoc. 1996;6:611-61.
9. Lal PR. Nutritional Recommendations for Indian Sports Persons-A Review. J Indian Dietetic Association. 2006;31(1&2):1-19.
10. Berning JR. Nutrition for exercise and sports performance. In: Krause's Food & Nutrition Therapy. Mahan KL and Stump SE eds. Missouri: Saunders Elsevier; 2008.
11. American Dietetic Association. Timely statement of the American Dietetic Association: nutrition guidance for child athletes in organized sports. J Am Diet Assoc. 1996;6:610-1.
12. Schoonen JC. Adolescence. In: Benardot D ed. Sports Nutrition. A Guide for the Professional Working with Active People. Chicago: The American Dietetic Association; 1993. pp.113-21.
13. Jennings DS, Nelson S. Play Hard Eat Right. Minneapolis, MN: Chronimed Publishing; 1995.
14. American Dietetics Association, Dieticians of Canada and the American College of Sports Medicine: Nutrition and athletic performance- Position Statement. J Am Diet Assoc. 2000;100:1543.
15. Spear BA. Nutritional management of the child athlete. In: Williams CP ed. Pediatric Manual of Clinical Dietetics. Chicago: TheAmerican Dietetic Association; 1998.pp.139-1448.
16. Committee on Sports Medicine 1986-88. Infant exercise programs. Pediatrics. 1988;82(5):800.
17. Steen SN. Nutrition for the school age child athlete. In: Berning JR, Steen S, eds. Nutrition for Sports and Exercise, 2nd ed. Gaithersburg, MD: Aspen Publishers; 1998.pp.199.
18. Nancy L, Nevin Folino. Sports Nutrition for children and adolescents. In: Handbook of Pediatric Nutrition, eds. Samour PQ, Helm KK, Lang CE. 2nd edn. Massachusetts: Jones and Bartlett Publishers; 2004.

Interaction of Nutrition and Infection in Children

INTRODUCTION

The fact that nutrition and infection act synergistically to worsen the clinical outcome of any disease, and conversely good nutrition status is essential for maintaining maximum resistance to infections and ability to recover from them, has been well established.[1] Infections have a deleterious effect on the nutritional status of the host through physiologic and anatomic changes. These changes become evident in such systemic reactions as fever, leukocytosis and stimulation of adrenal cortical activity. Local reactions include diarrhea, tissue inflammation and necrosis, increased mucus secretion, fatty liver and changes in skin and hair.

A well-nourished child has greater ability to fight infections due to his/her greater resistance and recovers faster as compared to a child with poor nutritional status and impaired resistance. The nutritional status is determined by diet and factors that condition the requirement, absorption, assimilation and utilization of nutrients including activity levels and environmental factors in particular infection and stress.

The effects of repeated infections become cumulative if sufficient intervals do not pass between two episodes and adequate time is not allowed for the dietary intake to optimum levels. The effect of chronic infections will depend upon their nature and severity and the pre-existing nutritional status of the host.

The mechanisms by which infection worsens nutritional status include:
- Reduced appetite
- Tendency of solid food to be discouraged
- Increased metabolic N losses
- Decreased N absorption especially in infections of the gastrointestinal tract.

Moderate to severe malnutrition can have serious consequences, especially in infants and children both short-term and long-term. In well-nourished children, the body reserves normal dietary intake and can avoid malnutrition unless they get prolonged infections.

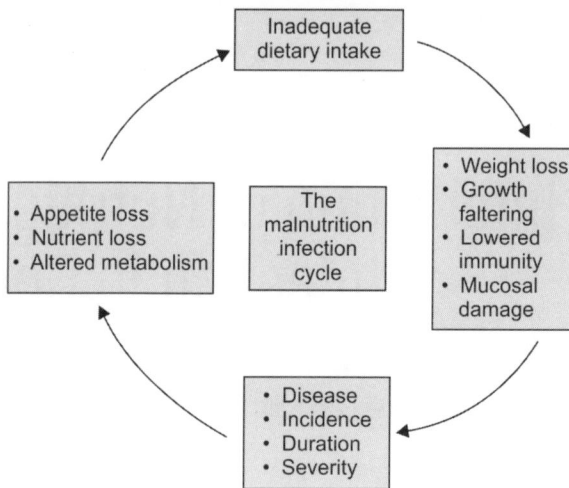

Fig. 10.1: Spiral of malnutrition and infection

Malnutrition and infection can however become a vicious cycle (Fig. 10.1). An inadequate dietary intake leading to weight loss, lowered immunity, mucosal damage, invasion by pathogens finally result in impaired growth and development in children.

A sick child's nutrition is further aggravated by diarrheas, malabsorption, loss of appetite, diversion of nutrients for immune response and urinary N loss, all of which lead to nutrient losses and further damage to defense mechanisms. These in turn cause decreased intake. Added to this fever may further increase both energy and micronutrient requirements. Infections like malaria and influenza have mortality rates proportionate to the degree of malnutrition.[2]

The observed effect of infection on nutritional status varies with time, place and person. The age or the physiological state of the host often determines whether nutritional deficiency will `be manifest or clinically unapparent under a given circumstance. Growing children and pregnant and lactating women are particularly vulnerable. An added stress, such as infection, often relatively innocuous by itself, may be sufficient to precipitate acute malnutrition.

SYNERGISM AND ANTAGONISM

Malnutrition is usually aggravated by infection, the consequences of which are bound to be more serious in a malnourished host than in a well nourished one. This effect of malnutrition being aggravated by infection leading to decreased immunity or infection aggravating malnutrition is termed as 'synergistic'. The simultaneous presence of malnutrition and infection resulting in an interaction is more serious for the host than would be expected from the combined effect of the two working independently. A state of vicious cycle is formed when an infection precipitates clinical malnutrition and which further becomes more and more severe in the malnourished host.

In a different situation when malnutrition is more likely to discourage multiplication of the agent than to affect the resistance mechanisms of the host, the action is termed as 'antagonistic', the combined effect being less than would have been expected.

Metabolism and Infection

Decreased Food Intake

In most infections some degree of anorexia is generally associated, and if this condition persists, it can account for a significant part of the adverse effect of infection on nutritional status especially in children. In addition to this, the normal dietary character is generally altered by either elders or caregivers with a view to exert lesser load on digestion in an already compromised system. This results in with holding certain foods from the diet, e.g. solid foods and their substitutes which are offered may not always be energy dense, e.g. sweetened gruels or beverages like tea, etc. These factors finally contribute to the development of clinically evident nutritional diseases. It is therefore very important to ensure adequate feeding which is possible to be given orally in most cases and to refrain from discouraging or withdrawing of specific foods from the diet. Prolonged administration of grossly inadequate diets leading to severe nutritional deterioration of patients is commonly encountered even in hospitalized patients who assume a critical condition at times, besides prolonging the length of hospital stay and early recovery.

Decreased Nutrient Intake

There is a considerable decrease in nutrient utilization especially in conditions of acute diarrhea due to decreased absorption of nitrogen (N), fat and carbohydrates. Studies have confirmed that moderate diarrhea in a young child may result in an increased caloric loss, almost more than 500–600 cals/d.[3] Similar effects of malabsorption of other micronutrients like vitamin A, iron, folate too have been observed. This is due to increased transit time and the direct effect of toxins produced in the lumen, besides bacterial overgrowth into the small intestine and flattening of the intestine villi and microvilli.

Effect of Malnutrition on Infection

Nutrition and disease (infection) are interconnected. Low nutritional status makes infections worse. A direct correlation has been observed between mortality from infections and nutrition for children, but not for breastfed infants. Malnutrition makes the host more susceptible to infectious diseases and when illness occurs, it is more severe, prolonged and carries increased risk of permanent damage or death. Malnutrition is also directly linked to the severity of the disease, e.g. diarrhea can become a life threatening disease due to dehydration. The duration of illness too is influenced by the state of nutrition resulting in longer duration and time taken for recovery.

Malnutrition directly affects all forms of immunity which may not be nutrient specific. Studies have shown that the defense mechanisms affected by nutritional status include interference with production of antibodies and bactericidal capacity of phagocytes, complement formation, number of T lymphocytes and T cells, subsets, the complement system and more.[4] Other factors apart from malnutrition influencing disease, are environmental, which coexist with malnutrition, leading to infection, e.g. over crowded housing, poor hygiene and sanitary arrangements which cause spreading of infection. Therefore, along with adequate nutrition, environmental and socioeconomic conditions need to be improved too.

Interaction between Malnutrition, Disease and Immunity

Nutrition deficiency affects immunity through specific mechanisms. Adequate nutrition is essential for adequate immune response, which is responsible for building resistance to infectious diseases in humans.[5] One effect of poor nutritional status is, reduced production of hydrochloric acid in the stomach, thus making the pH level higher than normal, allowing multiplication and passage into the small intestines of pathogens responsible for diarrheal disease. Deficiency of vitamins A and B are also known to impair immunity seriously.[6]

Infection worsens the nutritional status and malnourished children are more easily affected by the synergistic effect of these which further impairs immunity. The combination of infectious diseases, reduced food intake and altered metabolism is associated with hampering of growth and development in young children.[7] Infections like diarrhea are associated with decreased absorption of all major macro micronutrients: Carbohydrates, fats and proteins besides affecting vitamins and trace elements. Intestinal transit time is reduced which allows for less absorption time and pathogen-induced damage to the intestinal mucosa.[8]

Micronutrients and Immunity

Micronutrients are basic components of every cell in the body, serving as chemical messengers, building blocks and enzymes. For tissues to function efficiently, all of them need to be present in the right proportion. As these are not stored in the body in large amounts, regular daily intake is important to maintain tissue levels. An erratic or inadequate supply of these weakens the cells and forces them to 'limp along' thereby increasing vulnerability to disease. In the body, both the humoral and cellular components of the immune system are dependent on nutrition. Marginal deficiencies of micronutrients like vitamin A, E, C, B_6, B_{12} and folate and minerals like zinc, manganese, magnesium, copper and selenium can impair production of new white cells and their activity against foreign substances and cells.

Vitamin A

Vitamin A maintains the integrity of the epithelium in the respiratory tract and gastrointestinal tract (GIT). The WHO estimates that worldwide 100–140 million children are vitamin A deficit, thereby increasing the risk of diarrhea, *Plasmodium falciparum* malaria, measles and overall mortality.[9] As early as 1868, Scrimshaw had inferred that no nutritional deficiency is more consistently synergistic with infectious diseases than that of vitamin A.[1] In children, concentration of vitamin A in the blood are appreciably reduced in pneumonia, rheumatoid arthritis, tonsillitis and rheumatic fever.[10]

Intestinal absorption of vitamin A is also impaired in the presence of *Giardia lamblia*. In pathologic states, like obstructive jaundice, chronic nephritis and pneumonia, vitamin A is excreted in the urine. Children with meningitis, infantile diarrhea, chronic tuberculosis, measles, whooping cough and severe chickenpox frequently develop xerophthalmia,[1] thereby confirming that infection precipitates acute clinical avitaminosis A in children with latent deficiency. The deficiency of vitamin A in the form of xerophthalmia, keratomalacia and Bitot's spots are still commonly found among malnourished infants in the developing countries. Vitamin deficiency and measles are closely interacted. Measles in a child is more likely to exacerbate any existing deficiency and children who are already deficient in vitamin A are at much greater risk of dying from measles. Post-measles diarrhea is often very prolonged and has a very high mortality.[11] Since measles depletes the body reserves of vitamin A, vaccination against measles often includes a high dose of vitamin A. Supplementation of vitamin A reduces the risk of developing respiratory tract infections, reduces mortality from diarrhea and enhances immunity.

Vitamin C

Studies have demonstrated an increased loss of vitamin C in the urine during the height of the primary reaction to vaccination against small pox and to vaccination with attenuated measles virus, as well as during the acute clinical stages of measles and chickenpox. Clinical manifestations of ascorbic acid deficiency and low urinary excretion of this vitamin were reported for school children of Madagascar Island having severe ascariasis or other intestinal parasitic disease.[1]

Iron

Infections influence iron metabolism directly through loss of blood and a resulting anemia. An inadequate dietary intake of iron compensates for a mild to moderate hookworm infestation, thereby preventing iron deficiency anemia. Chronic malaria is also known to produce anemia due to significant losses of iron. Chronic infections of bacterial or viral origin produce 'anemias of infection,' a term coined due to the fact that it may interfere with iron binding capacity and erythrocyte life span. Some acute infections include hemolytic anemia.

Zinc

Zinc being a trace mineral, is required for activities of more than 300 enzymes, carbohydrate and energy metabolism, protein synthesis and degradation, nucleic acid production, heme biosynthesis and carbon dioxide transport. Deficiency of zinc can reduce nonspecific immunity, including neutrophil and natural killer cell function and complement activity; reduces numbers of T and B lymphocytes; and suppresses delayed activity, hypersensitivity, cytotoxic activity and antibody production.

Inadequate zinc prevents normal release of vitamin A from the liver and is associated with growth retardation, malabsorption, fetal loss, neonatal death and congenital abnormalities. Patients with Chron's disease, diarrheal illness and pneumonia have found to be having low concentrations of zinc. Supplementary zinc is associated with reduced duration of diarrheal diseases and pneumonia among children living in developing nations. Resistance to infection and improved appetite were found with continuous potassium and magnesium as well as zinc supplements.[12]

Effect of Infection on Malnutrition

Apart from malnutrition having an adverse effect on the severity or duration of infection, the opposite too can be equally contributory. Infection also can have an adverse effect on the nutritional status, which further contributes to growth faltering in children. Loss of appetite during infection can directly result in decreased intake leading to poor growth and high mortality. It was shown that even with minor infections, the rate of protein breakdown increases at the same time as appetite decreases and protein and other nutrient deficiencies are accelerated. An infection increases the basal metabolic rate, which may double the energy requirement. Increased demand for glucose can deplete glucose stores in muscle fat. Carbohydrate and fat metabolism are also affected. The outcomes of an infection can be more serious for a malnourished child, since the body reserves are depleted even under ordinary circumstances.

Intestinal Parasites

Parasitic infections like that of helminths are highly prevalent and known to influence the nutritional status in children considerably. *Giardia lambia* in children is another very common parasite encountered among children and contributing to log standing chronic malnutrition.

Systemic Infections

Measles: Other systemic infections like measles and tuberculosis are the commonest cause of influencing the nutritional status among children. The myths associated with measles as a curse of the goddesses, prohibit adequate feeding of children which results in considerable deterioration of their nutritional status. This further leads to protein–energy malnutrition, in which vitamin A and iron are commonly encountered in these post-measles children. A high mortality from measles in the developing countries is well known. This is attributable in part to the poor nutritional status of the children. Evidence from studies in Guatemala has shown that supplementary feeding alone can reduce fatalities significantly.[1] More complications were observed in malnourished than in well-nourished children in India.[1]

Tuberculosis: Tuberculosis is a frequent cause of malnutrition and vice versa where a malnourished child is more susceptible to contact the disease, given their low immunological status. Malnutrition alters the clinical manifestation in children and also impairs prompt recovery. It has been shown to be an independent predictor of death in hospitalized patients diagnosed with tuberculosis. Children with multi-resistant tuberculosis are mostly severely malnourished due to inadequate dietary intake and prolonged inflammatory process and long courses of toxic drugs. Drugs used to treat tuberculosis are commonly associated with gastrointestinal side effects and vomiting and these further impair food intake. Optimizing nutritional status of such children is bound to confer some benefit on the host and course of recovery. Nutritional intervention like nasogastric feeding where oral intake is compromised can confer significant benefits by improving the nutritional status and prevent growth failure.

HIV infections: HIV infections cause considerable weight loss and protein depletion and play a significant role in morbidity and mortality. The development of malnutrition in HIV/AIDS is multifactorial and includes disorders of food intake, nutrient absorption and intermediary metabolism. Some common causes of decreased food intake in HIV infections are nausea, vomiting, taste alterations, dysphagia, anorexia, early satiety, depression, food access or preparation problems and voluntarily reduced intake to avoid diarrhea. Interventions like nutritional counseling, oral supplements and nasogastric feeding where indicated, are known to improve nutritional status and faster recovery, besides reduced complications.[13]

Gastrointestinal infections: A number of studies from the developing world have established that acute diarrheal disease and upper respiratory tract infections occur more frequently and last longer among malnourished than among well-nourished children.[1] Intestinal parasites like hookworms and giardia may be associated with reduced intake, malabsorption, endogenous nutritional loss and anemia.[14] Parasitic infections are known to cause malnutrition, but the extent to which malnutrition can cause parasitic infections is not clear. Helminthic infection in school-aged children is associated with cognitive deficits.[1] Children free of parasites have better nutritional status, grow faster, learn more and are freer of infections than are children with parasites.

Infection and Protein Nutrition Status

Bacterial infections of the GIT have an adverse effect on protein nutrition which is of major public health importance especially in the developing countries. In children during the weaning period, where inadequate diets lead to malnutrition, like in typhoid fever there has been found to be a two to three fold increase in nitrogen excretion together with a decrease in urinary creatinine due to loss of muscle mass. A decrease in serum albumin is characteristic of acute infections. Acute bacterial infections like pneumonia produce marked changes in all blood serum components, especially a decrease in albumin and an increase in alpha and beta globulins.

Similarly in tuberculosis, it has been observed that urinary nitrogen excretion was markedly increased. Several reports from various authors have confirmed that tuberculosis can precipitate kwashiorkor in children already suffering from chronic malnutrition, due to the strongly negative effect on nitrogen balance.[1]

Therefore, it is clear that increased excretion of nitrogen and decreased intake of food associated with tuberculosis not only complicate clinical management, but also can pose an important public health problem in regions where protein-energy malnutrition is prevalent.

Apart from the above mentioned infections almost all bacterial infections produce an increased urinary excretion of nitrogen. Generally they also result in some decrease in protein intake. Both these effects depend upon the severity of the disease with respect to urinary nitrogen, on the nutritional state of the host as well. Acute episodes can often delay the clinical recovery from the illness.

Infection and Growth and Development

Besides altering absorption, metabolism and excretion of specific nutrients, infections also reduce food intake by an action on appetite. Moreover, it is common to withhold solid food or modify diet during any episode of infection, thereby reducing nutrient intake. Purgatives or other drugs administered as part of therapy also tend to interfere with nutrient intake. As a result severe or prolonged illness has an adverse effect on growth and malnutrition, especially in an already nutritionally compromised child.

REFERENCES

1. Scrimshaw NS, Taylor CE, Gordon JE. Interaction of nutrition and infection. WHO Monograph Series No.57. Geneva: WHO; 1968.
2. Muller O, Garenna M, Kauyate B, et al. The association between protein energy and malnutrition, malaria morbidity and all cause mortality in West African children. Trop Med Int Health. 2003;8:507-11.
3. Rosenberg IH, Solomons NW, Scneider RE. Malabsorption associated with diarrhea and intestinal infections. Am J Clin Nutr. 1977;30:1248-53.
4. Scrimshaw NS, San Giovanni JP. Synergism of nutrition, infection and immunity: an overview. Am J Clin Nutr. 1977;66(2):464S-77S.
5. Chandra RK. Nutritional regulation of immunity and risk of illness. Ind J Pediatrics. 1989;56(5):607-11.
6. Pollard John H. 'Morbidity and longevity' in Ross, John A (ed), International Encyclopedia of population. The free press, Macmillan, New York. 1982;2:452-8.
7. Scrimshaw NS, Taylor CE, John E. Intractions of nutrition and infection. Monograph Ser No. 37, World Health Organisation, Geneva.

8. Lunn P. 'Nutrition, immunity and infection' in Schofield R, Reher D, Bideau A (eds). The Decline of mortality in Europe. Clarendon Press; pp. 131-45.

9. Shank RE, Coburn AF, Moore LV, et al. The level of vitamin A and carotene in plasma of rheumatic subjects. J Clin Invest. 1944;23:289-95.

10. Neidecker-Gonzales O, Nestel P, Bouis H. Estimating the global cost of vitamin A capsule supplementation: a review of the literature. Food Nutr Bull. 2007;28: 307-16.

11. Tomkins A, Watson E. Malnutrition and infection-a review. Nutrition policy No.5,1989,http://www.unsystem.org/scn/archives/npp05/ch4.html. Accessed 31 March 2008.

12. Khanum S, Ashworth A, Hutley SRA. Controlled trial of 3 approaches to the treatment of severe malnutrition. Lancet. 1994;344:1728-37.

13. Heckler LM, Kotler DP. Malnutrition in patients with acquired immune deficiency syndrome. Nutr Rev. 1990;48:393-401.

14. Stolzfus RJ, Dreyfus ML, Chwaya HM. et al. Hookworm control as a strategy to prevent iron deficiency. Nutr Rev. 1997;55:223-32.

Vegetarianism in Children

INTRODUCTION

The term 'vegetarian' is commonly defined as a person who excludes meat, sea food and poultry from his/her diet. However, this term may further be categorized as lacto-ovo vegetarian or lactovegetarian or strictly vegetarian, depending upon the type of foods that are excluded from one's diet (Table 11.1).

The most common type is the lacto-ovo-vegan who includes dairy products and eggs in their diets. On the other hand, vegans are strictly vegetarians in the literal sense, since they exclude all animal products and by products including honey and gelatin besides milk and eggs.

An increasing popularity of vegetarianism is being observed since a decade or more globally. In general, the most frequently cited reason for doing so is health benefits and disease prevention.[1]

For pregnant women and parents of vegetarian children, moral and religious considerations are more commonly given as reasons for doing so.[2]

The seventh day adventist religion strongly encourages a lacto-ovo-vegetarian diet, while other religions like the Jains, Muslims, Hindus, especially

Table 11.1: Categories of vegetarian diets

Vegetarian type	Foods excluded	Protein source	Nutrient risk
Partial vegetarian	Red meat	Poultry, fish, eggs, milk, cheese, yogurt, beans, lentils	Iron
Lacto-Ovo-vegetarian	Red meat, fish, poultry	Milk, cheese, yogurt, eggs, lentils, beans	Iron
Lacto vegetarian	Red meat, fish, poultry, eggs	Milk, cheese, yogurt, lentils, beans	Iron, vitamin D
Vegetarian	Red meat, fish, poultry, eggs, milk cheese, yogurt	Beans, lentils, nuts	Proteins, energy, iron, fat-soluble vitamins, B_{12}, vitamin D, calcium, zinc

the Hare Krishna cult have prohibitions against eating some or all forms of animal foods.

ADEQUACY OF VEGETARIAN DIETS

The American Dietetic Association (ADA) and the American Academy of Pediatrics (AAP) have endorsed that well planned vegan and vegetarian diets can meet the nutritional need and promote normal growth of infants and children.[3,4]

In fact it has been observed that a vegetarian style of eating follows the dietary guidelines and meets the requirements of the recommended allowances for nutrients, if taken in a well balanced and planned way. A number of studies have shown that children and adolescents following a well-designed vegetarian diet grow and develop normally.[5,6] Birth weights of infants born to well-nourished vegetarian women have been shown to be similar to birth weight norms and to birth weights of infants born to nonvegetarian mothers.[7]

The nutritional advantages of vegetarian diets have been well established and it has been indicated that the style of eating can lead to lifelong healthy eating habits when adopted at a younger age. Children and adolescents on vegetarian diets are known to have a lower intake of cholesterol, saturated fats and total fats and a higher intake of fruits, vegetables and fiber than their nonvegetarian counter parts.[8,9] Vegetarian children are also known to have decreased risk for several chronic diseases like diabetes mellitus, cardiovascular diseases, hypertension, obesity and some other types of cancer.[10] Vegetarian diets are mainly rich in carbohydrates, omega 6 fatty acids, dietary fiber, carotenoids, folic acid, vitamin C, vitamin E, potassium and magnesium.[11,12]

It has been stated that lifestyle changes incorporating a low-fat vegetarian or vegan diet could not only prevent various degenerative diseases like coronary artery disease, but even reverse them.[13,14]

NUTRITIONAL RISKS

A vegetarian diet if not well balanced or planned can have negative effects since they may be low in vitamin B_{12}, calcium, omega 3 fatty acids, vitamin D, iron, zinc, niacin and iodine. However, if adequately balanced, it can meet all the nutrients and can be appropriate for all stages of the life cycle including pregnancy, lactation, infancy, childhood and adolescence.[11] It is likely that vegans may be associated with malnutrition where as children eating lacto-ovo-vegetarian diet consume diets closer to the recommended allowances than children whose diets include animal foods.[14]

Vegetarian mothers who breast feed their infants need to be careful to provide adequate vitamin D, calcium and iron sources so as to produce nutritionally complete breast milk for at least the first 6 months of life. In case of vegan mothers it would be worth considering supplementing of the above nutrients to avoid deficiency, which could result in neurological damage in infancy, especially due to vitamins B_{12} and folate (progressive myelopathy and neural tube defect).

In infants beyond 6 months of life, semi solids should be introduced gradually which may include cereals and pulses. However due to the high fiber content they tend to be bulkier. To reduce this bulk, addition of fats and sugars can help to increase the density of foods. Cereals and pulses in their finer form can be prepared like washed dals or suji, dalia, etc. Full fat dairy milk may gradually be introduced along with fortified soy-based foods.

The nutritional areas of concern for vegetarian children include:
- Providing sufficient energy and nutrients for normal growth
- Providing an adequate iron intake to prevent iron deficiency anemia
- Identifying adequate sources of vitamin B_{12} to prevent deficiency
- Obtaining sufficient vitamin D and calcium to prevent rickets
- Ensuring adequate provision of long chain (n-3) of acids from non-meat sources like seeds and nuts
- Consuming food in appropriate form and combination to ensure nutrients can be digested and absorbed by the child.

Energy

Without adequate energy the child can gradually lead to failure to thrive. Vegetarian diets being high in bulk (fiber), concentrated sources of energy like oils can be used to increase the energy content of the foods. Foods like seeds, nuts and peanut butter when incorporated in the dishes planned for toddlers can provide concentrated source of calories along with minerals and proteins.

Proteins

Vegetable and pulse proteins have a lower concentration and range of essential amino acids than those from animal or fish sources. The protein needs therefore may be slightly higher than the recommended allowances due to the lower biological value of some plant proteins. Vegetarian children can derive their required amount of protein if offered a variety, including pulses and grains and the frequency of feeding. Dairy products in lacto-ovo-vegetarian children or even those who are lacto-vegetarian, can provide ample amount of proteins in their diets.

Calcium

Milk and milk products are a natural source of calcium for infants and children for both vegetarian and nonvegetarian children. Vegans will need to derive their calcium from fortified sources like soya milk, tofu or other soya products. If consumed recommended amounts for specific age groups, the calcium requirement can be met easily.[15] It must be kept in mind that since toddlers need an adequate fat diet too for proper growth and development, the use of whole fat milk can be beneficial at least till the age of 2 years. Breastfeeding during the second year of life too can provide adequate fat. It is worth considering also that the same product from different manufacturers can differ by more than 100% of any nutrient per serving, e.g. chocolate milk or yogurt from two different manufacturers can vary in their nutrient content considerably.[15,16] The absorption rate ranges from 50% of the calcium in fortified orange juice to about 30% from other sources.[15]

Among the vegetarian sources green leafy vegetables like spinach, though containing a good amount of calcium, is rendered as poor source due to it being bound to the high oxalate content present in it, thus inhibiting its absorption. Similarly peanuts though a good source of calcium, are high in oxalates which make it a poor source for this nutrient. Foods like broccoli, cauliflower, sesame seeds and figs are also good sources of calcium for vegetarian children. Nuts like walnuts and almonds are also very rich in calcium (Table 11.2).

Table 11.2: Some good vegetarian sources of calcium[17]	
Food sources	*Calcium (mg%)*
Milk (cow's)	120
Milk (buffalo)	210
Curd (cow's)	149
Skimmed milk powder	1370
Soybeans	240
Rajma	260
Black channa (Horse gram)	287
Bengal gram, whole	202
Ragi	344
Beans, cluster	130
Beans, field	210
Lotus stem, dry	408
Fenugreek	395
Curry leaves	830
Mint	200
Mustard leaves	155
Spinach	73
Bathua	150
Walnuts	100
Almonds	230
Coconut, dry	400
Groundnuts	90
Figs	80
Lemon	70
Phalsa	129
Raisins	87
Apricot, dry	110
Dates, dried	120

Source: Gopalan C, Rama Sastri, SC Balasubramanian. Nutritive value of Indian foods, NIN, ICMR, Hyderabad. 2000.

Vitamin D

Vitamin D is found in liquid milk although not in all other milk products. Exposure to sunlight too is a good source of this vitamin for children who may expose their hands and feet for 20–30 minutes at least thrice a week.[18] As per literature available[19] specific age groups require a vitamin D supplement like.

- infants who are exclusively breast fed
- infants consuming <500 mL of vitamin D fortified milk per day
- children and adolescents who do not receive adequate sunlight exposure
- children who are not on any multivitamin containing atleast 200 IU of vitamin D.

An important factor to be kept in mind is the calcium balance bioavailability. Optimal calcium balance can be facilitated by adjusting other factors in the diet like sodium, oxalates, iron and proteins. Protein and sodium both increase urinary calcium loss. Since vegetarian diets are moderate in proteins, calcium absorption can be increased by powering the oxalates and phytate content of the diet.[15]

Iron

Iron is one micronutrient which needs careful consideration in a vegetarian or a vegan diet, since plant sources have lower iron content as compared to animal sources and even the bioavailability of iron from vegetarian sources is lower than as compared to the nonvegetarian sources. A number of studies have shown that vegans and other nonvegetarians were not found to suffer from iron deficiency any more than nonvegetarian children.[20,21] However, while one study agreed that iron deficiency anemia is not more common among vegetarians, they found 'vegetarian' children had reduced levels of hemoglobin and iron compared to 'omnivores' due to 'the absence of animal iron sources with high utilisability'.[22] Studies from India have confirmed that 'strict vegetarian' mothers as well as their newborns have a greater risk and incidence of anemia and iron deficiency.[23] Keeping in view the bioavailability of iron from vegetable sources, it is recommended that iron intake of vegetarian children be 1.8 times that of nonvegetarians.[11,22] Foods like cereals, nuts, seeds, legumes especially soy based are significant sources of iron (Table 11.3), so a well-planned vegetarian diet including these foods should not lead to iron deficiency anemia. However, fruits and raw foods should be avoided for infants and children.[11] An important point to be borne in mind while planning a diet with iron sources, is that, inhibitors and enhancers play an important role in the bioavailability of iron. For instance, ascorbic acid can enhance the bioavailability of iron while phytates like tannin in tea, wine or legumes can also inhibit iron absorption.[11]

Iron being an integral part of many proteins and enzymes which help in cell growth and differentiation and is involved in transporting of oxygen to the red blood cells, care should be taken to so plan a diet for vegetarian and vegan children, that it provides a good amount of bioavailable iron too.

Table 11.3: Vegetable food sources of iron	
Foods	*Iron (mg%)*
Bajra	8.0
Ragi	3.9
Wheat flour	4.9
Bengal gram flour	4.9
Bengal gram dal	5.3
Bengal gram roasted	9.5
Soybean	10.4
Horse gram, whole	6.7
Amaranth	18.4
Cauliflower greens	40.0
Colocasia leaves	10.0
Mint	10.2
Mustard leaves	16.3
Dates, dried	7.3
Custard apple	4.31

Source: Gopalan C, Rama Sastri, SC Balasubramanian. Nutritive value of Indian Foods, NIN, ICMR, Hyderabad. 2000.

Zinc

Overt deficiency of zinc in vegetarians has not been found to be greater than in nonvegetarians.[24] Phytates have been the main factor in inhibiting the availability of zinc from food.[11] High-fiber foods, processed foods like sprouted beans and leavening bread are also known to lower the phytate content of the diet. Therefore, some vegetarians may require a higher intake of zinc than the dietary reference intake for their specific age. Major plant sources of zinc include cooked dietary beans, sea vegetables, fortified cereals, soy foods nuts, peas and seeds, legumes and cheese.

Cobalamin (B$_{12}$)

B$_{12}$ is an important vitamin belonging to the B-complex vitamin group. It is necessary for cell division and blood formation. Lacto-ovo-vegetarians can obtain their requirement of B$_{12}$ from eggs and dairy products. Vegetable sources of this vitamin include cereals, bread, nuts and some fortified soy products.

It is important for vegan breastfeeding mothers to supplement vitamin B$_{12}$ or include sources which are rich in this nutrient, since a deficiency of this vitamin may lead to certain neurological disturbances that could occur in their baby.[25,26] Another factor causing B$_{12}$ deficiency may not be due to lack of the dietary source but due to limited absorption like that in those following a macrobiotic diet.[27]

Meal Planning for a Vegetarian Child

All infants begin life as vegetarians, since they are mainly breastfed for the first part of the year and even later are weaned on to formula milk or cereal-based semisolids. The milk produced by vegetarian mothers is nutritionally adequate and so the infants of such mothers also grow and develop normally.[27] But babies who have not received breastfeeds should receive appropriate cow's milk or soy-based formula to support normal growth.

Solid foods are added to the diet gradually as per the normal infant feeding guidelines (See Chapter 6). A vegetarian diet planned as per the dietary recommendations can meet the nutritional needs of toddlers and preschoolers and can aid in healthy growth and development.

In India, the problem of vegetarianism is not a 'grave' concern, since it is largely a lacto-vegetarian population followed by a significant number being lacto-ovo-vegetarians. Even among the nonvegetarian population, the consumption of nonvegetarian sources is not a daily routine followed in all meals and yet in most well to do families the vegetarian sources of foods are consumed in adequate amounts which take care of the nutritional requirements of the older population. However, in case of children, nutritional anemia is a very common feature observed in very well to do families. This is because of faulty feeding habits, mainly being prolonged breastfeeding with inadequate solid foods or excess consumption of milk or milk products which are low in iron. It is therefore very important that children of vegetarian families take special care to incorporate all those foods which can provide all the micronutrients besides adequate macronutrients. A healthy eating style of the vegetarian family as a whole can go a long way in inculcating good and healthy eating pattern in children too.

REFERENCES

1. Yankelovick, Clancy, Shulman. Survey of adult Americans, Time Magazine and CNN. April 1992.
2. Finley DA, Dewey KG, Lonnerday B, et al. Food calories of vegetarian and nonvegetarians during pregnancy and lactation. J Am Diet Assoc. 1985:678-85.
3. American Academy of Pediatrics Committee on Nutrition.1998. Soy protein based formulas: Recommendations for use in infant feeding. Pediatrics. 1998;101:148-53.
4. Messina VK, Burke KI. Position of the American Dietetic Association: vegetarian diets. J Am Dietet Assoc. 1997;97:1317-21.
5. Nathan I, Hackett AF, Kriby S. A longitudinal study of the growth of matched pairs of vegetable and omnivorous children, aged 7-11 years in the north west of England. Europ J Clin Nutr. 1997;51:20-5.
6. Sanders TAB, Reddy S. Vegetarian diets and children. Am J Clin Nutr. 1994;1176S-81S.

7. O'Connel JM, Dibley MJ, Sierra J, et al. Growth of vegetarian children. The Farm Study. Pediatrics. 1989;84:475-81.

8. Novy MA. Are strict vegetarians at risk of vitamin B_{12} deficiency? Cleveland Clinic J Med. 2000;67:87-8.

9. Sanders TAB, Manning J. The growth and development of vegan children. J Human Nutr Dietet. 1992;5:11-21.

10. Rajaram S, Sabate J. Health benefits of a vegetarian diet. Nutrition. 2000;16:531-3.

11. "Position of the American Dietetics Asociation and Dietitians of Canada: Vegetarian diets" http://www.adajournal'org/article. J Am Dietet Assoc. 2003;06

12. Key TJ, Appleby PN, Rosell MS. Health effects of vegetarian and vegan diets. Proceedings of Nutr Soc. 2006;65:34-41.

13. Ôrnish D, Brown SE, Sckerwitz LW, et al. Can lifestyle canges reverse coronary heart disease? The Lifestyle Heart Trial: Lancet. 1990;336;8708:129-33.

14. Alder M, Specher B. Atypical diets in infancy and early childhood. Pediatrics Annals. 2001;30(11):673-80.

15. Weaver CM, Plawecki KL. Dietary calcium: adequacy of a vegetarian diet. Am J Clin Nutr. 1994;(5S):1238S-41S.

16. Coughlin CM. Vegetarianism in children. In: Handbook of Pediatric Nutrition, eds. Samour PQ, Helm KK, Lang CE. Massachusetts: Jones and Bartlett Publishers; 2004; pp.1133-48.

17. Gopalan C, Rama Sastri, SC Balasubramanian. Nutritive value of Indian foods, NIN, ICMR, Hyderabad. 2000.

18. Mangels A, Messina V. Considerations in planning vegan diets: Infants. J Am Diet Assoc. 2001;101:670-7.

19. Gartner LM, Green FR. Prevention of rickets and vitamin D deficiency: new guidelines for vitamin D intake. Pediatrics. 2003;111:908-10.

20. Larsson CL, Johansson GK. Dietary intake and nutritional status of young vegans and omnivores in Sweden. Am J Clin Nutr. 2002;76:100-6.

21. Ball MJ, Bartlett MA. Dietary intake and iron status of Australian vegetarian women. Am J Clin Nutr. 1999;70:353-8.

22. Krajcoviova – Kudlackova M, Simoncic R, Bederova A, et al. Influence of vegetarian and mixed nutrition on selected hematological and biochemical parameters in children. 1997, http://www.adajournal.

23. Sharma DC, Kiran R, Ramnath V, et al. Iron deficiency anemia in vegetarian mothers and their newborns. Ind J Clin Biochem. 1994;9(2):100-2.

24. Freeland- Graves JH, Bodyz PW, Epright MA. Zinc status of vegetarians. J Am Diet Assoc. 1980;(77):655-61.

25. Graham SM, Arvela OM, Wise GA. Long-term neurological consequences of nutritional vitamin B_{12} deficiency in infants. J Pediatr. 1992,121(Pt 1):710-4.

26. Johnson PRJ, Roloff JS. Vitamin B_{12} deficiency in infant strictly breast fed by a mother with late pernicious anemia. J Pediatr. 1982;100:917-9.

27. Messina M, Messina V. The Dietitians guide to vegetarian diets. Issues and Applications. Gaithersburg, MD: Aspen Publishers; 1996.

Protein-Energy Malnutrition

"Health is not simply the absence of sickness"

—Hannah Green

INTRODUCTION

The health and well being of any individual is based on a combination of various factors. Besides diet and good nutrition, a host of contributory factors go a long way in preventing disease and malnutrition. These may be environmental, sociodemographic, immunization programs, provision of clean water supply and even psychosocial.

Environmental factors include parental education, socioeconomic status, living standards and child rearing practices.

Sociodemographic factors include breastfeeding practices, diet during illness for mother and child, maternal malnutrition, low-birth-weight babies, recurrent infections, etc.

According to WHO definition, malnutrition involves a cellular imbalance between supply of nutrients and energy and the body's demand for them to ensure normal growth, maintenance and specific tissue functions. Malnutrition accounts for more than 50% of all infant mortality in developing countries, especially in the below 5 year age group.

The most common form of malnutrition in children is protein-energy malnutrition (PEM), which earlier was also called protein-calorie malnutrition (PCM). It has also been defined as a pathological state characterized by inadequate intake of proteins and calories in varying degrees commonly associated with infections.[1] Children between 6–36 months old are generally at high risk of falling prey to this condition, since they are more vulnerable to infections, especially gastrointestinal and measles. Death rates are high among children with untreated PEM, and the risk of dying increase with severity of the condition. Electrolyte imbalance, hypothermia and complicating infections are some of the causes of mortality in these children.

CAUSES OF PEM

PEM occurs primarily due to food deprivation, but other factors play a major role also. These can be discussed as the following:

- *Low birth weight and infections:* Recurrent diarrhea, acute respiratory infections, other preventable infections like measles, tuberculosis, whooping cough and helminthes, can aggravate and complicate a preexisting condition of low birth weight. Again maternal malnutrition is an important cause of low birth weight
- *Food deprivation:* Poverty is one important cause of food deprivation in small children. Large families contribute to this problem and the priority of food distribution generally is for the male child followed by other male members in the family
- *Food taboos and myths:* Even where resources are not a limiting factor, very often self-imposed restrictions regarding intake of food, can affect provision of adequate nutrients to the child. Food fads and myths related to consumption of specific type of foods at different phases of pregnancy or lactation and subsequently weaning practices can be a sole cause of food deprivation. Very often these fads and myths are interlinked with various cultural beliefs and/or religious beliefs. A common observation made is pertaining to infant feeding practices, where, in most rural classes colostrums is discarded as it is considered poisonous for the baby. The maternal diet is also restricted keeping in mind 'hot' or 'cold' foods which may be 'unsuitable for the infant. All such practices can go a long way to adversely affect the availability of essential macro- and micronutrients required for adequate growth and development of the child
- *Ignorance:* Many rural and urban mothers are quite ignorant of their infant's need for adequate nutrition. It's a common belief that milk is the 'best and only' food for a child, even after he has crossed the first 6 months of his life. They continue to breast feed exclusively, well up to 12–24 months, making little effort to offer cereal supplements. Alternatively, if breast milk is inadequate, they will continue to feed diluted milk without introducing cereals. Even during illness of the child, solid food is withheld and the baby is kept on undiluted milk or tea with an occasional biscuit or so. Cereal, pulse base foods are considered 'heavy' for the child's liver. These factors further contribute to inadequate nutrient intake and subsequently growth failure.

PATHOGENESIS OF PEM

Gopalan in 1968 introduced a new hypothesis, that of 'adaptation'.[2] This was termed as 'dysadaptation', stating that kwashiorkor in fact was a failure of adaptation. This was explained on biochemical and hormonal factors. The malnourished child adapts himself to the unfavorable circumstances and to the calorie and protein gap. They reduce their activity, curtail their growth thereby bringing down the basal metabolic rate (BMR) and thus, save energy for survival.[3] This reduction in BMR and lack of insulating fat leads to hypothermia which may prove fatal.

The basic adaptation to explain the mechanism was that the gradual wasting of muscle and subcutaneous fat would also protect certain other metabolic processes. Like, the essential amino acids are made available, which it was assumed, would enable the liver to maintain the synthesis of components essential for homeostasis, like serum albumin and β lipoprotein. This could explain the absence of edema or fatty liver in marasmus.[4]

The high level of catabolic hormones including cortisol causes muscle and fat breakdown. The anabolic hormones like insulin and insulin-like growth factors maintain near normal anabolism to prevent edema and fatty liver by enabling the synthesis of albumin and β lipoproteins from the available pool of amino acids.

Another theory postulated in the pathogenesis of PEM is that of free radicals which are assumed to play a role in edema, skin changes and fatty liver. The free oxygen radicals which are toxic to cell membranes are produced during infections. In the malnourished child, deficiency of nutrients like vitamins A, C and E and selenium which are anti oxidants can result in the accumulation of toxic-free oxygen radicals. These further damage the liver cells resulting in kwashiorkor.

CLASSIFICATION OF PEM

Various parameters are used to classify PEM like, weight for age, height for age or weight for height. The most widely used accepted criterion is the weight for age. This has been done by various workers of different times. Besides Gomez and the IAP classification (Refer Chapter 3, Tables 3.2 and 3.3), two more classifications have been proposed:

- **Jelliffe's classification:** Proposed in 1965, it has been categorized into four classes as shown in Table 12.1[5]
- **Wellcome Trust or International classification:** This is based on clinical assessment as suggested by Wellcome Trust in 1970.[6] Besides weight for age, it also considers presence or absence of edema as seen in Table 12.2.[6]

Table 12.1: Jelliffe's classification of PEM

Nutritional status (PEM)	Wt. for age (Harvard) % of expected
Normal	>90
First degree	80–90
Second degree	70–80
Third degree	60–70
Fourth degree	<60

Table 12.2: Wellcome Trust classification		
Weight for age (Boston) % of expected	**Edema**	**Clinical type of PEM**
60–80	+	Kwashiorkor
60–80	-	Underweight
<60	-	Marasmus
<60	+	Marasmic kwashiorkor

SPECTRUM OF PEM

There are three forms of PEM recognized, based on the clinical presentations:

- Kwashiorkor
- Marasmus
- Marasmic kwashiorkor
  A picture of the various features of PEM can be had from Table 12.3.

Kwashiorkor

The word 'kwashiorkor' was first described by Dr Cicely Williams in 1933. The word originates from the African language—*Ga* of Ghana, meaning the 'red boy' due to the characteristic pigmentation. Other workers from the West Indies described this as 'sugar baby' due to the characteristic 'prominent cheeks' and edema. This deficiency is known to occur with the coming of the second sib, when the child is displaced from the breast by another child. This condition is seen mostly in children in their second year of life, following abrupt weaning. They appear to be apathetic, irritable, weak and inactive, with the presence of edema and fatty liver. The edema is detected by the production of a definite pit on exerting moderate pressure for 3 seconds with the thumb over the lower end of the tibia and dorsum of the foot.

Initially, parents may miss these features and on the contrary be satisfied by the false image of a 'fatty child' But what is not generally realized by the lay person is that this fat appears typically on the belly and is commonly referred to

Table 12.3: Clinical features of PEM		
Spectrum	**Clinical symptoms**	
	Always present	**Sometimes present**
Marasmus	Wasting	Hunger, wizened appearance
Kwashiorkor	Edema	Mental changes: Irritability, poor appetite Skin changes: Flaky paint dermatosis Hair: Sparse, loose, straight
Marasmic kwashiorkor	Wasting + Edema	Any of the above symptoms and signs

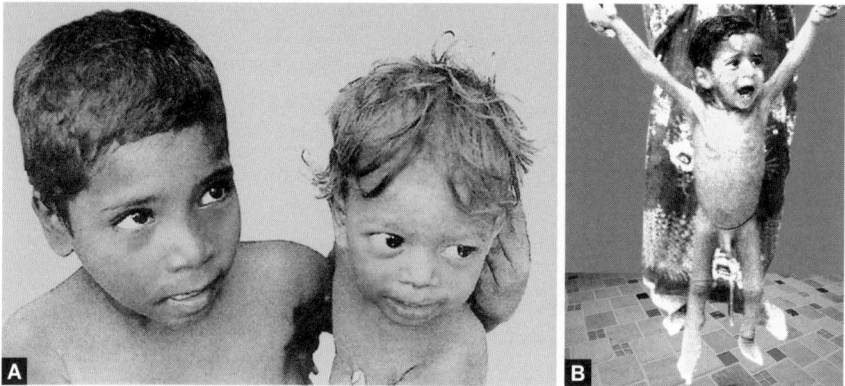

Figs 12.1A and B: (A) Child with sparse hair; (B) Child with pot belly

as 'pot belly', but from his buttocks would be flat and give a wasted appearance (Figs 12.1A and B).

The typical signs of PEM are described by the following associated abnormalities:

- *Body:* All body parts, especially buttocks, arms and legs have decreased subcutanous fat layer
- *Skin:* The skin appears dry and flaky (flaky paint dermatosis). Hyperpigmented plaques may be visible over areas of trauma
- *Hair:* It becomes thin, sparse and brittle. It also turns dull brown or red, giving an appearance of a 'flag sign'
- *Nails:* There will be fissures or ridges and increased fragility
- *Abdomen:* The presence of edema due to accumulation of ascitic fluid and also hepatomegaly (fatty liver), makes the abdomen appear distended
- *Mouth:* Signs of vitamin B group deficiency—Cheilosis, angular stomatitis and papillary atrophy are commonly present
- *Behavior:* The child neither appears irritable and avoids social interaction, nor responds socially. They have a poor appetite and refuse to eat
- *Deficiencies:* It is common to observe deficiency signs of vitamins, like, vitamin A, D and B group and minerals like iron and iodine.

Marasmus

The term marasmus is derived from the Greek 'marasmos' which means wasting. In this condition, there is gross wasting of muscle and subcutanous tissues, marked stunting but no edema. This picture can be seen in early infancy unlike in kwashiorkor (Fig. 12.2).

The marasmic condition is typical of sequel to prolonged starvation, chronic or recurrent infections and limited food intake. Marasmus represents an *adaptive* response to starvation, unlike kwashiorkor

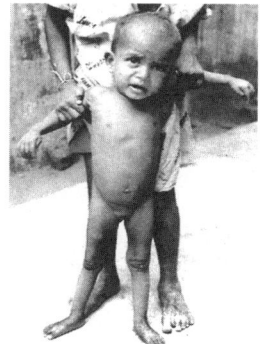

Fig. 12.2: Marasmic Child

which represents *maladaptive* response to starvation. In marasmus, the body utilizes all fat stores before using muscles. It is commonly seen in the first year of life due to lack of breastfeeding and the use of diluted animal milk. Poverty or famine like conditions and presence of diarrhea besides ignorance and poor maternal nutrition, are the precipitating factors. There is severe wasting of the shoulders, arms, buttocks and thighs with no visible rib outlines. The typical appearance of a marasmic child is described as follows:

- A 'thin old' man
- Baggy pants (the loose skin of the buttocks hanging down)
- Child may be alert despite his condition
- Absence of edema on the lower extremities
- Prominent ribs
- Large head with sunken eyes
- A hungry child
- Associated diarrhea or dehydration.

In marasmus there is a marked deficit of weight but not as much in height. The marasmic infant has a good appetite but may also appear irritable, fretful and apathetic as in cases of kwashiorkor. Though the skin might appear dry, the typical characteristic peeling or patchy hypopigmentation may not be there.

It is worth mentioning here that during the past decade or so, the profile of PEM presenting in our hospitals has gradually changed. Frank cases of kwashiorkor are rarely encountered, but the marasmic type of picture is frequently observed. The prevalence of clinical form of malnutrition has been reduced to less than 1%. Hospital statistics also show that in recent years, admissions due to severe PEM have come down significantly.[7]

Marasmic Kwashiorkar

This condition is intermediary between marasmus and kwashiorkor, since such children present with a mixed picture. The body weight is less than 60% of the expected along with the presence of edema. The degree of stunting seems greater in marasmic kwashiorkor, indicating that duration of illness in this condition is greater than in kwashiorkor.

MANAGEMENT OF PEM

Treatment of severe malnutrition is a challenging task and involves multipronged approach. Most of the cases of severe malnutrition are not without complications on presentation. Severe infection is one major complication to be tackled. Management of these children involves hospitalization in majority of the cases. Noncomplicated cases can be managed on outpatient basis in a hospital or any primary healthcare center. But children presenting with complications can be managed in a hospital setting alone. Initial approach involves treating the complications first which may be:

Resuscitation

This involves tackling the life-threatening medical emergencies on priority, which may include:

1. *Hypothermia/Hypoglycemia*—These are generally found together. The child is managed by keeping him warm and 'bedding in' with the mother is encouraged. Feeding if possible may be initiated. For hypoglycemia, the child is put on IV glucose 10%, if immediate feeding is not possible. Child is treated for sepsis.
2. *Infections*—Infections are a major cause of mortality in PEM. Appropriate antibiotic therapy is initiated.
3. *Anemia*—If not managed appropriately, severe anemia may lead to heart failure. If required blood transfusion is resorted to.

Deydration/Electrolyte Imbalance

Most often such children present with diarrhea. Depending upon the severity of stooling, ORS should be initiated. In moderate dehydration 70–100 mL/kg ORS in 4 hours is given by sips. In severe dehydration, 100 mL/kg normal saline or ringer lactate is given over 3–6 hours. Mostly hypokalemia is present which can be managed by potassium supplement.

Congestive Heart Failure

In case of presence of heart failure, fluid intake is restricted and kept on maintenance dose. Diuretics may be given to prevent fluid overload.

Vitamin Deficiencies

Deficiency of vitamins is a common feature among children with PEM. Vitamin A can be supplemented in all cases. Vitamin K also is given to those with florid PEM and accompanied by diarrhea. All B complex vitamins, vitamin C, E and D too are administered along with calcium and zinc. Magnesium also needs to be supplemented if seizures, tetany or apathy are present.

Dietary Management

Different workers have laid down special formulae for achieving high-energy intakes and to fulfill protein requirements for maximum catch up growth rates.

The general pattern followed by them was of providing first class protein, in the form of milk protein powder, oil for energy along with sugar for flavor as well as extra energy. Oil is used to increase the density of the feed without increasing the bulk. Medium-chain triglycerides are more desirable to enhance absorption and metabolism.

Almost all workers advocated regimens providing calories of around 150–200 per kg/d for maximum catch up growth. The protein requirements have been suggested around 3–4 g/kg/d. But certain workers preferred to maintain calories at around 100 cal/kg/d initially and gradually increased over a week till the full volume is tolerated. This is specially so in children with kwashiorkor until the edema disappeared.

WHO in 1999,[8] laid down guidelines for routine treatment of severe malnutrition where the nutrition component was also stressed as follows:

Stabilization Phase—Initiate Refeeding

Feeding should be initiated gradually as soon as possible after admission. It should be formulated to provide just sufficient calories and proteins to maintain basic physiological functions. The main features include:
- Small frequent feeds of low osmalarity (<350) mosm/L and low lactose (<2–3 g/kg/d)
- Oral or nasogastric feeds
- 100 cal/kg/d—not to exceed in initial phase
- 1.0–1.5 g prot/kg/d
- 130 mL/kg/d of liquid (may begin with 100 mL/kg/d if edema present)
- Feed should be of low viscosity, easy to prepare and socially acceptable
- Continue breastfeeding if already doing so.

The above regimen is achieved using the F-75 formula which is designed to provide 75 cals/100 mL and 0.9 g pro/100 mL of the feed (Table 12.4).[8] These should be fed by cup and spoon. The recommended schedule suggested is as shown in Table 12.5.[9]

For children with good appetite, without edema, the schedule can be completed in 2–3 days. Careful monitoring should be done for the following:
- Amounts offered and left over
- Vomiting
- Stool frequency and consistency
- Daily body weight.

There may be accompanying diarrhea in some children, in which case milk-based feeds can be replaced with soya-based or any lactose-free feeds till such time the stools settle down. Gradually low lactose feeds like curd may be initiated, and if tolerated, the amounts increased, and even milk-based cereal feeds can be initiated.

In both types of PEM, basal energy expenditure increases gradually during refeeding. As the child loses weight, total body water as percentage of body weight increases and the child becomes relatively over hydrated. In children with edema, initiation of nutritional recovery is characterized by a progressive loss of extracellular fluid resulting in an initial loss of weight, followed by stabilization for 10–12 days and again followed by weight gain.[10]

Methods of feeding should be ideally from a cup and spoon along with continuation of breast feeds. Even when breast feeds are inadequate, nonnutritive sucking should be encouraged which itself can enhance lactation. In case oral feeds are difficult to achieve, tube feeding can be resorted to for a few days till such time oral feeding is restored adequately.

Table 12.4: Recipes and composition of starter formulae and catch up formula

Ingredients	Starter formula (F 75)	Starter formula with cereal (F75)	Catch up formula (F 100)
Dried skim milk (g)	25	25	80
Sugar (g)	100	70	50
Cereal flour (g)	-	35	-
Vegetable oil (mL)	27	27	60
Electrolyte mineral solution (mL)	20	20	20
Water: To make up to final soln. (mL)	1000	1000	1000
Contents per 100 mL			
Calories (kcal)	75	75	100
Protein (g)	0.9	1.1	2.9
Lactose (g)	1.3	1.3	4.2
Potassium (mmol)	4.0	4.2	6.3
Sodium (mmol)	0.6	0.6	1.9
Magnesium (mmol)	0.43	0.46	0.73
Zinc (mg)	2.0	2.0	2.3
Copper (mg)	0.25	0.25	0.25
% energy from protein	5	6	12
% energy from fat	32	32	53
Osmolality (mOsm/L)	413	334	419

Source: WHO 2000.

Table 12.5: Feeding schedule for children with severe malnutrition

Days	Frequency (hrly)	Vol/kg/feed (mL)	Vol/kg/d (mL)
1–2	2	11	130
3–5	3	16	130
6–7+	4	22	130

Source: WHO, seer malnutrition. In: Pocket Book of Hospital Care for Children, guidelines for the management of common illnesses with limited resources. WHO, 2005.

A weight gain of 0.5 kg/week in children and 70 g/kg/week in infants is the goal. With recurrent infections this goal may be difficult; therefore control of infections is very important.

Catch-up Growth

This is the rehabilitation phase, when the appetite of the child is restored within 8–10 days, return of social smile and the child begins to take interest in the surroundings. These are the first signs of recovery in a child with PEM. The increase in the feeds should be done gradually at this point to avoid risk of heart failure. To achieve the catch-up growth the transition made is as follows:

- Replace F-75 by F100 which contains 100 cal. and 2.9 g protein per 100 mL. This can be achieved by incorporating oil and sugar with milk or using milk cereal based preparations (Table 12.4)
- Subsequently, the feeds are increased by 10–20 mL and finally 25–30 mL/kg/feed. This can provide up to 200 cal/kg/d
- Monitoring for respiration and pulse rates are done regularly. The volume of feeds needs to be decreased as also the frequency (4 hourly) in case increase in respiration is observed. Once stabilized:
  - Increased amounts of F100 formula at least 3–4 hourly can be started
  - Calories given—150–200 kg/d
  - Proteins increased—4–6 g/kg/d
  - Continue breastfeeding
  - Ensure administration of 6 monthly vitamin A dose.

The Indian Academy of Pediatrics in 2006 formed a working committee to bring out a revised consensus on the management of severely malnourished children in the Indian context,[11] which were adapted from the WHO guidelines of 2000 mentioned earlier. These guidelines are based on the hospital management of such children.

The modified formulae recommended for F 75 and the catch-up formula F 100 are as given in Tables 12.6[11] and 12.7.[11]

The cereal-based low lactose (lower osmolarity) diets are recommended as starter diets for those with persistent diarrhea.[12] Lactose-free diets are rarely needed for persistent diarrhea as most children do well on the above mentioned, low lactose F-75 diets. Children with persistent diarrhea, who continue to have diarrhea on the low lactose diets, should be given lactose (milk) free starter diets, as shown in Table 12.8.[11] They can be followed on to lactose-free catch-up diets as shown in Table 12.9.[11]

Table 12.6: Starter diets F 75[11]			
Diet contents (per 100 mL)	F-75 starter	F-75 cereal based-(1)	F-75 cereal based-(2)
Cow's milk (mL)	30	30	25
Sugar (g)	9	6	3
Cereal puffed rice (g)	-	2.5	6
Vegetable oil (mL)	2	2.5	3
Water—to make up to 100 mL	100	100	100
Calories (Kcal)	75	75	75
Proteins (g)	0.9	1.1	1.2
Lactose (g)	1.2	1.2	1.2

- Egg white can be replaced by 3 g of chicken or commercially available casein
- Powdered puffed rice can be replaced by commercial rice or precooked rice (in same amounts)

Table 12.7: Catch-up diets F 100[11]

Diet contents (per 100 mL)	F-100 Catch-up	F-100 Catch-up (cereal based) Example 1
Cows milk/toned dairy milk (mL)	95	75
Sugar (g)	5	2.5
Cereal: Puffed rice (g)	–	7
Vegetable oil (g)	2	2
Water to make (mL)	101	100
Energy (kcal)	100	100
Protein (g)	2.9	2.9
Lactose (g)	3.8	3

Source: AP 2006 (11).

Table 12.8: Starter lactose-free diet[11]

Egg white *(g)	5
Glucose (g)	3.5
Cereal flour: Powdered puffed rice** (g)	7
Vegetable oil (g)	4
Water to make (mL)	100
Energy (kcal)	75
Protein (g)	1
Lactose	-

* Egg white may be replaced by 3 g of chicken or commercially available pure protein like casein
**Powdered puffed rice may be replaced by commercial pre-cooked rice preparations (in same amounts)
Source: IAP, 2006

Table 12.9: Catch-up lactose-free diet[11]

Egg white *(g)	20
Glucose or sugar (g)	4
Cereal flour: Puffed rice** (g)	12
Vegetable oil (g)	4
Water to make (mL)	100
Energy (kcal)	100
Protein (g)	3
Lactose (g)	–

*Egg white may be replaced by 3 g of chicken or commercially available pure protein like casein
**Powdered puffed rice may be replaced by commercial pre-cooked rice preparations (in same amounts)
Source: IAP, 2006

Table 12.10: Low-lactose catch-up diets (F 100)[11]		
Catch-up low-lactose diets	*Example 1*	*Example 2*
Milk (cow's milk or toned dairy milk)	25 mL	25 mL
Egg white *(g)	12	–
Roasted powdered groundnut	–	5 g
Vegetable oil (g)	4	
Cereal flour: Powdered puffed rice** (g)	12	12
Energy (kcal)	100	100
Protein (g)	2.9	2.9
Lactose (g)	1	1

* Egg white may be replaced by 3g of chicken or commercially available pure protein like casein
**Powdered puffed rice may be replaced by commercial pre-cooked rice preparations (in same amounts)
Jaggery could be used instead of glucose/sugar
Source: IAP, 2006.

The low lactose catch-up diets F 100, can be started at the rehabilitation phase as shown in Table 12.10.[11]

Complementary foods should be added as soon as possible to prepare the child for home foods at discharge. They should have comparable energy and protein concentrations once the catch-up diets are well tolerated. Khichri, dalia, banana, curd-rice and other culturally acceptable and locally available diets can also be offered liberally.

Nutrition recovery syndrome is a condition encountered generally during the rehabilitation phase of a child with severe PEM. It is marked by heptomegaly, gynecomastia, abdominal distension, ascites, splenomegaly, etc. This is attributed to sudden increase in energy and protein intake by these children. It is mostly self limiting and might also be associated with tremors (kwashi shake) during treatment. Protein restriction during this period was generally advocated. But recently it has also been thought to result of excess hormones secreted during recovery phase.[13]

REFERENCES

1. WHO Technical Report Series, No. 522, FAO Nutrition Meetings Report Series, No 52, Energy and protein requirement. Report of a Joint FAO/WHO, Adhoc Committee, WHO, Geneva, 1973.
2. Gopalan C. In: Calorie Deficiencies and Protein Deficiencies. McCance RA, Widdowson EM (Eds). Edinburgh and London: Churchill, Lvingstone; 1968. p. 49.
3. Gopalan C. Calorie deficiencies and protein deficiencies. In: Kwashiorkar and Marasmus: evolution and distinguishing features. Mc Cance RA, Widdowson EM (Eds). London: Churchill Livingstone; 1967.
4. Alleyne GAO, Hay RW, Picou DI. Stanfield. New Delhi: JP Brothers.
5. Jelliffe DB. WHO Monog Ser. No.53. 1966.
6. Wellcome Trust Working Party. Classification of infantile malnutrition. Lancet. 1970;2:302-3.

7. Reddy V. Protein energy malnutrition. Textbook of Human Nutrition. Mahatab S Bamji, N Prahalad Rao, Vinodini Reddy (Eds). Oxford and IBH Publishing Co Pvt Ltd, 1996;pg 252-65.

8. WHO. Management of the child with a serious infection or severe malnutrition. Guidelines for the care at the first referral level in developing countries. Geneva: WHO; 2000.

9. WHO, Severe malnutrition. In: Pocket Book of Hospital care for children, Guidelines for the management of common illnesses with limited resources. WHO, 2005.

10. Viterri FE. Primart protein energy malnutrition: Clinical, biochemical and metabolic changes. In: Suskind RM ed. Textbook of Pediatric Nutrition, New York: Raven Press, 1981:189-215.

11. Bhatnagar S, Lodha R, Chowdhary P, Sachdeva HPS, et al. IAP guidelines 2006 on hospital based management of severely malnourished children (Adapted from WHO guidelines). Ind Pediatr. 2007;44:443-61.

12. Bhatnagar S, Bhan MK, Singh KD, Saxena SK, Shariff M. Efficiency of milk based diets in persistent diarrhea: A randomized controlled trial. Pediatrics. 1996;98:1122-6.

13. Elizabeth KE. Protein energy malnutrition. In: Nutrition and Child Development, 3rd Ed. Paras Medical Publishers; 2004. pp.133-7.

Childhood Obesity

"One should strive to maintain good health by taking balanced diet and exercising regularly"

—**Atharva Veda**

INTRODUCTION

At one time the term childhood obesity was rarely seen in our country. The main nutritional problems in children focused around malnutrition which was in the form of undernutrition, anemia and vitamin A deficiency. However, gradually, over a period of a decade or two, the other aspect of malnutrition, that of over nutrition in the form of childhood obesity has emerged as a major health problem in India too. In the USA, childhood obesity has increased at least by 50% since 1976. It is well known that 80% of obese adolescents become obese adults. Over weight in adolescence predicts a broad range of adverse health affects that are independent of adult weight after 55 years of follow-up.[1]

Effective treatment and prevention of obesity must begin in childhood. However, studies indicate that care providers recommend initiation of treatment for only less than 20% of obese children.

The causes of higher rates of fatness in developing countries are poorly studied, but could be due to the extreme and rapid changes in lifestyle, physical activity and diet that accompany urbanization and rapid economic development. The results of such lifestyle are already being seen. Most cardiovascular disease deaths, generally associated only with Western industrialized countries now occur in developing countries.[2]

Common childhood and adolescent medical consequences of obesity include increased growth, then stunting, increased fat free mass, early menarche, hyperlipidemia, increased heart rate and cardiac output, hepatic steatosis with elevated transaminases and abnormal glucose metabolism.[3-5]

The various causative factors attributed to the increasing prevalence of obesity in the Indian scenario may perhaps be attributed to the lifestyle changes of the families. Increased purchasing power, better and comfortable living thanks to the improving technology, increased variety and availability of food products in the market and increased hours of inactivity have all been blamed for the changing trends. Television, video games and computers have replaced the hours of outdoor games and other activities leading to childhood obesity.

It is thought that the tendency of adults becoming obese is determined by genetic, intrauterine, childhood and adolescent condition. Critical periods for the development of obesity and its sequel have been postulated, including period of gestation, the period of adiposity rebound (between 5 and 6 years) and adolescence. Studies have also demonstrated that an active lifestyle in childhood is more likely to be reflected in more active adolescents and adults. Although 10% weight loss in adults can improve the comorbidities of obesity, most comorbidities are irreversible.[6]

DEFINITION OF CHILDHOOD OBESITY

Obesity actually can be viewed as the energy balance of any individual. Energy expended should be equal to that of energy consumed. Therefore, basically it can be defined as energy expended to be equivalent to energy consumed. In other words it means that the energy balance should not be tilted. A positive energy balance will probably lead to overweight and finally obesity.

Overweight and obesity are both labels for ranges of weight that are greater than what is generally considered healthy for a given height. The terms also identify ranges of weight that have been shown to increase the likelihood of certain diseases and other health problems.

For adults, overweight and obesity ranges are determined by using weight and height to calculate a number called the body mass index (BMI). BMI is used because, for most people it correlates with their amount of body fat.
- An adult who has a BMI between 25 and 29.9 is considered overweight
- An adult who has a BMI of 30 or higher is considered obese.

WHAT IS BMI

Body mass index (BMI) is a number calculated from a child's weight and height. It does not measure fat directly, but research has shown that BMI correlates to direct measures of body fat. Moreover it is a simple and inexpensive method of screening for weight categories that may lead to health problems. For children and teens, BMI is age and sex specific and is often referred to as BMI for age.[7]

WHAT IS A BMI PERCENTILE

After BMI is calculated for children and teens, the BMI number is plotted on the CDC BMI-for-age growth charts, either for boys or girls, to obtain a percentile ranking (Refer Chapter 3, Figs. 7, 8). The percentile indicates the relative position of the child's BMI number among children of the same sex and age. The growth charts show the weight status categories used with children and teens (underweight, healthy weight, a risk of overweight and overweight).

Table 13.1: BMI for status categories and percentile[7]	
Weight status category	*Percentile range*
Underweight	Less than the 5th percentile
Healthy weight	5th percentile to less than the 85th percentile
At risk of overweight	85th to less than the 95th percentile
Overweight	Equal to or greater than the 95th percentile

BMI for age weight status categories and the corresponding percentiles are shown in Table 13.1.

BMI is used as a screening tool to identify possible weight problems for children. CDC and the American Academy of Pediatrics (AAP) recommend the use of BMI to screen for overweight beginning at 2 years of age. It is used to screen for overweight, at risk of overweight, or underweight. But it definitely is not a diagnostic tool. High BMI for age and sex in a child may not necessary determine if excess fat is a problem. For this some other parameters like skinfold thickness measurements, evaluation of diet, physical activity, family histories, etc. are also required.

The BMI for age percentile is used to interpret the BMI number because BMI is both age and sex specific for children and teens. These criteria are different from those used to interpret BMI for adults, which do not take into account age or sex. Age and sex are considered because
- The amount of body fat changes with age
- The amount of body fat differs between girls and boys.

The CDC BMI-for-age growth charts for girls and boys take into account these differences and allow translation of a BMI number into a percentile for a child's or teen's sex and age.[7]

BMI is now a universally accepted standard to measure childhood obesity. A consensus proposed the use of a BMI above the 85th percentile as a screening index for overweight and a BMI above the 95th percentile as an index of excess adiposity in adolescents.[8,9] In other words, when the weight exceeds 110% of the standard weight or when the skin fold thickness is more than 30 mm. Obesity is considered when the weight exceeds 120% of the standard weight. Super obesity has been described when the weight for height above the 95th percentile on the growth charts from NCHS, and weight in excess of 140% of the median weight for a given height.[10]

Measuring skin fold thickness (SFT) can help distinguish patients who are over fat from those who are over weight due to increased muscle and bone. SFT provides direct measure of body fat. It can be measured at several sites, including triceps, biceps axilla, mid abdominal, subscapular and supra iliac. SFT above 85th percentile for age and sex suggests obesity and above 95th percentile for age suggests super obesity. The trunk skinfold measurement, subscapular, axilla, supra iliac and abdominal may be suitable indicators of abdominal adipose tissue in children.[11,12]

However, at the Workshop on Childhood Obesity in 1999, views from participants were presented, where the use of SFT for measuring obesity in children was debated. It was remarked that the validity of SFT measurement in different populations has not been carefully explored. Further no evidence suggests that SFT measurements predict hyperinsulinemia, hypertension or other illness in children better than does BMI. Results from several data suggest that childhood BMI remains stable into adulthood, better than does SFT. This observation may reflect measurement error in SFT changes in fat distribution.

The group noted that circumference (e.g. waist or hip) may reflect morbidity in adults, but the relation between visceral fat and morbidity in children and adolescents has not been clarified.[13]

PATHOGENESIS OF CHILDHOOD OBESITY

Genetic Factors

Hereditary or genetic factor also has been recognized for obesity. It considers expression of a complex interaction between genetic and environmental factors including food intake. Parental obesity has been considered as a strong predictor, especially when both parents are obese. The resting energy expenditure (REE) and metabolic rate are known to be based on heredity.

Genetic factors have also been linked to birth weight in the pathogenesis of obesity. This has now been recognized as the Barker's theory.[14] This theory is supported by studies suggesting that a low birth weight is adversely associated with a greater risk of cardiovascular disease and type II diabetes in adult life. The relationship between birth weight and adult fatness is affected by many confounding factors, such as gestational age, parental factors and socioeconomic classes.[15]

Many studies have observed that familial aggregation of obesity can be traced through three generations as shown by a report indicating that the grandparents' obesity is related to that of the parents' BMI and also to obesity indices in grandchildren.[16] It has also been shown that familial factors with regard to eating habits also influence the children's eating behavior and consequently obesity. Similarly, a strong relationship was also found between the level of parental physical activity and that of their preschool children.[17]

Early Feeding vs. Obesity Risk

Scientists have shown that perinatal nutrition is related to obesity risk in young adulthood. In a study during the Dutch famine of 1994–45, significantly lower obesity rates were observed in young adults exposed to famine conditions in the last trimester of gestation and the first months of postnatal life, compared to controls that were not exposed perinatally to the famine.[18]

The feeding of children during the early infancy on breast or formula milk has been found to influence overweight or obesity in them. Previously breast fed children are less likely to be overweight or obese at school entry than children who were previously formula fed. Breastfeeding for at least 6 months was found to be associated with a risk reduction for overweight and obesity of >30% and >40%, respectively.[19]

Metabolic Factors

There can be syndromic obesity which basically is due to certain metabolic diseases. Such obesities are commonly found in children, e.g. Praden Willi syndrome, Beckwith-Widemann syndrome, Lawrence-Moon-Biedi-Bardet syndrome, etc.

Environmental/Lifestyle Factors

The most commonly observed form of childhood obesity is due to environmental factors, which are linked to high fat, high sugar foods, junk foods, aerated sweetened beverages, long hours of television viewing or computer/video games and above all sedentary lifestyle.

Other Factors

Constitutional obesity is known in children and perhaps the commonest type. This is basically a result of excess caloric intake.

Endocrine disorders is also known to cause obesity in children, e.g. in Cushings syndrome or Turner syndrome. Hypothyroidism and growth hormone deficiency can also lead to obesity.

Polycystic ovarian syndrome is one typical example of obesity in adolescent girls and this is considered to be lined with excess calorie intake also.

There are certain conditions related to neuropsychiatric disorders which can result in obesity. These include bulimia nervosa and other conditions like hypothalamic, pituitary and other brain lesions like craniophyaryngioma. The mechanism involved is thought to be of disregulating appetite.

ASSESSMENT OF OBESITY

The general approach to assess obesity involves:

History

A detailed history is of utmost importance to evaluate obesity. This includes:
- Family history
- Lifestyle pattern
- Dietary history
- Anthropometry
- Laboratory investigations.

Family History

It is generally observed that parents of overweight or obese children are also inclined to be overweight or obese. Heredity or genetic factors might have some role in contributing towards obesity in children, as mentioned earlier in this chapter.

Lifestyle Pattern

This is a major contributing factor in the etiology of obesity. Therefore, a detailed history of the complete daily routine of the child is essential which includes hours of sleeping, waking, time spent in commuting to school and mode of transport, outdoor activities involving aerobic games, etc., and number of hours of television viewing or involvement in video games. Besides this, frequency of dining out, type of meals taken at school, frequency of celebrations/feasts at home involving food and in between munching are also significant indicators to ascertain their lifestyle.

Dietary History

This involves a detailed dietary intake of the child/adolescent for the whole day (See Chapter 3).

Anthropometry

Assessing BMI of these children and evaluating them on the growth charts is used to determine the extent of obesity in various age groups of children. Indian Academy of Pediatrics (IAP) has recently published revised growth charts for children aged 5–18 years, while for children from 0 to 5 years, the existing CDC growth charts are followed (See Chapter 3).

Clinical/Laboratory Investigations

These involve bone age which is suggestive of hypothyroidism and may be confirmed by T3, T4 and TSH estimation in serum. A detailed clinical examination can be done which include checking of blood pressure, sugar and lipid profile.

MANAGEMENT OF CHILDHOOD OBESITY

Management of childhood obesity involves multifactor intervention which includes dietary, physical activity, behavioral/psychotherapy, drug therapy and ultimately may be surgical approaches. The factors responsible for the etiology of obesity are also the ones which can be influenced in the treatment or even prevention of obesity. Therefore, exploring the impact of the home environment is crucial to design effective programs to help children establish healthy eating patterns and lifestyle.

Socioeconomic Status

Socioeconomic status (SES) is thought to influence management of obesity indirectly. It is known that adults of lower SES and lower educational qualifications have less healthy diets and are less likely to participate in physical activities like sports. Hence, their children if predisposed to adiposity are likely to live in environments that promote obesity. According to Epstein,[20] if socioeconomic levels are related to parent management success, then families with fewer children also may be of higher SES and may benefit more from parent than do larger families in lower socioeconomic levels. Effective programs emphasize parental attention as an important motivational factor for weight loss. Therefore, parental availability is the key to successful management.

Food Consumption and Eating Pattern

It has been worked out that increasing energy intake by as 150 calories per day above the RDA for weight maintenance would result in a significant weight gain over one year.[21]

Besides our social interaction in any sphere of work or area, encourages and facilitates a way of life that promotes weight gain gradually leading to obesity. This imposes a great challenge on the part of the individual to resist or adapt to a criteria of eating behavior to enable them to maintain the required energy balance. Food composition varies from place to place and from family to family. This may also influence adiposity. High fat/sugar diets are generally energy dense and palatable. Therefore, it is important to effectively maintain the energy balance. Food choices need to be strictly monitored. Changes in the recipes can be effected at the same time retaining the palatability. In case of children, care needs to be taken that emphasis is laid on home-based diets. This can be facilitated by encouraging home environments to suit the needs of the child's requirements in terms of optimal growth without tilting the positive energy balance. Social events can incorporate home-based foods with a variety of food choices and preferences. The increasing culture of dining out in the younger age groups is setting a negative trend with regard to eating behavior. School canteens can be supervised to ensure healthy foods and stress should be made on children getting home packed tiffin. These too can be supervised and monitored by the authorities. Parent–teacher meets can be made more meaningful by involving parents in activities like competitions, etc. on healthy packed tiffin. Current dietary recommendations according to American Academy of Pediatrics advocate reducing fat intake and increasing consumption of complex carbohydrates and fiber containing foods including vegetables and fruits.[22]

The early exposure that children have to fruits and vegetables and to foods high in energy, sugar and fats, may play an important role in establishing an hierarchy of preferences and selection. It was shown that children consumed more fruits and vegetables at schools where more of these items were served and the extent to which these are made available and accessible to children may shape their liking for and consumption of these foods.[23] In view of the rising incidence of childhood obesity in India, the Government of India has also recently proposed introduction of guidelines banning all kinds of junk foods in school canteens and eating facilities.

Food Availability

Generally the access to food is controlled by parents and older siblings. The types of food that are stored at home by them influence the younger child's food consumption and preferences. Therefore, parents and elders can be instrumental in providing and facilitating the right type of healthy foods. Junk foods or other energy dense foods should be in restricted access and portion size of such foods if available may be suitably divided. However when storing the month's ration one should take care to avoid storage of such food which are calorie dense and likely to be a source of temptation for youngsters, and easy susceptibility to obesity.

Food Preferences and Child Feeding Practices

Observations from familial eating patterns suggest that it is the parents who are more likely to over indulge and prompt eating in obese children, compared to the lean ones whose parents are more selective in choosing food varieties for them. Most authors are of the view that children should be allowed to choose from foods that they are offered and control the amounts they choose to eat.[24-26]

It has been seen that children are quite responsive to parental attempts to control their intakes. However, it is also established that on the contrary, stringent parental control can exert a negative impact also. They (children) tend to make just the opposite choices and prefer high-fat, high-calorie foods. Children have also been known to learn to dislike foods when they are encouraged to eat for rewards or when they are bribed into eating. It has been suggested that parental and child feeding practices play a crucial role in the development of individual food preferences and control of food intake.

Social Learning Environment/Early Learning

It is well accepted that the family plays a pivotal role in providing a social learning environment. Certain behaviors, meal patterns and leisure activities that are associated with the development and persistence of obesity are often modeled and reinforced by parents and older siblings at home. Parents who overeat or eat very fast or ignore their internal satiety cue, set a poor example to the children. The onus lies on the parents to present healthy eating styles at home, as well as in external social environments where the family interacts and to model a healthy selection and consumption of foods and regular physical activity. It is a common observation that obese families appear to store more food in all the targeted areas of the home. Since children tend to influence parental habits and even modify them, they can play an active role in the transmission of messages in the home which focus on healthy eating patterns.

The first choice of flavor in a child's diet is either breast milk or formula milk. The perception of flavor in milk also is one of human infant's earliest sensory experiences; and there is evidence to show that this early experience with flavors has an effect on milk intake and later on food acceptance.[27] It has been reported that flavors in breast milk influence infant's consumption.

Early experience with a variety of flavors leads to more ready acceptance of new foods later. Studies in rats have shown that because of repeated early experiences with flavors of the maternal diet present in the mother's milk, rat pups learn to prefer their mother's diet. In humans, formula fed infants have experience with only a single flavor, whereas breast fed babies are exposed to a variety of flavors from maternal diet that are transmitted to the milk. It is postulated that varied flavor experience of breast fed infants can facilitate acceptance of solid foods during the weaning period, with breast fed infants showing greater initial acceptance of new foods than formula fed infants.[27] Infants and children do not accept new flavors instantly with the exception of sweet or salty foods; but after repeated exposures to new foods, preferences for new foods generally increases, providing increased intakes, although 5–10 exposures may be required.[28]

Physical Activity

Sedentary lifestyle with low activity levels is known to promote childhood obesity. Therefore, increasing physical activity preferably the aerobic type can prove very beneficial in the treatment of obesity in children. Exercise showed a beneficial effect when combined with reduced energy intake programs, dietary and behavioral management techniques or as part of a multi component program.[29] Targeting either sedentary behavior or promoting increased physical activity was associated with significant decrease in percent overweight and body fat and improves aerobic fitness. The American Academy of Pediatrics has recommended limiting television viewing to 1–2 hours a day. Limiting television watching and playing video and computer games appears to compel the choice of other pastimes. The couch potato culture among young children and adolescents, if curtailed can give more options and time for them to go for outdoor activities.

Parental Role

The role of parents in making the food choices is also significant. When parents participate actively in their child's weight program, they are expected to modify their own behaviors that contribute to the child's condition and to model eating and exercise behaviors in ways that promote weight loss. They are also expected to work towards accepting new habits and lifestyles. When parents are targeted and provided with reinforcing intervention to promote weight loss, the results are more effective. When parents involved in such programs are supportive and the child motivated enough, long-term success is more likely. Therefore, for effective weight loss programs, it is the whole family that should be targeted, rather than just the child alone.

Some authors have found greater success with involving just the parents and excluding the obese child. According to them, this strategy also inculcates healthy eating behavior in the child rather than the conventional dietary interventions that target the child alone.[30,31]

In this model, change is delivered through the parents instead of the obese child. This approach is basically to target a healthy lifestyle and not just weight reduction. This approach seems more rational, since parents are the ones who can play authoritative role models, at the same time provide a family environment, which provides healthy practices related to weight control issues. Moreover it was observed that this approach was more suitable for the young children as compared to the older ones, since the former seem to be more receptive.

Parental involvement without the obese child is thought to help by prompting change in two areas. Firstly, parental cognition and behavior is involved by increasing nutrition/health skills, regular exercise and improved parenting skills. They are encouraged to provide company at meal times and promote participation of all family members in meals. Secondly they are involved to follow regular meal times and scheduled snacks, thereby setting standards for day-to-day eating practice.

Parents are advised to serve meals to the members individually rather than self helping, teach portion sizes and provide alternate leisure time activities. The second area involves environmental changes so designed to facilitate a healthy lifestyle, rather than relying in individual self control in eating. They are encouraged to create opportunities for physical activities. Healthy eating is encouraged and inappropriate foods are kept out of reach or sight. At the same time restriction on the amount of food eaten by the child is avoided. The instructions given to parents are as follows:

1. To avoid mixed messages and unintentionally reinforce undesired behavior.
2. To use praise and corrective actions that are directed to the child's behavior rather than pinpointing at his personal attributes.
3. To identify ways to help children develop independence and initiative.
4. To regulate and empower children to make decisions about selected issues and to cultivate friends and outlets in the community.
5. To promote positive attitudes and self acceptance and to strengthen self confidence and self esteem.

CONCLUSION

- Obesity has been recognized as a major public health problem by WHO, but childhood obesity also has posed an equally challenging role for nutritionists and pediatricians. Obese children are at an increased risk of becoming obese adults and the risk is higher if both parents are obese
- Exclusive breast feeding in the early months may have a protective role against childhood obesity. Early introduction to a variety of flavors introduced through breast milk can indicate healthy food preferences in the child
- Education regarding choice of healthy foods, i.e. low-fat, low-sugars and high-fiber foods like fruits and vegetables needs to be imparted from early years of childhood. This can help instill healthy food preferences

- Management of obesity in children should be with the involvement of the family without focusing on the child in isolation
- Behavioral and lifestyle modifications with the help of the dietician, pediatrician and a counselor in collaboration with the family can give encouraging results.

REFERENCES

1. Popkin BM. The nutritional transition in low income countries: An emerging crisis. Nutr Rev. 1994;52:285-98.
2. Pearson TA. Cardiovascular disease as a growing health problem in developing countries. The role of nutrition in the epidemiological transition. Public Health Rev. 1996;24:131-46.
3. Gidding SS, Bao W, Srinivasan, et al. Effects of secular trends in obesity on coronary risk factors in children. The Bogalusa Heart study. J Pediatrics. 1995;127:868.
4. Arab M. Diabetes mellitus in Egypt World Health Stat Q. 1992;45:334.
5. Burns TL, Moll PP, Lanner RM. Increased familial mortality in obese school children: The Muscatine Ponderosity, Family Study. Pediatrics. 1992;39:262.
6. Schonfeld-Warden N, Warden CH. Pediatric Obesity. An overview of etiology and treatment. Ped Clinics of N America. 1997;44(20):339-61.
7. National Center for Chronic Disease Prevention and Health Promotion, Division of Nutrition, Physical Activity and Obesity. 2000.
8. Himes JH, Dietz WH. Guidelines for overweight in adolescent prevalence services: recommendations from an expert committee. Am J Clin Nutr. 1994;59:307-16.
9. Must A, Dallal GE, Dietz WH. Reference data for adiposity: 85th and 95th percentiles of body mass index wt/ht^2 and triceps skinfold thickness. Am J Clin Nutr. 1999;53:839-46.
10. Kanders BS. Weighing the options. Criteria for evaluating weight management programs. In TPR (Ed):Pediatric Obesity. Washington DC: Academy Press; 1995;p.210.
11. Brambilla P, Mauzoni P, Simon S, et al. Peripheral abdominal adiposity in childhood obesity. Int J Obe Adol Metab Disord. 1994;18:793.
12. Goen MI, Kaskaun M, Shiman WP. Intra abdominal adipose tissue in young children. Int J Obes Relat Metab Disord. 1995;19:279.
13. Mary C, Bellizi and Williams H Dietz. Workshop on Childhood Obesity: summary of the discussion. Am J Clin Nutr. 1999;70:1735-55.
14. Barker DJ. Fetal origin of cardiovascular disease. Ann Med. 1999;31(Suppl.1):3-6.
15. ParsonsTJ, Powen C, Logan S, Summerbell CD. Childhood predictors of adult obesity: a systematic review. Int J Obes. 1999;23(suppl8):S1-107.
16. Guillaume M, Lapidus L, Beckers F, et al. Familial trends of obesity through three generations, the Belgian-Luxembourg child study. Int J Obes. 1995;19:55-9.
17. Moore LL, Lombardi DA, White MJ, et al. Influence of parents' physical activity levels or activity levels of young children. J Pediatr. 1991;118:215-9.
18. Ravelli ACJ, van der Meulex JHP, Osmond C, et al. Obesity in young men after famine exposure in utero and early infancy. N Engl J Med. 1976;295:349-53.
19. von Kries R, Koletzko B, Saurerwald T, et al. Breast feeding and obesity: cross sectional study. BMJ. 1999;319:147-50.
20. Epstein LH, Koeske R, Wing RR, et al. The effect of family variables on child weight change. Health Psychol. 1986;5:1-11.

21. Rosenbaun M, Leibel RL. The physiology of body weight regulation: relevance to the etiology of obesity in children. Pediatrics. 1998;101:525-39.
22. American Academy of Pediatrics. Committee on Nutrition Statement on cholesterol. Pediatrics. 1992;90:469-73.
23. Hearn MD, Baranowski T, Baranowski J, et al .Environmental influences on dietary behavior among children: availability and accessibility of fruits and vegetables enable consumption. J Health Educ. 1998.
24. Evers C. Empower children to develop healthful eating habits. J Am Diet Assoc. 1997;97(suppl 2):S116-8.
25. Birch LL. Development of food acceptance in first years of life. Proc Nutr Soc. 1998;57:617-24.
26. Birch LL, Fischer Lo. Development of eating behaviors among children and adolescents. Pediatrics. 1998;101:539-49.
27. Sulivan SA, Birch LL. Infant dietary experience and acceptance of solid foods. Pediatrics. 1994;93:271-7.
28. Carpretta PI, Petersik IT, Steward AI. Acceptance of novel flavors is increased after early experience of diverse tastes. Nature. 1975;254:689-91.
29. Epstein LH, Valoski AM, Vara LS, et al. Effects of decreasing sedentary behavior and increasing activity on weight change in obese children. Health Psychol. 1995;14:109-15.
30. Golan M, Weizman A, Apter A, et al. Parents as the exclusive agents of change in the treatment of childhood obesity. Am J Clin Nutr. 1998;67:1130-8.
31. Golan M, Fainaru M, Weizman A. Role of behavior modification in the treatment of childhood obesity, with parents as the exclusive agents of change. Int J Obes. 1998;22:1217-24.

Nutritional Anemia in Children

"Health is not valued till sickness comes"

—Dr Thomas Fuller (1732)

IRON DEFICIENCY ANEMIA

Iron deficiency anemia (IDA) has been considered as one of the major national nutritional problems in our country. In view of the various consequences of inadequate iron stores in children, it poses a major health problem for all pediatricians and dieticians. The incidence is found to occur in significant proportions among both urban and rural populations. Because of the fact that mild to moderate forms of anemia are not recognized by parents, it goes untreated for a considerable length of time, till the child is brought to a clinician for any other illness or just for inadequate weight gain. Most often, among the rural groups or the lower socioeconomic population, children are not taken for a regular routine check up and therefore the problem, even if existing in milder forms may go unnoticed. Even if they are taken for the routine immunization schedule, clinical examination is often missed out.

A number of studies at various times have demonstrated that IDA is one micronutrient deficiency, the prevalence of which is up to 53% of children surveyed.[1] Prevalence rates are generally found to be more among girls compared to boys among older age groups but among the below 6 year age group, it has been found to be as high as 64.8% in most of the cities in India.[2]

It has been well documented that breastfeeding exerts a protective effect in preventing or reducing the incidence of iron deficiency. The fact that exclusive breastfed babies maintained higher Hb levels than infants on formula feeds, has been well established. This is because the maternal stores of iron are adequate to suffice for their needs till 6 months through the breast milk. But beyond 6 months these stores are inadequate and serial supplements are required to meet the increased demands of the infant.

Moreover, the bioavailability of iron in human milk is also superior compared to other milk sources which can take care of the growth needs of the child. But a premature infant is unable to assimilate adequate iron from breast milk and hence, have to be given iron supplements by 6–8 weeks of age. This is adequately absorbed when given along with breast milk.

There are studies to show that infants when fed whole cow's milk, the risk of gastrointestinal bleeding can cause loss of iron, therefore unmodified cow's milk is best avoided in early infancy.

FUNCTIONS OF IRON IN THE BODY

Iron is widely distributed in the body. About 55–60% of iron is in the blood; about 3% exists in the muscle tissue while a variable amount is stored in the liver, spleen, kidney and bone marrow, ranging from 1 to 2 g.

In The Blood

Iron is located in the form of erythrocytes in the red blood cells. Hemoglobin is the compound formed by the union of an iron-containing pigment, heme and the protein globin. Iron is incorporated into hemoglobin after its absorption. Hemoglobin is involved in the function of carrying oxygen from the lungs to the tissues.

About 0.2% of iron exists in the blood plasma, which is in transport form. Plasma iron comes from

1. That absorbed from the gastrointestinal tract.
2. That salvaged from the breakdown of hemoglobin.
3. That released from the stores in the body.

It is estimated that about 27–28 mg of iron per day is derived from hemolysis (destruction of red blood cells), whereas only 1 mg comes from dietary source. Under normal conditions, the plasma iron level may vary from 50 to 180 mg per 100 mL of plasma. In iron deficiency anemia, this level is reduced.

In Muscle Tissue

Iron is present in the muscle tissue in the form of

1. Myoglobin.
2. As a constituent of a combination of an iron pigment and a protein and is a carrier of oxygen. The iron containing enzymes in muscle tissue makes possible the oxidation of carbohydrates, fat and protein within the intact cell. Iron serves in a double capacity in cellular oxidation, it carries oxygen to the cells and makes possible oxidation in the cells through the iron containing enzymes.

DEFINITION

IDA has been defined when the Hb concentration of the blood is lower than the given standard for the specific age and sex group. As per WHO,[3] IDA is

Table 14. 1: WHO criteria for diagnosis of anemia	
Age/sex group	*Hb (g/dL)*
Children 6 mths–6 years	<11
Children 6–14 years	<12
Adult males	<13
Adult females (nonpregnant)	<12
Adult females (pregnant)	<11

(Source WHO, 1968)

categorized into 3 groups based on the level of Hb present in the blood for all age groups and both sexes as seen in Table 14.1.

Iron deficiency is actually the end result of a well-defined sequence of changes that account for iron depletion. These are as follows:

1. Disappearance of storage forms from bone marrow (iron ferritin) and the reticuloendothelial tissues.
2. A decrease in serum iron level and simultaneous increase in the serum iron binding protein transferritin.
3. A decrease in the mean red cell volume and increase in free erythrocyte porphyrin levels.
4. A decrease in concentration of hemoglobin.

CLINICAL FEATURES OF IRON DEFICIENCY ANEMIA

As mentioned earlier in this chapter, mild to moderate forms of anemia may go unnoticed by parents or other caregivers. This is because the fall in the Hb level is usually gradual and by the time it actually falls very drastically, it generally comes to severe type.

Some of the common features encountered are as follows:

- Pallor, irritability, anorexia
- Palpitation, fatigue, shortness of breath
- Decreased exercise intolerance, congestive heart failure
- Koilonychia (spoon-shaped nails)
- Vitamin B deficiency signs in severe chronic conditions
- Pica (craving to eat clay, laundry starch, etc.)
- Alterations in small bowel mucosal functions
- Lowered IQ and decreased attentiveness are also frequently observed in children with anemia.

IMPLICATIONS OF IRON DEFICIENCY ANEMIA

Iron being an integral component of several enzymes which have an important role in metabolic processes and cell proliferation, a number of variable changes are observed in various organs and systems. Some significant adverse affects observed on various systems are as follows:

Failure to Thrive/Growth Retardation

This is a common finding in most iron-deficient children and could be due to the existing anorexia and altered intestinal functions. It is observed that very often children who are anemic are predominantly milk fed on prolonged breastfeeding without adequate cereal supplementation. Milk being a poor source of iron, the child's reserves gradually gets depleted resulting in loss of appetite. This becomes a vicious cycle that of faulty feeding leading to anemia and this condition further resulting in loss of appetite. Iron supplementation is the only way to break this cycle which further helps in return of appetite.

Activity

Another very obvious outcome of iron deficiency anemia is decrease in work capacity and this is directly proportionate to the severity of iron deficiency. Studies from Hyderabad have shown that school children, who were anemic, did poorly in physical activity.[4]

Ever among housewives early signs of anemia can be foreseen by symptoms like easy fatigue ability during the course of routine household chores or weakness or loss of energy at the calves of their legs.

Temperature Regulation

Children with anemia are known to experience hypothermia and feel uncomfortably cold at normal temperatures too.

Mental and Psychomotor Response

It is well established that children who are inclined to be anemic, also show poor mental performance, are not able to concentrate or even comprehend in academics and suffer from loss of memory. Studies have shown that children with anemia are unable to meet the desired standards of scholastic tests besides having impaired motor development.

Immune Response

Iron deficiency leads to defect in cell-mediated immunity which could result in recurrent infections. The leucocytes are adversely affected and unable to kill ingested microorganisms. They are also known to have depressed skin test response to common antigens.

Maternal Iron Deficiency

Maternal iron deficiency adversely affects fetal outcome. WHO studies have demonstrated that 20–40% of all maternal deaths ascribed to childbirth every year, are due to anemia among the pregnant mothers.[5]

Infants born to anemic mothers have less than half the reserves compared to those born to nonanemic mothers. They are likely to remain deficient in iron during their early years and suffer from long-term consequences.

Gastrointestinal Affects

Children with anemia are also likely to suffer from increased acid production leading to atrophic gastritis encouraging further infections.

ETIOLOGY OF IRON DEFICIENCY

Iron deficiency can occur due to three main mechanisms which may be either solely responsible or in combination. These are as follows:

Inadequate Intake or Absorption

Adequate supply of iron to the body stores is essential to meet the demand of the body from time to time, under variable conditions. It is well known that for an infant breast milk can provide adequate stores of iron till 6 months of age. But beyond that it fails to meet the increasing demands of growth of the baby. Firstly because after 6 months, the iron stores in the breast milk diminish and secondly because the demand increases. Therefore, cereal pulse supplements are strongly advocated after 6 months, so that the iron requirements can be met with (Refer Chapter 2, Table 2.1). However, we also know that absorption of iron from cereals and pulses is not very good. Addition of green leafy vegetables can improve the iron content of the diet. Therefore, if in a vegetarian diet the quantity of cereals, pulses and green leafy vegetables is increased and used in combination, the absorption is likely to increase by about one third. Intake of nonvegetarian foods like fish, meat or egg yolk, not only help increase the available iron in the diet but also increases the absorption. The bio availability of iron from these sources is about 20–30% and they also help in better absorption from other food sources.

Very often it is observed that children are continued to be exclusively breast fed well up to even one year. Even if they do supplement their diet, it is very insignificant, in the form of biscuits, rusks or very small quantities of cereals, pulses or vegetables which hardly contribute any iron. Milk being a very poor source of iron, the child if fed predominantly on it, either breast or formula or even dairy source, can gradually be left with very poor of iron stores leading to nutritional anemia.

Besides poor intake, there are other factors which may inhibit the absorption of dietary sources like the presence of phytates which when bound with iron may make it unavailable. Similarly the presence of tannin in tea can also inhibit its absorption from food. Therefore, it is very important that children should be strongly discouraged to have tea especially with meals. A common practice observed in the northern part of the country, is that mothers generally tend to feed the infant with tea right from 6 to 12 months of age.

Tea is considered as beneficial in providing relief from colds and coughs and even digestion, therefore widely encouraged. On the contrary, the prolonged consumption of tea can make the children addicted to it, to the extent of causing gastritis and loss of appetite.

On the other hand, cooking of infant feeds in iron pans can help in better absorption from the dietary sources.

The food intake of children can also be compromised with the existence of infections. Any infection, whether respiratory or gastrointestinal decreases the appetite leading to inadequate intake. Again mothers tend to feed them with milk or tea. 'Starving a fever' is a very common belief which contributes to poor food consumption, thus indirectly being a causative factor for anemia.

Increased Losses

Even if the intake or supply of iron from the diet is adequate but if there are simultaneous losses, IDA can occur. The losses can be in the form of parasitic infestations which can result in gastrointestinal bleeding, e.g. hookworm infestations in which case blood losses can vary from 2 to 100 mL/day depending upon the severity of infection.[6]

Another common cause of iron losses in children is malabsorption which can be due to defective absorption of iron, folic acid, B_{12} or pyridoxine.

Other sources of blood loss can be due to bleeding from any other source like gums, piles and fissures, polyps, peptic ulcers which could be drug induced or otherwise or in any other conditions like esophageal varices, ulcerative colitis, dysentery, etc.

Increased Demands

There can be certain physiological conditions when despite adequate intake and no losses or adequate absorption, the body demands increase like in pregnancy and in children during the growth period, i.e. during infancy and childhood. All the conditions mentioned in the earlier two causative factors can indirectly exert increased demands on the body reserves of iron.

TREATMENT OF IDA

In children, reversal of the iron deficiency state is generally achieved by iron supplementation orally. However, diet counseling regarding adequate cereal and pulse, green vegetables, etc. is also reinforced for long-term management. Infants and children being fed on excessive milk are advised to restrict the milk intake, not exceeding 500 mL per day which is even otherwise the recommended allowance. Iron-rich dietary sources like ragi, wheat, whole pulses especially black gram, green leafy vegetables are advised. Jaggery and dates are good sources which can be complemented in the routine meals of children. A list of iron-rich sources are given in Table 14.2.[7]

Table 14.2: Iron content of common foods

Foods	Iron content (mg %)		
	Poor <2.0	Average >2–4	Rich >4.0
Bajra			8.0
Ragi		3.9	
Wheat flour whole		4.9	
Bengal gram dal			5.3
Bengal gram washed			9.5
Black gram dal		3.8	
Soyabean			10.4
Rajmah		5.1	
Other dals		2–4 mg	
Amaranth			18.4
Beet greens			16.2
Celery leaves			40.0
Colocasia leaves			10.0
Mustard leaves			16.3
Root vegetables	0.5–2.0		
Other vegetables	0.5–2.0		
Onion stalks			7.43
Plantain green			6.27
Almonds			5.09
Walnut		2.6	
Peaches		2.4	
Pineapple		2.4	
Raisins			7.7
Custard apple (seethaphal)		4.31	
Watermelon			7.9
Dates (dried)			7.3
Apricot (dry)			4.6
Other fruits	0.6–1.5		
Fish (hilsa)		2.1	
Pomfret (black)		2.3	
Sardine		2.5	
Surmar (dried)		2.0	
Egg (hen)		2.1	
Liver (sheep)			6.3
Milk	0.2–0.3		
Jaggery (cane)		2.64	

Source: NIN, ICMR, Hyderabad, Nutritive value of Indian Foods. Revised and updated by Narsingha Rao BS, Deosrhal IG and Pant KC (2002). Gopalan C, Rama Sastri BV and Balasubramanian SC.

Nonvegetarian foods like meat, fish and egg yolk are better sources of iron, besides having higher bioavailability in the body.

There are certain foods which act as iron enhancers, i.e. they promote better absorption in the body. These are ascorbic acid and nonvegetarian foods.

Ascorbic acid when ingested with a highly available iron salt can increase the bioavailability by almost 33%. Moreover, added in the food, it also lessens the inhibitory effect of other compounds present in the food. This is due to its reducing effect and preventing the formation of insoluble ferric hydroxide. Iron absorption, as we know, is always in the ferrous form. It also helps in formation of soluble complexes with both ferrous and ferric forms at low pH, which then preserves iron solubility at the more alkaline duodenal pH.

Meat, Fish and Amino Acids

The enhancing effect of meat and fish is well known. Unlike other enhancers, meat and fish increase the absorption of both heme and nonheme iron though the mechanism may differ in both. For nonheme iron, it is unlikely to be due to protein presence, as egg albumin has been shown to have no promoting effect. It is thought that it could be linked to amino acids composition. Amino acids like cysteine, histidine and lysine have also been known to enhance iron absorption. The action of cysteine is thought to be due to its chelating and reducing powers.

PREVENTION OF IRON DEFICIENCY

In the light of the issues discussed above, it seems obvious that the problem of IDA, which is widely prevalent among the preschool and older children, needs to be tackled right from the beginning with a right guidance and counseling to the parents related to good diets. Prevention is better than cure, so if certain preventive steps are taken into account the prevalence of anemia can be avoided to a large extent.

These may be summarized as follows:

Enhancing/ Inhibitory Factors

As discussed earlier due to high iron requirements in infancy and a rather monotony of the infant diet, i.e. predominately milk, which is a poor source of iron, this deficiency is widely prevalent in the developing world.

We know, that bioavailability of iron from different foods varies widely. Iron enters into two common pools that differ in their mechanism of absorption—the heme and the nonheme iron pools. Heme iron present in the hemoglobin and myoglobin is well absorbed and even helps absorption from nonheme sources. The nonheme iron which is present in vegetables, cereals and pulses, etc is poorly absorbed and is greatly affected by enhancing or inhibiting factors in the diet (Table 14.3). Since most food iron is nonheme, the presence or absence of these substances play a vital role in the availability of dietary iron.

Table 14.3: Factors affecting bioavailability of nonheme iron

Enhancing	Inhibiting
Meat, fish, chicken	Carbonates, oxalates, phosphates, phytates
Ascorbic acid	Bran, vegetable fiber
Certain amino acids	Tea
	Egg yolk

Breastfeeding

Infants can be prevented from falling into the pit of iron deficiency anemia right from birth itself thanks to nature's greatest gift to them that of breast feeds. It is well established now that breast milk though low in iron has a superior bioavailability compared to cow's milk. But this is only up to 6 months of their life. Beyond this breast milk is inadequate to meet the increasing demands and it is here that introduction of iron-rich foods need to be introduced. So till 6 months an exclusively breastfed child can be prevented from developing anemia. Infants on cow's milk or other dairy milk run high risk of iron depletion thus, leading to anemia. Again when solid food is introduced, care should be taken to take into consideration the enhancers or inhibitors of iron bioavailability. In most of the northern rural areas and even in a large section of the urban population, offering tea is a common practice. It is infact given as a medicinal drink to children suffering from respiratory problems, fevers, indigestion, etc. Thus, practice of feeding tea to children should be avoided.

In our own country cooking food in iron pans is very common. This is a good practice as it is known to enhance the iron content of the food cooked in them. Children can be fed food cooked in these pans.

Another common practice among Indians is use of lemon or tomatoes in the cooking practice. This also can help enhance the iron bioavailability of the food cooked this way. Consumption of citrus fruits or fruit juice is another simple way of enhancing iron bioavailability. Nonvegetrian families can take the advantage of using fish or meat preparations in the diets of their children to enhance the bioavailability even from non heme iron sources.

Avoiding Excess Iron Losses

In infants and children the commonest source of iron losses is through parasitic infections. Infants with acute or chronic diarrhea may also lose significant amounts of blood. The cumulative loss of iron occurring from repeated episodes of gastrointestinal infections can be very significant. Therefore, prevention of such infections through better sanitary conditions can significantly help in preventing iron deficiency anemia. Another contributory factor for iron losses is use of cow's milk in early infancy which in some can cause gastrointestinal bleeding. Therefore, avoiding use of cow's milk or any other dairy milk in early infancy can help prevent bleeds and hence, iron losses.

Food Fortification

Food fortification serves as the most preferred and simple method of preventing iron deficiency anemia. Today, we can see a range of products especially the baby foods fortified with iron. Some of the infant formulae available in the market are fortified with iron which can take care of a good percentage of infants or children and help prevent anemia.

A suitable vehicle is required to do the fortification and ensure palatability and acceptance. Foods commonly preferred for fortification are either salt or cereal flour. Though not yet practiced routinely, in common household foods, extensive studies need to be undertaken to successfully make sure their availability. It is important to ensure good bioavailability, of our fortified product without compromising on the color, taste or shelf life of the food product.

FOLATE AND B_{12} DEFICIENCY—MEGALOBLASTIC ANEMIA

Besides iron deficiency anemia, another common type of anemia observed among infants and children is the folic acid deficiency. Also known as megaloblastic anemia and B_{12} deficiency which manifests as pernicious anemia (a genetic disorder) due to the absence of the intrinsic factor in the gastric secretion. Intrinsic factor is a protein that facilitates vitamin B_{12} absorption. The name 'megaloblastic' is due to the fact that the peripheral smear exhibits large oval red cells and hypersegmented nuclei in polymorphs.

Folate Deficiency

This is a very common cause of megaloblastic anemia in children. Initially, the infants needs are adequately met by human or cows milk but babies fed on goats milk generally tend to get deficient, due to negligible content of folic acid in it. This type of anemia is also termed as 'goat's milk anemia'.

Causes of Deficiency

Food folate is susceptible to heat and cooing processes, therefore, pasteurized milk reheated several times for sterilization can get deficiency in folic acid. Fresh uncooked fruits and vegetables and juices, etc. when added to the diet of children fed on pasteurized milk helps in preventing this deficiency. All unprocessed and raw foods are good sources of folic acid.

Inadequate absorption

Absorption of folic acid occurs from the upper third of the small intestine. Therefore, any destruction (structural or functional) of their area can result in megaloblastic anemia.

Certain food compounds like those found in beans which when activated by heat inhibits absorption of folic acid.

Some drugs are also known to block folate absorption like the anticonvulsants dilantin. Most children on such drugs tend to be deficient in folate. But treating them with B_{12} can antagonize the effect of the anticonvulsant action and thereby increase the tendency for recurrent seizures.

Increased requirements

Requirements are known to increase during infancy which is the period of rapid growth and particularly so in the mature infants. Conditions causing an increase in metabolic rates, e.g. hyperthyroidism can also exert an increased requirement of folate. Children with sickle cell anemia, in which in there is increased hematopoiesis, also tend to have increased requirements. In conditions like tropical sprue also the requirement increase since the plasma levels of both vitamin B_{12} and folic acid are low, deficiency is commonly found.

Increased excretion

In conditions like renal dialysis or recurrent episodes of vomiting, folate deficiency is usually found due to the reduced ability to incorporate folate into the cells due to lack of vitamin B_{12} It is both heat labile and water soluble.

Increased destruction

Oxidative destruction can diminish the levels of folate but they can be preserved by use of reducing substances. In scurvy, folate deficiency can be observed since low vitamin C foods are also low in folates.

Clinical Manifestation

Classical manifestations of folate deficiency existing along with leucopenia are thrombocytopenia since folic acid deficiency affects all proliferating cells in the body rather than red cells alone. There may be presence of smooth and sore tongue. About 10% of them might have hyperpigmentation splenomegaly and or low-grade fever. Features of mental changes and other neurologic signs like irritability, forgetfulness and sleeplessness may exist but these can also be found in vitamin B_{12} deficiency.

Vitamin B_{12} Deficiency/Cobalamin (Pernicious Anemia)

Vitamin B_{12} is also termed as cyanocobalamin due to the fact it is composed of cyanide group and cobalt. It is slightly water soluble, therefore likely to be leached out during prolonged cooking processes. Deficiency of B_{12} is not routinely found in infants and children since maternal stores are adequate to take care of requirements during the first year of life. Moreover, human or cows milk also does provide small amounts. Beyond 6 month when cow's milk is increased the requirements are usually met (Refer Chapter 2, Table 1 for requirements of B_{12} and folic acid).

However, in mothers from families who are strict vegetarian, i.e. not even consuming milk this deficiency may be encountered. B_{12} producing micro-organisms and animal foods are the sole source of vitamin B_{12}. So a diet devoid of even milk can produce manifestation of megaloblastic anemia of B_{12} deficiency.

B_{12} the extrinsic factor (provided by diet) absorption takes place in the presence of another protein called the intrinsic factor, a glycoprotein which is present in the gastric secretion produced by the gastric parietal cells. In pernicious anemia, vitamin B_{12} is not absorbed due to the atrophic changes in the stomach wall and scanty secretion of the intrinsic factor. The absorption of B_{12} takes place in the ileum in pH 6–8 in the presence of a divalent ion like calcium. Therefore, in conditions like ileal inflammation due to tuberculosis or resection of the ileal malabsorption or absorption can be impaired. However, diffuse absorption does occur throughout the length of the small intestine.

Clinical Manifestations

Deficiency of vitamin B_{12} generally occurs due to the absence of the intrinsic factor of the stomach leading to malabsorption of orally consumed vitamin B_{12}. Specific manifestations of B_{12} deficiency occurs in the form of hematological and neurological changes.

The hematological changes are evident by macrocytic anemia wherein the blood smear shows variation in size and shape of the red cells. Neurological changes generally manifest in the form of spinal cord degeneration. These are however, not very common among children. Mental changes like, depression psychosis and loss of mental energy may be seen in some cases which respond to B_{12} therapy.

Treatment involves intramuscular injection of B_{12} in therapy doses.
Household tips to enhance iron absorption in diets of children
  1. Use jaggery in place of sugar in porridge or any other sweet preparation. Groundnut with jaggery laddoos are a good example.
  2. Cook dry vegetables like spinach, methi, radish, brinjal, bitter gourd, okra in an iron skillet (kadhai), as it enhances absorption of iron from these iron-rich foods.
  3. Use coriander and mint leaves in the form of chutneys and seasoning to increase iron availability.
  4. Use dates and figs as fruits or in other preparations as they are rich in iron.
  5. Use lentils like black gram or chick pea (white channa), soya bean, tofu (soya paneer) black gram, kidney beans (rajma), sprouts, etc. along with other foods as snacks or main meals.
  6. Use methi leaves, spinach or radish leaves as a curry or in, khichdi, paranthas or rotis—ideal for children who are fussy about vegetables. Broccoli and potato are good source of iron and hence, can be incorporated in any form in a child's diet.
  7. Tamarind pulp can be used in various preparations or as chutneys in sandwiches or any cereal preparation. It is rich both in iron and ascorbic acid and hence, well absorbed in the body.
  8. Fruits like gooseberries (amla), guava or citrus fruits and strawberries, along with other iron rich foods can enhance iron absorption to optimum level.

9. Black chocolate too is rich in iron and so can be offered to children after a meal, rather than the milk chocolate.
10. Egg yolk is good in iron with better availability and hence, a good option for those who can consume them.
11. Cereals like ragi, whole wheat flour, jowar and bajra are good sources of iron, and if taken with acidic foods like citrus ones or amla or tamarind can enhance the availability of iron from foods.
12. Commonly used snacks and sweets like jaggery and peanut laddoos or barfi, chikki, sweet rice preparation using jaggery, ragi porridge or upma and use of seeds like sesame (til) or pumpkin seeds and other dry fruits like almonds, walnuts and raisins in any food preparation can enhance iron content of the foods consumed.

Annexure

Iron-rich Recipes

Gram Ladoo

Wheat flour	250 g
Roasted gram flour	75 g
Soya flour	25 g
Roasted groundnut powder	25 g
Oil/Ghee	25 mL
Jaggery	250 g

Method
- Mix the three flours, add ghee and sauté till light brown and gives out a light aroma
- Add roasted groundnuts to the above, mix well in the previously made jaggery syrup
- Let cool and make even-sized laddoos and store.

Energy Bar

Khas khas	50 g
Dates	300 g
Almonds (roasted)	50 g
Sesame seeds (roasted)	50 g
Roasted gram flour	50 g
Roasted groundnut powder	50 g

Method
- Mix all the ingredients and grind them in a mixer
- Pour the mixture on a greased plate and allow to cool and set. Cut into rectangular pieces and store.

3 Palak Barfi

Milk	150 mL
Sugar/Jaggery	10 g (2 tsp)
Groundnut powder	10 g
Gram flour	25 g
Palak	100 g
Oil	5 g (1 tsp)
Skimmed milk (SM) powder	10 g

Method
- Wash and chop the palak, suate it in oil for 2–3 minutes and blend
- Boil milk till it is reduced to half the quantity and thickens
- Add SMP into the milk along with the palak puree and cook it
- Add sugar or jaggery to the above mixture till it thickens and binds
- Add roasted gram flour slowly and mix well to avoid lumps
- Pour the above mixture on a greased plate and let cool and set
- Cut evenly into barfi shape and store.

Kathi Rolls

Radish leaves	20 g
Broccoli	25 g
Spinach	10 g
Nutri nuggets	2–3 tsp
Flax seed powder	1 tsp
Green stalk onion	10 g
Green peas	10 g
Wheat flour	30 g
Oil	2 tsp

Method
- Chop all green vegetables and onion stalk finely
- Crush broccoli finely
- Soak nutri in water for 10 minutes in a pan
- Saute all the vegetables with nutria in some oil in a pan
- Add salt and spices and mix well to form a coarse mixture
- Make a dough with flour and flax seed powder and make medium size balls
- Roll out chapattis and fry lightly on both sides
- Place vegetable mixture on the chapatti and roll it tighty
- Cut into equal pieces and sere hot with green chutney.

Sattu Drink

Roasted gram flour	20 g
Mint leaves chopped	1 tsp
Roasted cumin seed powder	1/4th tsp
Onion finely chopped	1/4th tsp
Lemon juice	1 tsp

Black salt	A pinch
Green chillies (optional)	As desired
Water	200 mL

Method

- Add roasted gram flour, chopped onion, lemon juice, black salt, roasted cumin seed powder in a glass of water and stir well
- Refrigerate and serve with chopped mint leaves.

Ragi Pancake

Ragi	50 g
Onion	1 medium
Peanuts	10 g
Oil	1 tsp
Salt	To taste
Water	To mix

Method

- Mix ragi, salt, chopped onions and peanuts (coarsely ground) in a bowl
- Add water and mix to make a thick batter
- Heat a pan, add oil and spread the batter evenly on it
- Bake lightly on both sides till golden brown and serve hot.

REFERENCES

1. Indian Council of Medical Research Studies on Pre School Children. Technical Report Series No.26, New Delhi, ICMR, 1977.
2. Report of the Working Group on Fortification of Salt with Iron. Use of common salt fortified with iron in the control and prevention of anemia. A collaborative study. Am J Clin Nutr. 1982;35:1442-5.
3. Nutritional Anemias': Report of a WHO Scientific Group. WHO Technical Report series No.405, Geneva, World Health Organization, 1968.
4. Satyanarayana K, Pradhan DR, Ramnath T, Prahlad Rao W. Anemia and physical fitness of school children of rural Hyderabad. Ind Pediatr. 1990;27:715-21.
5. World Heath Organization. Causes of death. Anemias. Wld Hlth Stat Q. 1962;15:594-604.
6. Layrisse M, Rocke M. The relationship between anemia and hookworm infestation. Amer J Trop Med Hyg. 1964;79:279-301.
7. Narsingha Rao BS, Deorshall IG, Pant KC. Nutritive Value of Indian Foods. National Institute of Nutrition, ICMR, Hyderabad, 2002.

Nutrition in Diarrheal Diseases

Diarrheal diseases have been recognized as a major public health problem in the developing world. According to WHO estimate, every child under the age of 5 years in the developing world suffers from, on average 2–3 episodes of diarrhea per year. In the first two years of life as many as 20 per 1000 children may die from diarrhea.[1]

This means that the acute diarrheal diseases cause an estimated 750–1000 million episodes of illness and some 4–5 million episodes of death per year in children under the age of 5 years. In India, diarrhea is the third leading cause of childhood mortality and 13% of all deaths per year in children under 5 years of age, killing an estimated 300,000 children each year.[2] This gravity of the problem assumes more significance in the light of the fact that repeated attacks of diarrhea-exposed children to the diarrhea–malnutrition cycle, which can have long lasting effects on the quality of life of the child.

RISK FACTORS OF DIARRHEA IN CHILDREN

Diarrhea is a prominent clinical feature of childhood malnutrition and is mostly associated with infections and infestations. These are generally a result of multiple pathogens which may be associated with other systemic infections especially the respiratory tract. The chief contributory factors leading to this preventable disease are as follows:
- Poor sanitation and unhygienic practices by the mother/caregiver
- Low socioeconomic status
- Low birth weight
- Inadequate breastfeeding
- Low birth weight
- Illiteracy of the mother
- Mode of water transportation and poor handling at the household level
- Inadequate refuse storage, collection and disposal
- Indiscriminate stool disposal by mothers

- Lack of hand washing before feeding their children or not washing using soap.

INTERACTION BETWEEN DIARRHEAL DISEASES AND MALNUTRITION

Mechanisms causing diarrhea in malnourished children can be grouped into those associated with structural damage to the intestinal mucosa and those due to changes in the intra luminal environment. Structural damage occurs characteristically with entero invasive bacteria or enteric viruses, e.g. *E. coli*, which cause intestinal fluid secretion, stimulated by entero toxins and mediated by enzymatic processes within the enterocytes. Microbial contamination of the upper intestinal secretions is a feature of childhood malnutrition and has damaging effects on intestinal digestion and absorption. The intestinal mucosa itself is extremely damaged in children with malnutrition and this contributes to the diarrhea–malnutrition cycle.

The adverse affects of diarrhea are as follows:

- *Reduced food consumption:* Most often diarrheal disease affects the appetite which may be due to presence of vomiting, dehydration, fever and discomfort. To add to this, it is the prevailing food myths and false beliefs regarding different foods and their affects on digestion and absorption, which prevents the intake of adequate food intake, during acute attacks of diarrhea

- *Reduced absorption of nutrients:* Besides inadequate food intake, there is reduced absorption of macronutrients. The enterotoxins released by adhesion of bacteria to the mucosa, damage the enterocyte and crypt cells which results in diminished capacity of absorption of macro- and micro-nutrients. The recovery, of the mucosa takes almost 6–8 weeks to recover, only after which some absorption can gradually begin to occur

- *Increased secretion:* The damage to the villous tips and the immature crypt cells left due to replacement of absorptive surfaces, results in increased secretion of water from the infected segment of the small intestine into the lumen. This hypersecretory state results in important deficits in sodium, potassium, chloride and water and also certain minerals and vitamins

- *Nutrient losses:* Most often being in the diarrheal state due to the *Rotavirus*, *Shigella* and *Campylobacter*, there is an increased loss of proteins from the mucosa which can lead to a protein deficient state like in kwashiorkor. Other metabolic alterations like negative nitrogen balance, decreased magnesium, potassium and phosphorous also are found to occur

- *Effect on growth and development:* Diarrhea induces acute weight loss and arrests linear growth just like in any other infection. But a negative affect of diarrhea on growth has been described in a number of studies. The wasting and stunting have been found to be more pronounced in children who have had marked fetal retardation. They are prone to suffer from a more severe course of diarrhea and also have a higher risk of mortality. Therefore diarrhea, be it due to any cause has a malnourishing effect, which in turn enhances the risk of dying from infection, thus causing a vicious cycle.

Diarrheas may broadly be looked into from two aspects:
- Acute diarrheas (AD)
- Persistent/Protracted diarrhea (PD).

Acute Diarrheas

Acute diarrheas can be a result of acute infections as mentioned earlier in this chapter and is likely to resolve within a few days. But repeated episodes of AD can result in poor appetite, reduced intake and hence, reduced absorption of nutrients. Nutritional management therefore, is of prime importance to prevent the child from slipping into the cycle of infection and malnutrition.

Nutritional Management of AD

A common practice observed in the developing countries during acute episodes of diarrhea is to withhold feeding. This leads to increased losses which are not able to be met. It also delays the repair of the intestinal mucosa and reversal of digestive enzymes, besides malabsorption of important micronutrients. The concept that feeding increases the stool volume and length of illness is totally unfounded. A number of studies have demonstrated the beneficial effects of early feeding during the course of the illness and the resulting shorter duration of hospital stay.[3,4]

Oral Rehydration Therapy

The first step to consider in the management of AD is to tackle the dehydration if existing. Oral rehydration therapy (ORT) is the mainstay of the initial treatment. The oral rehydration solution (ORS) recommended by WHO contains 20 g glucose, sodium chloride, 3.5 g, sodium bicarbonate 2.5 g or sodium citrate 2.9 g and potassium chloride 1.5 g to be mixed in 1 liter of water.[5] However, it was found that this composition of ORS proved to be hyperosmolar most of the time since the electrolyte content of non cholera stool is such that it contains only about 56 mmol/L of sodium and potassium of about 25 mmol. By using this ORS, a state of hyperosmolarity may be achieved which can only worsen the diarrhea. Some authors have also termed this solution as oral dehydration solution (ODS) instead of ORS.[6] Therefore, it would be prudent to assess the type of diarrhea before choosing the type of ORS. A more user friendly ORS has been formulated—the hypo-osmolar ORS and the super ORS, which is rice based.

Among the hypo osmolar solutions available, two are more common:
1. With sodium 75 and glucose 75 mmol/L.
2. With sodium 60 and glucose 24 mmol/L.

The super ORS solution contains starch 40 g instead of 20 g of glucose per packet.[6] The advantage of using super ORS is that it decreases the stool output by 25%, besides avoiding nutrient compromie in the child during the diarrheal episode. Normal feeding is otherwise affected during acute episodes, resulting in significant nutrient losses. By using super ORS which is rice based, some amount of feeding can be ensured. This has been aptly demonstrated by various studies, where a decrease in stool output too was reported by 28% and ORS consumption too decreased by 27%.[7]

Dietary Management

Adequate feeding during the episodes of diarrhea can not be over emphasized. Anorexia is a common feature observed during any illness but may vary on the type of illness. Febrile illnesses are more prone to lead to decreased intake especially in children. In diarrheal episodes, though there may not be frank anorexia, children and even mothers themselves, prefer to feed only plain liquids more than solids, e.g. weak tea, milk or even fruit juice. Infants on breast feeds must be allowed to continue on the same. In fact, it has been demonstrated that infants fed on breast milk during AD, gain weight better and are prevented from going into a state of malnutrition. Moreover, cessation of breast feeds is known to exert a deleterious effect on the nutritional status of the child, besides increasing the risk of dehydration 5 times as compared to breast fed infants.[8]

In the acute diarrheal episode most children may be lactose tolerant, therefore, withdrawing of milk from their diet should be avoided, unless and until the child has had a history of lactose intolerance earlier. Bhan and his team have had a vast experience on the management of such children and have recommended a calorie intake of at least 125% of the normal required with nutrient dense foods and should be continued till the child achieves the preillness weight and normal nutritional status.[9]

WHO has formulated some guidelines for the feeding schedule of infants and children during AD episodes, which is tabulated as in Table 15.1.[10,11]

Table 15.1: Feeding during acute diarrhea

Stage of hydration and feeding pattern	Recommended schedule of feeding
During rehydration phase • Breastfed infants • Non-breastfed infants • In severely malnourished children	Continue breastfeeds Preferably give ORS till rehydration Beyond 4 hours, animal milk/food Offer some food as soon as possible
After rehydration phase • Breastfed infants • Non-breastfed infants • Infants 4–6 months • Older children	Continue breast feeds more frequently Offer undiluted animal milk/formula as before Add energy dense cereal/pulse supplements Give energy dense thickened feeds with oil-pulse (K rich) and green leafy vegetables, carrots, etc. Encourage feeding 6 times a day

Source: WHO, 1991.

As evident from this table, stress has been made on continuation of breast feeds in young infants. This also helps maintenance of lactation in the mother for a longer duration and also ensures better milk production due to the sucking stimulus. For older children or the non breast fed infants, animal milk can be offered but, it should be full strength, as soon as dehydration is corrected, as has been advocated by numerous authors.[11,12]

Older children can be fed on a mixed diet of cereal, pulse and vegetables, with addition of oil/ghee/butter for increasing the density without increasing the bulk. Milk cereal combinations are also well tolerated even among the slightly lactose intolerant children. Amylase rich factor (ARF) can be made use of to reduce the viscosity of the feeds (Refer Chapter 5).

Nutritional Management of Persistent Diarrhea

Persistent diarrhea (PD) or protracted diarrhea is defined when the duration of passage of stools exceeds 14 days. The state of hydration may or may not be preserved. Growth faltering and severe malnutrition are characteristic features in this condition. This is due mainly to inadequate intake and in most cases with malabsorption.

Pathogenesis of Persistent Diarrhea

The pathogenesis in PD may involve digestion and absorption of all the nutrients—Carbohydrates, proteins and fats.

In carbohydrate malabsorption usually there is disaccharide deficiency due to the decreased luminal amylase resulting in impaired exocrine pancreatic function. Lactose enzyme is the one which is mostly affected, leading to secondary lactose intolerance. This condition is frequently encountered following rota viral diarrheas where the villous tip cells are partially damaged. Lactose enzyme being the first to be affected is also the last to be restored for adequate absorption of lactose.

Sucrase enzyme too can be affected leading to malabsorption of sucrose in protracted diarrheas. These can lead to ineffective villous repair or prolonged mucosal injury in malnourished children. This in fact also can be the cause of PD.

Steatorrhea is often associated in PD due to insufficient pancreatic lipase or due to the defect in bile acid metabolism. Similarly protease activity in the pancreatic secretion may also be compromised, especially in children with PD.

Cow's milk protein intolerance (CMPI) is sometimes associated with PD and can be seen in children below 6 months of life. The β lactoglobulin fraction in cow's milk is the cause for CMPI in such children. Milk antibody and IgE are increased in the mucosa in this condition, and this itself can lead to PD also. Such children may also be known to be intolerant to soya protein and may present with blood and mucus.

Finally, PD can also result from abnormal bacterial colonization in any part of the gastrointestinal tract. Breast fed babies are however, prone to be protected from such attacks. It is mostly the older children who are on mixed diet or formula feds, who may be affected by such over growth of bacteria. Common examples are the *Clostridium difficle* and bacteriodes.

Dietary Management

As emphasized earlier, infants below 6 months already on breast feeds should be continued on the same. Older infants will however not be satisfied with breast milk alone nor will their nutritional needs be met with only breast milk.

Dietary manipulation in older children presenting with diarrhea depends upon the malabsorptive state of the child. They may be partially lactose intolerant to sucrose besides lactose. Children presenting with PD generally might already have been fed on milk-based diets for the first week or ten days. In such children the lactose load can be decreased by substituting curd for milk or buttermilk too can be offered. For older infants beyond 6 months, cereal and milk-based formulae can be used where the total quality of milk used is quite less. Rice is the most preferred cereal used. Rice can be made into flour which makes it easier to cook into porridge or gruel form. Some of the formulae used have been recommended by the Indian Academy of Pediatrics[13] as shown in Tables 15.2 and 15.3. These provide approximately 80 cals/100 mL and about 2.5 g/100 mL of protein.

These feeds can be given by nasogastric route also in cases where oral feeding is difficult to achieve. It is generally observed that children who are difficult to feed and are put on tube feeding, generally regain their appetite within 5–6 days and if oral feeding is restored over a period of time nasogastric feeds can be stopped.

At this stage, the feeds can be made slightly thicker, to make them more calorie dense, by either increasing the amount of cereal or addition

Table 15.2: Low-lactose diets for infants (milk with rice) (4–12 Months)

Ingredients	Amount	Calories (%)	Proteins (g%)
Milk	75 mL	52	2.6
Rice	5 g	17	0.4
Sugar	2.5 g	10	-
Water	100 mL		
Total		79	3

Lactose content 4.5 g%
Source: IAP, 2006.

Table 15.3: Curd with rice feed

Ingredients	Amount	Calories (%)	Protein (g%)
Curd	75 mL	45	2.3
Rice	5 g	17	-
Sugar	2.5 g	10 mL	-
Water	100 mL		
		72	2.7

of oil proportionately. Coconut oil, a good source of medium-chain triglyceride (MCT), can be used successfully to avoid further deterioration of malabsorption. Older children can be given a mixed cereal pulse based family diet, e.g. 'khichdi', which is traditionally used even otherwise in Indian families. Banana is a good calorie dense supplement and also potassium rich, and hence can be used for most children.

There is also a considerable percentage of children who may not tolerate lactose-based diets and may need to be taken off milk/curd completely. This is evident from the perianal excoriation seen in children with continuous purging. In such cases, a total milk/curd-free feed is advised, where in cereal pulse based diets like blenderised khichdi can be fed. Some of these feeds are shown in Tables 15.4 and 15.5.

Egg white based feeds along with rice powder, glucose and oil has also been formulated by WHO,[11] but in the Indian context, due to certain religious and cultural constraints, it may not be well accepted.

Only rice-based formulae can be used for infants below 6 months of age at this stage. The gut malnutrition in terms of enzymes is more efficient after the age of 6 months and secondly too early introduction of variable proteins may also lead to hypersensitization in some cases. Rice is considered the least allergenic among the cereals, therefore, it is better to begin first with rice-based feed alone and then gradually add other protein sources. An example of rice-based formula is given in Table 15.6. This formula is slightly low in calories and also in proteins, but the energy can be increased by addition of more oil, preferably MCT, and the protein content can be enhanced by addition of

Table 15.4: Lactose-free diets cereal pulse based feeds (sweet)

Ingredients	Amount	Calories (%)	Protein (g%)
Rice	15	48	1.2
Moong dal	5	17	1.1
Sugar	2.5	10	-
Oil	2.5	22	-
Water	100		
		97	2.3

Table 15.5: Cereal pulse-based feeds (salty)

Ingredients	Amount	Calories (%)	Proteins (g%)
Rice	4.0 g	13.8	2.7
Moong dal	6.0 g	21.0	14.7
Oil	5.0 mL	45.0	-
Water	100 mL		
		80	1.7

Table 15.6: Rice gruel (sweet)

Ingredients	Amount	Calories (%)	Proteins (%)
Rice	5.0 g	17	0.3 g
Sugar	4.5 g	18	–
Oil	3.0 g	27	–
Water	100 mL		
		62	0.3

any commercially available protein supplement like protinex. Most of the supplements available are skim milk based, therefore care should be taken to read the labels before using them in such feeds. Other lactose-free commercial supplements available are soyal, prosoyal, zerolac nusobee and Simyl MCT. These contain in addition some essential micronutrients, like vitamins and minerals and varying amounts of taurine, carnitine and MCT.

It has been observed that some children, who are lactose intolerant, are also intolerant to soya protein, and therefore these children can not be offered such feeds. In such situations, the only option left is to use rice-based feeds and pulses can be added in older infants.

A small percentage of infants may not respond to even lactose-free diets as they may be intolerant to sucrose also. In such cases, lactose- and sucrose-free formulae have to be used which are available commercially. These have been tried successfully in many centers.

Some centers also use comminuted chicken for lactose- and sucrose-free diets (Table 15.7), but due to religious issues, these are not very commonly popular.

Once the child is put on any of the above mentioned feeds, the quantity can be gradually increased. Small frequent feeding, about 5–6 times a day helps ensure adequate nutrient intake and also faster recovery. Older children can be fed with the home-based solid diets without including lactose. It may be borne in mind, that once the child slips into a state of PD, the recovery also is a slow process. The lactose enzyme which is the first to be affected is also the last to return to normalcy. It is usually about 4–6 weeks by the time lactose foods can be reintroduced successfully. Therefore, low lactose diets may

Table 15.7: Comminuted chicken feed

Ingredients	Amount (g)	Calories	Proteins (g)
Chicken	100	110	26
Glucose	50	200	–
Coconut oil	50	440	–
Water	1000		
		750	26

(Per 100 mL of feed contains 75 cal. and 2.6 g of protein)

first be introduced, like curd, which can be tried initially and gradually milk-based porridge or gruels can be initiated. The amounts may be small first and gradually increased as tolerance improves.

In case if a child with chronic or intractable diarrhea fails to respond to the above regimen, parenteral nutrition (PN) needs to be considered. The major part of energy is provided by the fat emulsion mixture, containing essential fatty acids. However, PN has its own disadvantages, if used over a prolonged period. Hence, it should be given only till the oral intake is restored.

Preventive Measures against Childhood Diarrhea

- Ensuring exclusive breastfeeding for first six months of life and continuing for 2 years or more along with complementary feeding
- Improving sanitation conditions among the underprivileged population
- Providing clean drinking water
- Provision of open defecation by ensuring clean toilets and feces disposal mechanisms in all households
- Ensuring feeding children even during illness
- Elimination of vectors in the surroundings by improving environmental hygiene
- Provision of ORS in nearest health centers and educating mothers regarding importance of adequate hydration and feeding during illness
- Dispelling any prevalent local myths regarding diarrheal diseases by educating and creating awareness through social media.

National Guidelines for Managing Diarrheas in Children

The National Task Force for Feeding Guidelines on the Management of Diarrheas, May 2006 held under the IAP Action Plan 2006,[12] has recommended specific guidelines, as summarized below.

1. Low osmolarity ORS (without added probiotics and minerals) to be prescribed by all physicians for all ages in all types of diarrheas.
2. Zinc supplementation to be given to all children in addition to zinc—uniform dose of 20 mg of elemental zinc older than 6 months, to be started at onset of diarrhea and continued for 14 days. Children aged 2 months to 6 months to be given 10 mg elental zinc for a period of 14 days.

REFERENCES

1. Synder JD, Merson MH. The magnitude of the global problem of acute diarrheal disease: a review of acute surveillance data. Bull WHO. 1982;60:605-13.
2. Bassani DG, Kumar R, Awasthi S, Morris SK, Paul VK, et al. Millions Death Study Collaborators. Causes of neonatal and childhood mortality in India. A nationally representative mortality survey. Lancet. 2010;376:1853-60.
3. Brown KH, Gastanaduy AS, Saavedra JM, et al. Effect of continued oral feeding on clinical and nutritional outcomes of acute diarrhea in children. J Pediatr. 1998;112:191-200.

4. Ornestein SR. Enteral vs. parenteral therapy for intractable diarrhea of infancy. A prospective randomized trial. J Pediatr. 1981;99:360-1.

5. Mahalanbis D, Bhan MK. Development of an improved oral rehydretion solution, Ind J Pediatr. 1991:58:757-61.

6. Elizabeth KE. Diet in various diseases. In: Nutrition and Child Development, 3rd Ed. Paras Medical Publishers; 2004.pp.224-30.

7. Molla AM, Ahmed SM, Greenough WB III. Rice based oral rehydation solution decrease the stool volume in acute diarrhea. Bull WHO. 1985;63:7556.

8. Faraque AS, Mahalanabis D, Islam A, Hoque SS, Hasnat A. Breastfeeding and oral rehydration at home during diarrhea to prevent dehydration. Arch Dis Child. 1992;67:1027-9.

9. Arora NK, Bhan MK. Nutritional management of acute diarrhea. Ind J Pediatr. 1991;58:763-7.

10. Jelliffe DR, Jelliffe EFP. Dietary management of young children with acute diarrhea, 2nd Ed. Geneva: WHO; 1991.pp.3-26.

11. World Health Organisation. The management and prevention of diarrhea. Practical Guidelines. 3rd Ed. Geneva: WHO; 1993.pp.1-4.

12. Bhan MK, Arora NK, Khoshoo V, et al.Comparison of a lactose free cereal based formula and cow's milk in infants and children with acute gastroenteritis. J Pediatr Gastroenterol Nut. 1998;7:208-13.

13. Bhatnagar S, Lodha R, Choudhary P, Sachdev et al. IAP National task Force for Framing Guidelines on the Management of Diarrhea, May 2006 held under IAP Action Plan 2006. Indian Pediatr, Vol 44, May 2007.

Vitamin A Deficiency in Children

INTRODUCTION

Vitamin A deficiency affects more than 127 million preschool children.[1,2] It is estimated that 20-50% of infant mortality can be reduced by improving the status of vitamin A levels in this group of population.[3] Deficiency of vitamin A can extend through school age and adolescent years into adulthood. In India, the prevalence is more than the WHO critical limits in most states. However, as per the National Nutrition Monitoring Bureau (NNMB) estimates it is higher in the states of Andhra Pradesh and West Bengal.[3]

Surveys carried out by NNMB in India, and Integrated Child Development Services (ICDS) indicate that the prevalence of Bitot's spot (the common indication of vitamin A deficiency) in preschool children (1-5 years) ranges between 1-5% in different parts of the country. Incidence of corneal lesions is uncommon. Corneal xeropthalmia is reported to be about 0.05-0.1 per 100 preschool children in South India.[3] As per their estimates about 50,000 children become blind every year in India due to vitamin A deficiency.

The main causes of vitamin A deficiency in children are known to be:

MOTHER DEFICIENT IN VITAMIN A

Maternal vitamin A deficiency exists in a good magnitude with serious and long-term implications. Infant and maternal morality is a common outcome of this deficiency. Deficient mothers obviously will produce breast milk low in vitamin A, thus adversely affecting the health of the offspring. The main cause of maternal deficiency in women is consumption of diets poor in this vitamin besides prolonged breastfeeding due to high fertility rates. In addition to consuming diets low in vitamin A, women in developing countries spend a substantial proportion of their lives breastfeeding, when vitamin A requirements are very high. In industrialized countries, women have on an average 1.6 babies and breast feed them for 5 months. These women spend 8 months or 2.2% of their 30 reproductive years (ages 15-45) breastfeeding. But, in the lesser developed countries, women have on an average 5 children and breast feed each for 2 years. Therefore, rural Bangladesh women spend one third of their reproductive years breastfeeding, when their dietary intake of vitamin A provides less than one third of their RDA.[4,5]

Maternal vitamin A deficiency although has little impact on the fetus, during lactation, healthy mothers transfer about 250 μmol of vitamin A (130 lt. of breast milk consumed, containing 1.92 μmol of vitamin A per lt.), where as women in underdeveloped countries transfer only about half that amount, since the average milk vitamin A concentrations are about 1.05 μmol/l.[6,7] Therefore, all babies are physiologically depleted of vitamin A at birth.

But, during lactation, breast fed babies of well-nourished women accrue adequate stress, whereas babies of poorly nourished mothers remain depleted. In addition, if weaning foods are poor in vitamin A than the breast milk, the child's risk of deficiency increases further when breastfeeding stops.

POOR DIETARY SOURCE OF VITAMIN A IN CHILDREN

A major factor of vitamin A deficiency in children is their poor dietary sources. In general, children in the developed countries receive a major percentage of their vitamin content from animal sources, where as poor children from the developing countries, consume mostly less expensive and poor plant sources. Studies from Egypt, Mexico and Kenya[8] and India[9] have shown that median intakes of animal sources of vitamin A were 174, 119, 50 and 33 μg/d, respectively providing only 11–58% of the RDA and leaving these children largely dependent on the plant sources. In a study from Bangladesh where the only source of vitamin A (preformed) was breast milk, weaned children consumed only negligible amounts of vitamin A from animal sources.[10]

CHILDHOOD ILLNESS AND INFECTIONS

It is well known that illness worsens vitamin A status primarily by reducing intake due to anorexia and malabsorption and increasing utilization through greater catabolism and urinary loss. Anorexia is a major determinant of reduced dietary intake during episodes of diarrhea. Studies have shown that malabsorption of vitamin A can occur during diarrheal illness and lower respiratory infection.[11]

The two most common childhood diseases, chicken pox and measles, can severely compromise vitamin A status. Measles results in markedly depressed circulating vitamin A concentrations and can precipitate xerophthalmia.[12]

Vitamin A supplementation during acute measles episode consistently and dramatically reduces their fatality rates. Therefore, high-dose vitamin A is recommended for treatment of all cases of severe measles in places where measles case fatality rate exceeds 1%.

IGNORANCE AND POVERTY

Lack of awareness among the rural illiterate regarding the importance of supplementing essential vitamins and minerals along with a healthy diet is another factor for deficiency in the rural masses especially in the underprivileged classes.

Poverty and poor purchasing power in most communities prevents them from processing adequate food especially the healthy foods like dairy products and other animal foods which are rich in preformed vitamin A. They are mainly dependent on preformed vitamin A in the form of plant sources.

FUNCTIONS OF VITAMIN A

Vitamin A is a group of compounds that play an important role in vision, bone growth, reproduction, cell division and cell differentiation. It also helps regulate the immune system which helps prevent or fight off infections. It also helps lymphocytes fight infections more efficiently.

Growth

Lack of vitamin A prevents normal growth, as the bony structure will suffer a growth failure before the soft tissues manifest the stunting effect. The cessation of bone growth can lead to overcrowding of the brain and the central nervous system. At times there can be pinching of the optic nerve, leading to blindness.

Role in Monitoring Healthy Epithelial Tissues

Vitamin A has a crucial role in maintaining the healthy epithelial lining. It helps the skin and mucus membrane function as a barrier to bacteria and virus. In the absence of vitamin A, the specialized functions of the tissue are suppressed and is transformed to a keratinized (dry horny) type of epithelium. Excessive dryness of the skin may fail to secrete normally and becomes less resistant to bacterial invasion.

Red Cell Production

The red blood like all other cells are derived from precursor cells called the stem cells. These are dependent on retinoids for normal differentiation into red blood cells.

Antioxidant or Immune Functions

Vitamin A is also commonly referred to as an antioxidant for normal immune functions. As mentioned earlier in this chapter, retinol and its metabolites are required to maintain the integrity and function of the cells that line the airways, digestive tract and the urinary tract, and thus function as a barrier against any infections. Vitamin A and retinoic acid (RSA) is known to play an important role in the development and differentiation of white cells like lymphocytes, which play a critical role in the immune response. Activation of T-lymphocytes, the major regulatory cells of the immune system appears to require all trans RA binding of RAR.

PATHOGENESIS

The pathology involves dryness of the cornea, since the tear glands fail to secrete, causing severe ulcer-like lesions. If untreated this can lead to blindness. The retina is the light sensitive inside layer at the back of the eye. There are two kinds of receptor cells in the retina—the 'rods' which function in dim light and the 'cones' that function in bright light and color vision in rods and rhodopsin in cones. In bright light, rhodopsin changes to retinene plus protein with a possible loss of some vitamin A to resynthesise rhodopsin, vitamin A is reoxidized to retinene and combined with a special protein opsin. In the absence of adequate vitamin A, night blindness may occur. This is a condition characterized by inability to see in dim light and the necessity of a prolonged time to adjust to dim light after exposure to bright light (Fig. 16.1). 'Night blindness' is a stage prior to complete blindness where inadequate retinol available to the retina results in impaired dark adaptation. This is then followed by total blindness, where inadequate retinol available to the retina results in impaired dark adaptation. This is then followed by total blindness, if left undiagnosed.

In ancient Egypt, it was known that night blindness could be cured by eating liver, which was later found to be a rich source of the vitamin.[13] Majority of the cases occur in children of 2–6 years of age. Initially, the condition may be left undiagnosed, when the child begins to stagger and find difficulty in seeing after dusk. This is characterized by mothers typically describing that the child has to grope his way towards evening or in dim light and needs help to find his way. Initially parents may over look these signs and by the time the child begins to literally lose vision, do they realize the gravity of the disease. Therefore, early intervention helps in not only reversing this condition, but also prevents from total loss of vision.

90% of vitamin A is stored in the liver with small amounts in the lungs, body fat and kidneys. The stores being nil at birth, increase gradually with age. These stores are dependent on the amount absorbed from the diet. It has been estimated that a normal liver may contain as much as 600,000 IU of vitamin A enough to supply vitamin needs of one year.[14]

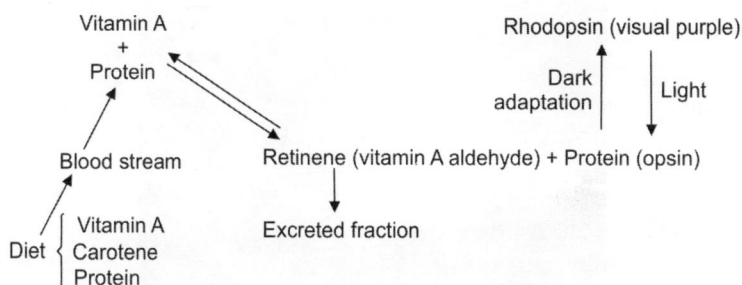

Fig. 16.1: Diagram of formation of rhodops in xerophthalmia
Source: Eddy and Dalldorf. The Avitaminosis. Baltimore: The Willims & Wilkin Co.;1944.p.66.

DEFICIENCY SIGNS OF VITAMIN A

Nutritional deficiency of vitamin A leading to blindness has been regarded as a major national health problem. WHO has recommended the following classification of xerophthalmia, a term covering all ocular manifestations of vitamin A deficiency.[15] These include structural changes affecting conjunctiva, cornea and at times the retina including the biophysical disorders of retinal rod and cone function.

- Night blindness (XN)
- Conjunctival xerosis (XIA)
- Bitot's spots (XIB)
- Corneal xerosis (XZ)
- Corneal ulceration/Keratomalacia (<1/3 corneal surface x 3A)
- Corneal ulceration/Keratomalacia (>1/3 corneal surface x 3A)
- Corneal scar (XF)
- Xerophthalmia fundus (XN).

Night Blindness (XN)

This is the first sign of vitamin A deficiency observed in children and history can be elicited by detailed questioning of the parent giving history of the child groping in dim light or they are unable to see the food in their plate in front of them.

Conjuctival Xerosis (XIA)

This is seen as dry patches on the conjunctiva. The tears in the child appear to emerge like sand at receding tide. There may be varying degrees of thickening, wrinkling and pigmentation of the conjunctiva.

Bitot's Spots (XIB)

This is an extension of the xerotic process. The spots are raised, muddy, and dry with triangular patches (Fig. 16.2). These spots are very early diagnosed, and may tend to remain as sequale of earlier corrected vitamin A deficiency even after therapy.

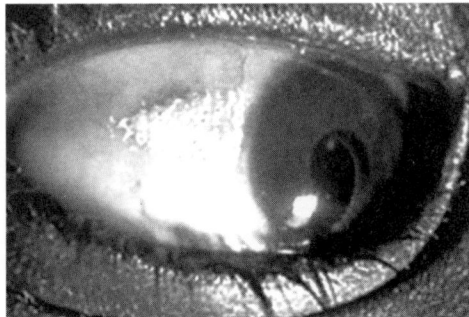

Fig. 16.2: Eye with Bitot's spot

Corneal Xerosis (X2)

This is diagnosed by the presence of haziness or dryness of cornea on clinical examination. The cornea gives the appearance of ground glass followed by corneal ulcers. Treatment reverses these symptoms except in cases where the stoma is deep rooted which can lead to blindness.

Keratomalacia (X3B)

This is the last stage, if left undiagnosed leading to irreversible blindness. It is marked by progressive necrosis and death of tissue affecting the full thickness of the cornea (Fig. 16.3).

VITAMIN A DEFICIENCY IN SPECIFIC CONDITIONS

There is increased interest in the early forms of vitamin A deficiency described as storage levels of vitamin A that do not cause obvious deficiency symptom. This mild degree of vitamin A deficiency may increase children's decrease likelihood of survival from serious illness.[16] In the United states, children are considered to be at increased risk for subclinical vitamin A deficiency in the following conditions:

- Toddlers and preschool age children
- Children living at or below poverty level
- Children with inadequate health care or immunization
- Children living in areas with known nutritional deficiency
- Recent immigrants or refugees from developing countries with high incidence of Vitamin A deficiency or measles
- Children with diseases of the pancreas, liver or intestines or with inadequate fat digestion on absorption.

Vitamin A deficiency can occur when there are losses through chronic diarrhea or when the total dietary intake is inadequate as in PEM. It has been suggested that vitamin A deficiency can also occur due to inadequate intake of protein, calories and zinc, since these nutrients are needed to make retinol

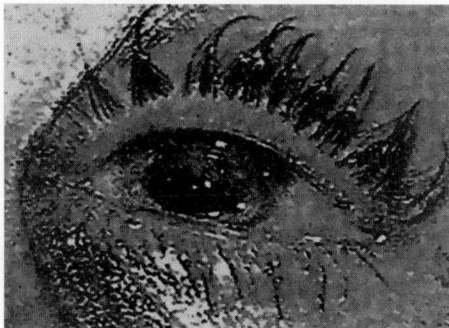

Fig. 16.3: Eye with keratomalacia

binding protein (RBP). Iron deficiency too can affect vitamin A metabolism. It is seen that iron supplements provided to iron deficiency individuals may improve body stores of vitamin A and iron.[17]

Hypervitaminminosis A

Excessive consumption of vitamin A may lead to toxicity called hypervitaminosis. Acute toxicity although rare, is marked by symptoms like nausea, headache, fatigue, anorexia, dizziness, dry skin and cerebral edema. Bone and joint pain may also be present. In infants, symptoms of toxicity include bulging fontanels. Severe cases of hypervitaminosis may result in liver damage, hemorrhage and coma. However, such signs are associated only with long-term consumption of the vitamin and in excess losses. On the other hand the toxicity can also occur by consuming large doses of preformed vitamin A over a short period. Such incidents generally tend to occur when taken as supplements. Dietary sources alone do not run the risk of toxicity.

TARGET GROUP FOR VITAMIN A SUPPLEMENTATION

The WHO and the United Nations Children Funds (UNICEF) recommend vitamin A administration for all children where vitamin A deficiency is a serious problem and where death from measles is greater than 1 percent. In 1994, the American Academy of Pediatrics recommended vitamin A supplements for two sub groups of children likely to be at high risk for subclinical vitamin A deficiency; children aged 6 to 24 months who are hospitalized with measles, and hospitalized children older than 6 months.[18]

Fat malabsorption can result in diarrhea and prevent normal absorption of vitamin A gradually leading to vitamin A deficiency. Some of the conditions involved would be as follows:

- *Celiac disease*: Genetic disorder where patients are allergic to the gliadin fraction of wheat protein
- *Chron's disease*: This is an inflammatory bowel disease characterized by fat malabsorption and malnutrition
- *Pancreatic disorders*: These include conditions like cystic fibrosis where due to the deficiency in enzyme secretion, fat malabsorption occurs causing huge losses of vitamin A. Supplementation of vitamin A helps prevent deficiency
- *Vegetarians*: Strict vegetarians not consuming eggs or even dairy products run the risk of developing of this vitamin A.

Requirements

The RDAs for vitamin A for infants and children are calculated on the basis of vitamin A intake through breastfed infants and extrapolated for children.[19] The daily intake of vitamin A by Indian infants through breast milk is about 140 µg during the first 6 months of life.[20] Since it was observed that children of such communities often develop deficiency signs during early childhood, intakes of 140 µg/d seem to be inadequate. Therefore, based on the observations of breast milk intake by well-nourished mothers, the expert group[21] has recommended a daily intake of 350 µg retinol up to 6 months of age. The same level is recommended for the next 6 months also, i.e. the later half of infancy, since no specific data is yet available on the needs of this group.

In view of the high incidence of vitamin A deficiency signs in and low-serum levels among Indian children with dietary intake less than 100 µg, the daily intake for pre-schoolers has been fixed at 400 µg and 600 µg for school children and adolescents. Table 16.1 gives the requirements suggested for different age groups of children and pregnant and lactating mothers, including the conversion factor of β carotene to vitamin A. Studies have shown that when vitamin A was supplemented with a total of 300 µg/d over a period of 6 months, serum vitamin levels were found to be around 30 µg/dL and clinical deficiency signs were absent.[22]

PREVENTION OF VITAMIN A DEFICIENCY

'Prevention is better than cure', so it is said and rightly so.

Deficiency of vitamin A is one disease which can easily be prevented. Education and awareness of the gravity of the problem, if explained to the parents can definitely help avoid this preventive disease with grave consequences. Nature has a bounty of food sources to provide vitamin A, both as preformed vitamin and β carotene, the precursor of the vitamin. Mostly all colorful fruits and vegetables, especially the yellow and the green ones provide the provitamin A, i.e. the carotenoids. These can be converted into the retinol form for absorption in the body. Common provitamin A carotenoids found in foods that come from plants are beta carotene, alpha carotene and beta cryptoxanthin. Among this β carotene is most easily converted into retinol. Some of the provitamin A carotenoids have been shown to function as antioxidants also. Dark green leafy vegetables like spinach, etc. are affordable good sources. Retinol is found in foods that come from animal sources like,

Table 16.1: Recommended intake of vitamin A (µg/dL)		
Group	*Retinol*	*β Carotene*
Adult men and women	600	2400
Pregnant women	600	2400
Lactating women	950	3500
Infants 0–6 months	350	1400
Infants 6–12 months		
Preschool children 1–5 years	400	1600
School children 7–12 years	600	2400
Adolescents 13–18 years	600	2400

Source: ICMR (1990).[19]

whole eggs, milk and liver. Most fortified foods like butter, margarine and breakfast cereals and fats and oils are converted to retinol.

Vitamin A sources from animal origin are absorbed more efficiently by the body. A list of vitamin A and provitamin sources are given in Tables 16.2 and 16.3.[23]

Table 16.2: Animal food sources of vitamin A (µg %)		
Foods	*Retinol*	*β carotene*
Animal sources		
Milk (cows)	53	
Curd (cows)	31	
Cottage cheese (cow milk)	110	
Cheese	82	
Butter	960	
Ghee (cow)	600	
Ghee (buffalo)	270	
Refined oil (fortified)	750	
Egg (hen)	420	
Liver (sheep)	6690	

Table 16.3: Vegetable food sources of vitamin A			
Foods	*Retinol*	*Carotene*	
		Total	*β*
Vegetable sources		15,700	
Colocasia leaves		15,000	5,920
Coriander leaves		42,000	4,800
Drumstick leaves		11,800	19,690
Fenugreek leaves		7,000	9,100
Lettuce		18,950	1,100
Mint		13,000	5,480
Radish leaves		9,400	2,200
Spinach		8,840	2,740
Carrot		2,100	6,460
Pumpkin		2,430	1,160
Chillies green		690	1,007
Chillies giant (capsicum)		400	140
Guava (country)		2,210	0
Mango (ripe)		2,240	1,990
Orange		2,740	190
Papaya (ripe)		3,010	880
Tomato (ripe)			590

Source: ICMR 1990.

Other strategies which can help prevent vitamin A deficiency are periodic supplements to the vulnerable groups and fortification of food products which are widely consumed. Nutrition counseling is simultaneously required to create awareness among the masses especially the lower socio economic sections. Education regarding making use of low cost, seasonally available fruits and vegetables can go a long way in prevention of the serious consequences of deficiency of this vitamin.

Another point to be stressed during education is the right cooking methods to be used while preparation of foods rich in vitamin A. Being fat soluble vitamins, it is important that for these foods deep frying for prolonged duration be avoided, since maximum losses can occur during this process.

TREATMENT

Treatment involves administration of large doses of vitamin A for all stages of active xerophthalmia including corneal lesions.

For the children aged 1–6 years, an oral dose of 200,000 IU or oil miscible vitamin A is administered. This is followed by another dose of 200,000 IU, one to four weeks later. For infants below 12 months of age weighing less than 8 Kg the same schedule is followed using half the dose of the vitamin. Children suffering from associated problems like diarrhea, acute respiratory infections and measles should be monitored closely and treated as medical emergency.[24]

SOME CONTROVERSIES ABOUT VITAMIN A

Vitamin A, beta Carotene and Cancer

Studies exist to suggest role of vitamin A rich diets in lowering risk of many types of cancer.[25]

However, there are other studies which contradict these observations. In fact, in one of the studies, where researchers provided supplements to subjects with lung cancer, they found a 46% higher risk of deaths occurring among them, therefore this study had to be abandoned.[26]

It was hence felt that beta carotene supplements are not advisable for general population, except in those with inadequate vitamin A.[17]

Vitamin A and Osteoporosis

There is no evidence of an association between beta carotene intake, especially from fruits and vegetables, and increased risk of osteoporosis. Current evidence suggests a possible association with vitamin A as retinol only. Similarly no association was found between blood levels of beta carotene and risk of hip fracture. However, it was also observed by some researchers that retinol intakes greater than 2,000 µg/d were associated with an increased risk of hip fracture as compared to intakes less than 500 mg.[27]

REFERENCES

1. West KF. Extent of vitamin A deficiency among pre school children and women of reproductive age. J Nutr. 2002;132:28575-665.
2. Humphrey JH, West KP Jr, Sommer A. Vitamin A deficiency and attributable morality among under 5 year olds. Bull WHO. 1992;70:225-32.
3. Vijayaraghavan K. Vitamin A deficiency. In: Textbook of Human Nutrition. Bamji MS, Prahlad RN, Reddy V (Eds). New Delhi: Oxford and IBM Publishing Co. Pvt Ltd; 1996. pp 287-97.
4. UNICEF (200). State of the world children 2000. www.unicef org/sowc002000 UNICEF New York.
5. WHO (1998) Complementary feeding of young children in developing countries: a review of current scientific knowledge. WHO Geneva, Switzerland. Publ No WS 13098 Co; 1998.
6. Walling Ford JC, Underwood BA. Vitamin A deficiency in pregnancy, lactation and the nursing child. Bauerufeind J (Ed.). Vitamin A Deficiency and its control. New York: Academic Press; 1986. pp. 101-52.
7. Chappel JE, Francis T, Clandinin MT. vitamin A and E content of human milk at early stages of lactation. Early human Dev. 11:157-167.
8. Calloway DH, Murphy SP, Beaton GH, Lien D. Estimated vitamin A intakes of toddlers: predicted prevalence of inadequacy in village population in Egypt, Kenya and Mexico. Am J Clin Nutr. 1993;58:376-84.
9. Ramakrishanan U, Martorell R, Latham MC, Abel R. Dietary vitamin A intakes of pre school age children in south India. J Nutr. 1999;2021-7.
10. Zeitlin MF, Megawangi R, Mara Kramer E, Armstrong HC. Mother's and children's intakes of vitamin A in rural Bangladesh. Am J Clin Nutr. 1992.
11. Sivakumar B, Reddy V. Absorption of labeled vitamin A by children with diarrhea during treatment with oral rehydration solution. Bull WHO. 64. pp.721-4.
12. Reddy V, Bhaskaram P, Raghuramula N, Milton RC, Rao U, Madhusudan J, Krishna KV. Relationship between measles, malnutrition and blindness : a prospective study in Indian children. Am J Clin Nutr. 1986;44:924-30.
13. Gerster H. Vitamin A functions, dietary requirements and safety in humans. Int J Vitam Nutr Res. 1997;67:71-90.
14. Wilson ED, Fisher KE, Fuqua HE. Introduction to the vitamins and the fat soluble vitamins. In: Principles of Nutrition. Wiley Eastern Pvt. Ltd; 1968.
15. Tielsch JM, Sommer A. The epidemiology of vitamin A deficiency and xerophthalmia. In: Annual Review of Nutr. 1984;4:183-205.
16. Stephens D, Jackson PL, Gutierrey Y. Sub clinical vitamin A deficiency: A potentially unrecognized problem in the United States. Pediatr Nutr. 1996;22:377-89.
17. Institute of Medicine. Food and Nutrition Board. Dietary reference intakes for vitamin A vitamin K, arsenic, boron, chromium, copper, iodine, iron, manganese, molybdenum, nickel, silicon, vanadium and zinc. Washington DC: National Academy Press; 2001.
18. Committee on Infectious Diseases. Vitamin A treatment of measles. Pediatrics. 1993;91:1014-5.
19. ICMR, Nutrient requirement and recommended dietary allowances for Indians, A report of the expert group of the ICMR, 1990, NIN, Hyderabad.
20. Belavady B, Gopalan C. Chemical composition of human milk in poor Indian women. Ind J Med Res. 1959;47:234.

21. WHO, Requirements of vitamin A, thiamine, riboflavin and niacin, 1967; WHO Tech Rep Sr no 362.
22. Reddy V. Vitamin A deficiency and blindness in Indian children. Ind J Med Res. 1978;68(suppl):26.
23. Gopalan C, Rama Sastri BV, Balasubraminiam SC. Nutritive Value of Indian Foods, National Institute of Nutrition, ICMR, Hyderabad, 1990.
24. Vijayraghavan K. Vitamin A deficiency. In : Textbook of human Nutrition, Ed. Bamji MS, Rao NP, Reddy V. Oxford and IBH Publishing Co. Pvt Ltd; 1996.
25. Fontham ETH. Protective dietary factors and lung cancer. Int J Epidemiol. 1990;19:532-4.
26. Pryor WH, Stahl W, Rock CL. Beta carotene: From biochemistry to clinical trials. Nutr Rev. 2000;58:38-53.
27. Feskanich D, Singh F, Willet WC, Colditz CA. Vitamin A intake and hip fractured among post menopausal women. JAMA. 2002;287:47-54.

Zinc in Infant Nutrition

INTRODUCTION

Zinc is one of the numerous trace elements which are known to have a significant role in the growth and development of an infant. In fact its role has been attributed right from the antenatal period, as deficiency of this micronutrient can have a crucial bearing upon the health of the new born. Prasad defined the role of zinc in human nutrition in 1991. It was the observation between increased susceptibility to infectious diseases and nutritional zinc deficiency which led to the increased interest in the importance of this trace element.[1]

Zinc is required in over 200 enzymes and hence, likely to affect a number of various systems in the human body. Severe to moderate zinc deficiency has been found to cause oxidative damage to the proteins, lipids and DNA in rat testes[2] which may be due to iron accumulation or a reduction in zinc-dependent antioxidant processes.

Zinc is present in all organs, tissues and other body fluids. It is primarily an intercellular ion with intracellular zinc contributing to more than 95% of the total body zinc. Skeletal muscle and bone together contain 80% of the total body zinc. It is widely distributed within the cells bound to protein. It governs a wide range of body functions:

1. **Cell division and growth:** Zinc has vital role in cell division and growth. It governs cellular growth and differentiation. Early zinc deficiency reduces cell division which in turn affects growth as an adaptive mechanism.
2. **Membrane function:** Zinc has an important role in the stabilization of biomembranes by binding sulfhydryl groups and forming mercaptides. Decrease in biomembrane zinc is suggested as one of the early biochemical lesions of zinc deficiency.
3. **Protection against free-radical change:** Zinc is believed to have a role as an antioxidant against free-radical related diseases. Liver injury, chronic inflammatory conditions, essential fatty acid deficiency, cancer and radiation damage are all associated with decreased levels of zinc in the body.

4. ***Zinc and sex hormones:*** Deficiency of zinc is known to impair testosterone production in humans. In pregnant females difficult labor is believed to be a manifestation of zinc deficiency.
5. ***Zinc and immune functions:*** Animal studies have confirmed the role of zinc in maintaining the immune levels in the body. This is considered to be due to its role in cell proliferation and other cellular functions. Zinc is essential for the function of many enzymes, which are vital for the growth, and regulation of immune cells.
6. ***Zinc and mental development:*** In experimental animals it has been demonstrated that zinc deficiency has an impact on the fetal outcome. This affect is however, dependant on the degree and duration of deficiency. The adverse affects on fetal outcome could be in the form of congenital malformation and fetal resorption. In humans however, such affects are not well established in case of mild or borderline deficiency states.
7. ***Zinc and brain development:*** Deficiency of zinc is known to have adverse affects on the cerebral morphology and also on behavioral development of animals.
8. ***Zinc and vitamins:*** Zinc is present in high concentration in the retina and other ocular tissues, therefore considered to be interrelated with vitamin A metabolism especially in relation to vision. Its deficiency can also affect night vision despite adequate amounts of retinol concentration.
9. ***Zinc and metals:*** Zinc is considered to be adversely affected by interaction by certain metals like iron, calcium and copper if present in excess.

METABOLISM

Zinc is absorbed from the proximal bowel. 60% of the circulating plasma zinc is found loosely bound to albumin and amino acids, while the remaining 40% is tightly bound to alpha globulins and is not free to diffuse into the tissues. The total zinc content in the human body is about 2–3 grams. Almost 50% of the total body zinc is in bone and is not readily available for metabolic needs. Zinc is not stored as such in the body which implies that there has to be a continuous provision of this micronutrient through the diet for tissue growth and repair.

Excretion of zinc is mainly through the stool. In fact the total zinc content is around 54 mg, 60% of which is passed to the fetus in the last trimester at the rate of about 30 micrograms per kg. of body weight per day. Inadequate amounts of dietary zinc or increased losses may place the infant at increased risk of developing deficiency.

The zinc content of breast milk is quite high, the concentrations in Indian mothers being about 36.1 μmol/L during the first week of lactation and gradually decreases to 24.4, 22.6 and 20.2 μmol/L by 3, 6 and 9 months, respectively.[3]

This concentration can vary from one mother to another although not significantly. The average daily intake of zinc in an infant works up to about 1.75 mg at 4 weeks, 0.83 mg at 12 weeks and 0.40 mg at 24 weeks.[4]

ZINC REQUIREMENTS

Zinc deficiency in humans is mainly due to a lack of bioavailable zinc in the diet, general malnutrition or malabsorption.[5]

Nutritional zinc requirements are influenced by many dietary factors that affect its bioavailability and physiological requirements which vary greatly between different age groups. On the basis of current evidence, the suggested recommended dietary intake of zinc during the first half of infancy is 3–4 mg/d, between 6 and 12 months is 6 mg/d and during later childhood it becomes 10 mg/d.[6] The requirements increase in the preterm low birth weight and children recovering from malnutrition. These requirements are considered for Indian children as well. For adults the zinc requirement has been set as 15.5 mg/d[7] which are in accordance with the values suggested by WHO.[8]

IMPLICATIONS OF ZINC DEFICIENCY

Zinc is perhaps one trace element, the deficiency of which has been implicated with a wide variety of problems like acrodermatitis enteropathica, sickle cell anemia, immunological disorders, and neurological disorders and even in the outcome of pregnancy. Its role has been well described in the treatment of diarrheas, infections and protein–energy malnutrition.

In children, moderate to severe zinc deficiency is known to depress skeletal growth and gonad development which were found to reverse on zinc therapy.[1,9]

ZINC STATUS IN PREGNANCY

Zinc deficiency in pregnancy not only affects the mother, but it also has immunological consequences for the fetus. Various immune defects have been reported in animal studies. One of the earliest and clinically most relevant signs of maternal zinc deficiency are low levels of natural immunoglobulins including a persistent defect in IgM and transiently diminished levels of IgA and IgG2 in neonates. The explanation proposed for this is diminished transport of immunoglobulins. Besides, the reduction in total amount of antigen, there is in addition, depressed repertoire of antigens recognized by these antibodies. This effect has been described even in mild transient deficiency.[10]

Prenatal zinc deficiency might also have an important effect on child immunity as observed in animal studies. Hypogammaglobulinemia together with altered antibody repertoire and decreased T cell proliferation in response to T-cell-dependent antigens may lead to impaired success of vaccination in the infant, which in turn can have important consequences for the health status of the population. In humans, immunological defects may possibly have a bearing on subsequent generations as suggested by animal studies which may be irreversible.[11]

Supplementation trials on pregnant women who can be at risk of zinc deficiency have not been conclusive. Controversy exists between different authors regarding the role of supplementation in this group, therefore no extra dose, is required except, when there might be some definite indication for deficiency.

ZINC AND CHILDHOOD INFECTIONS

Zinc and diarrhea: Zinc deficiency has been associated with high rates of infectious diseases including skin infections, diarrhea and respiratory infections besides malaria and delayed wound healing. In the developing countries, extensive studies have been done regarding diarrhea and respiratory infections. These trials were done in pre-school children who were representative of poor country population. The results from all the groups showed that zinc supplemented children have lower rates of diarrhea than those of normal children.[12] Trial studies of zinc supplementation during acute persistent diarrhea have shown consistent benefits of zinc supplementation. These benefits were in the form of shorter episode duration of diarrhea. More significantly, there were large reductions in the rate of 'treatment failure' or death in these trials.

Zinc supplementation is known to significantly reduce lactulose excretion in persistent diarrhea and this effect was seen to be more marked in malnourished children. Therefore, zinc has a significant effect on intestinal integrity and is likely to contribute to a better recovery. Besides, children with diarrhea who received supplementation 15 mg of zinc acetate per day had significantly greater gains in height and weight in the following 9 weeks than unsupplemented children.[13] It was therefore suggested that for preventive use of zinc, there is need to evaluate various ways to improve the zinc nutriture in children in developing countries. These include dietary sources and availability of zinc, fortifying foods with zinc and supplementation programs.

Zinc and respiratory infections: Several field studies have shown that zinc supplementation is beneficial in preventing pneumonia in children in developing countries. A pooled analysis (Zinc Investigators Collaborative Group, 1999) has shown that zinc supplemented children have a 41% reduced rate of pneumonia compared to the controlled group.[14]

Zinc in protein-energy malnutrition: Rehabilitation from severe protein-energy malnutrition requires the provision of adequate quantities of macro- and micronutrients. Zinc deficiency has been implicated as a limiting factor in recovery[15] and WHO recommends that all severely malnourished children be treated with zinc along with other micronutrients.

A study from India[16] has shown that though there was no difference in weight gain between zinc supplemented and placebo group, the former showed an increase in plasma zinc which rose to normal levels. In the latter group, the plasma zinc decreased significantly during the period of rapid growth. This indicates that though dietary zinc may be sufficient for efficient weight gain, it is not able to compensate for the extra requirements demanded in the process of new tissue deposition.

Zinc and cognitive development: The role of zinc in the cognitive development and behavior of a child has been explained based on its critical role in the function of several structural regulatory and catalytic proteins. It is present in the brain bound to proteins and is important for its structure and function.[17,18] There is also some evidence to suggest that zinc deficiency results in lowered levels of ω-3 and ω-6 chains possibly causing impaired fatty acid metabolism in the neurons.[19]

Moreover, it seems to be important for neurogenesis, neural migration and synaptogenesis and its deficiency could interfere with neurotransmission and subsequent neurophysiological development. Besides zinc is also understood to be involved in the metabolism of thyroid hormones, receptor functions and transport of other hormones that could influence the central nervous system.[20]

Findings from studies in monkeys suggest that the zinc deprived group showed progressive decline in day time activity and attention performance. The study also indicates that zinc deprived adolescents may be more susceptible to behavioral changes before the onset of growth retardation.[21] Studies from India have shown a positive association between zinc deprivation and activity in malnourished children. Reduced activity inhibits exploration which may contribute directly to diminished cognitive development. It was observed from this study that children randomized to receive 10 mg/d of zinc gluconate in addition to the vitamins A, B_1 B_2, B_6, D_3, E and niacinamide, spent 72% more time performing high movement activities like running. The effects were greater in boys and this could be due to extra zinc requirement in them. Among the zinc supplemented group, the activity rating was 12% and 8% higher by a previously validated children's activity rating and the energy expenditure score, respectively.[22]

There is evidence to prove the association between zinc status and neurophysiological behavior also. Supplementation with zinc have resulted in alteration in fetal neurobehavior, better motor development in very low birth weight infants, more vigorous physical activity in malnourished infants and toddlers and improved neuropsychological functions in school-age children.

Zinc deficiency affects cognitive development by alterations in attention, activity, other features of neuropsychological behavior and motor development. These effects vary by age and may be influenced by the care giving environment, particularly the behavior of the mother and the social context.[23]

Acrodermatitis enteropathica: The most extreme forms of zinc deficiency can be studied in zinc specific malabsorption syndrome 'acrodermatitis enteropathica'; a rare autosomal recessive inheritable disease[24] which appears to be more common in girls.

This disorder manifests insidiously from the age of weaning, characterized by severe skin lesions, alopecia, failure to thrive and diarrhea. The lesions appear typically on the cheeks, knees and elbows. The hair becomes reddish in color. Even ocular manifestations in the form of photophobia, conjunctivitis and corneal dystrophy can be observed. Associated characteristics like chronic diarrhea, stomatitis, glossitis, personality changes, intercurrent bacterial infections are also commonly seen. Administration of oral zinc therapy in doses of 50–150 mg/d reverses the symptoms dramatically.

A possible role of zinc involving metabolic interrelationship with other micronutrients has also been postulated.[25] Some of these are as follows:

- Zinc deficiency may lead to poor mobilization of hepatic stores of vitamin A and thus, cause hypovitaminosis
- Zinc absorption may be affected by inorganic iron
- Zinc may also depress copper absorption which can lead to biochemical evidence of copper deficiency.

ZINC TOXICITY

Although toxicity of zinc is not common, it is known to occur if ingested in large quantities in the form of inhaled fumes of zinc. Vomiting follows about 3 hours after ingestion of excess zinc. Dehydration, electrolyte imbalance, abdominal pain, nausea, dizziness and lethargy are some of the other symptoms known to occur if taken in large amounts. If taken over a prolonged period, it interferes with copper metabolism which results in severe anemia, neutropenia reduced serum levels of iron and even immunosuppression. If taken in excess during pregnancy, it can adversely affect the fetus too.[24]

Dietary Sources of Zinc

If a normal balanced diet is taken the requirements are generally met with. Good sources of zinc are whole pulses, nuts like almonds and cashew, oilseeds like gingelly, mustard, safflower and poppy seeds.

CONCLUSION

As per evidence available from Indian data, it was suggested that since isolated zinc deficiency rarely exists in pregnancy or in newborns' and older children, routine supplementation of zinc is not warranted. However, during treatment and rehabilitation phase of severe PEM or persistent diarrhea, zinc supplementation in the required doses is justified, where even other micronutrient supplement is also given in view of coexisting deficiencies.

REFERENCES

1. Prasad AS. Discovery of human zinc deficiency and studies in an experimental human model. Am J Clin Nutr. 1991;53:403-12.
2. Oteza PJ, Olin KL, Fraga CG, Keen CL. Zinc deficiency causes oxidative damage to proteins, lipids and DNA in rat testes, J Nutr. 1995;125:823-9.
3. Bhaskaram P, Hemalatha P. Zinc status in breast fed infants. Lancet. 1992;2:1416-7.
4. Zlotkin SH. Assessment of trace element requirements (zinc) in newborns and young infants, including the infant born prematurely. In: Trace Elements in Nutrition of Children-II Ed. Chandra RK. Nestle Nutrition Workshop New York, Raven Press. 1991;23:49-77.

5. Prasad AS. Zinc: an overview. Nutrition. 1995;11:93-9.
6. Hambidge KM. Zinc in the nutrition of children. In: Trace elements in Nutrition of children-II Ed. Chandra RK. Nestle Nutrition Workshop, New York, Raven press. 1991;23:9965-77.
7. ICMR, Nutritional requirements and recommended dietary allowances for Indians. A Report of the Expert Group of the Indian Council of Medical Research. 2002;41-2.
8. World Health Organization. Trace Elements in Human Nutrition (WHO Tech Rep Sr No. 532).
9. Agget PJ, Severe zinc deficiency In: Zinc in Human Biology. Ed. Mills CF. Berlin: Springer Verlag; 1988.pp.259-79.
10. Prasad AS. Discovery of human zinc deficiency and studies in an experimental human model. Am J Clin Nutr. 1991;53:403-12.
11. Shankar AH, Prasad AS. Zinc and immune function: the biological basis of altered resistance and infection. Am J Clin Nutr. 1998;68:447S-63S.
12. Beach RS, Gershwin ME, Hurley LS. Persistent immunological consequences of gestational zinc deprivation. Am J Clin Nutr. 1983;38:579-90.
13. Sazawal S, Black R, Bhan M, et al. Zinc supplementation in children with acute diarrhea in India. N Eng J Med. 1995;333:839-44.
14. Behrans RH, Tomkins AM, Roy SK. Zinc supplementation during diarrhea: A fortification against malnutrition. Lancet. 1990;2:442-3.
15. Zinc Investigators Collaborative Group. Prevention of diarrhea and pneumonia by zinc supplementation in children in developing countries: pooled analysis of randomized controlled trials. J Pediatr. 1999;135:689-97.
16. Hemalatha P, Bhaskaran P, Khan MM. Role of zinc supplementation in the rehabilitation of severely malnourished children. Eur J Clin Nutr. 1993;47:395-9.
17. Fierka C. Function and mechanism of zinc. J Nutr. 2000;130:1437S-46S.
18. Hambidge M. Humanzinc deficiency. J Nutr. 2000;130:13445-95.
19. Wauben PM, Wainwright PE. The influence of neonatal nutrition on behavioral development: a critical appraisal. Nutr Rev. 1999;57:35-44.
20. Morley JE, Gordan J, Hershman JM. Zinc deficiency, chronic starvation and hypothalamic pituitary-thyroid function. Am J Clin Nutr. 1980;33:1767-70.
21. Golub MS, Takeruchi PT, Keen CL, Hendricks AG, Gershwin EM. Activity and attention in zinc deprived adolescent monkeys. Am J Clin Nutr. 1996;64:905-15.
22. Sazawal S, Bentley M, Black RE, Dhingra P, George S, Bhan MK. Effect of zinc supplementation on observed activity in preschool children in an urban slum population. Pediatrics. 1996;98:1132-7.
23. Black MM. Zinc deficiency and child development. Am J Clin Nutr. 1998;68(Suppl):464S-9S.
24. Bhaskaram P, Krishnaswamy K. Trace elements of clinical significance. Zinc and Selenium. In: Textbook of Human Nutrition Eds. Bamji MS, Rao NP, Reddy V. New Delhi: Oxford & IBH Publishing Co Pvt Ltd; 1996.
25. Gopaln C. Micronutrient deficiencies- Public Health Implications. NFI. 1994;15:1-6.

Iodine Deficiency Disorders

Iodine is an essential micronutrient that occurs in soil and seawater in the form of iodides. It is oxidized by sunlight to iodine, which is a volatile substance. The concentrate of iodine in sea water is only 0.05 mg/L. If there are excessive losses of this nutrient from the sea without any correction, it may ultimately lead to deficit in the soil which can persist indefinitely. Crops grown in soil or water produced from such areas then tend to be deficient in iodine. Consumption of food produced form such crops can lead to deficiency of iodine, which is responsible for an array of disorder commonly termed as iodine deficiency disorder (IDD). Goiter and cretinism are the two clinical manifestations of endemic iodine deficiency, prevalent in many parts of the developing world.

Hetzel first used the term iodine deficiency disorder (IDD) in 1982 to denote all the effects of iodine deficiency on a population growth and development, which could be totally prevented by correction of the deficiency.[1] Though these effects can be evident in all stages of life, the most affected stages of human life are the fetus, neonate, infancy and pregnancy also to some extent.

Estimates exist, that about 800 million people living in iodine deficient environment throughout the world are exposed to the risk of IDD. Out of them 190 million are known to suffer form goiter and another 3.15 million from cretinism.[2]

FUNCTIONS OF IODINE

Iodine is considered an essential micronutrient due to the fact that it is a constituent of the thyroid hormone, thyroxin T4 and triiodo thyroxin T3, essential for normal mental and physical development in humans and animals and also for development of the brain and maintenance of body temperature. Deficiency of the hormone can lead to severe retardation and growth maturation of almost all organ systems. The total iodine content in healthy adult man is about 15–20 µg, 70–80% of which is present in the thyroid gland. Daily requirement of iodine is about 150 µg.[2]

In Energy Metabolism

The thyroid hormone has an important role in the rate of oxidation in the cells of the body. An increased secretion of thyroxin speeds up the rate of energy metabolism. On the contrary, lack of it can retard the rate. Besides basal metabolic rate as a method for assessing the state of thyroid function, there are two other parameters used to assess the thyroxin function which are as follows:

1. Determining the protein-bound iodine (PBI) in the blood serum.
2. Observation on the utilization of radioactive iodine.

The PBI is chiefly thyroxin. It is found to be low in hypothyroidism and elevated in hyperthyroidism.

Growth and Development

Thyroxin is essential for the normal growth and development of the young. Inadequate levels can lead to growth retardation, which if severe and prolonged results in failure to mature physically and mentally. In children, this form of growth retardation is known as 'cretinism'. Besides as shown in Fig. 18.1[3] arrested growth, their facial features appear coarse and swollen, the skin is thick, dry and pasty in appearance and deeply wrinkled. The tongue is enlarged and lips appear thickened and stay ajar usually.

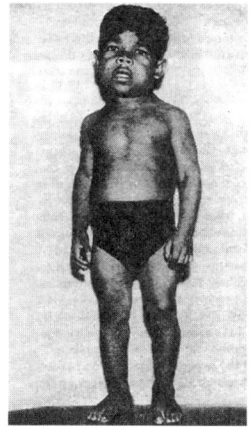

In adults, thyroxin deficiency is known as 'myxoedema'. The skin and subcutaneous tissue, particularly of the face and extremities are thickened and puffy. The face is characteristically expressionless and the person appears lethargic and inactive.

Fig. 18.1: A child suffering from cretinism
Source: Scrimshaw NS. Endemic goiter. Nutr Rev. 1957;15:161.

IDD has been described as the world's single most significant cause of preventable brain damage and mental retardation. It affects about 14% of the world's population and 834 million persons are affected by goiter. There exist 43 millions cases of preventable brain damage caused by iodine deficiency.[4]

In Pregnancy and Lactation

Iodine has an important role in normal reproduction in both sexes. Goiter is generally known to occur in pregnancy, indicating a greater need for the thyroid hormone.

METABOLISM OF IODINE

Iodine is readily absorbed both in organic and inorganic form. Most of the iodine is absorbed from the small gut and excreted by the kidney. Iodine enters the circulation and is taken up by the thyroid gland and other tissue. The thyroid gland concentrates the element and serves as a storehouse for it.

Iodine is oxidized by hydrogen peroxidase from the thyroid peroxidase system. This oxidized iodine combines with the amino acid 'tyroxine' present in the thyroglobulin to form monoiodotyrosine (MIT) and diiodotyrosines (DIT)

By the coupling of the MIT and DIT, T4 and T3 are formed. The iodized thyroglobulin is absorbed back into the thyroid cells, where it undergoes proteolysis, releasing T4 and T3 into the blood. This entire process of absorption, synthesis and release of thyroxin is regulated by thyroid stimulating hormone (TSH) secreted by the pituitary gland.

The body can autoregulate its iodine supply. When thyroxin levels are down, it is assumed that some of the iodine is saved for reuse. This salvaged iodine joins that absorbed form the gastrointestinal tract (GIT) in a common pool for use.

SPECTRUM OF IDD

As mentioned earlier some stages of life are affected adversely by the deficiency of iodine. There can be grouped as follows:

Fetus   : Abortions
Stillbirths
Congenital anomalies
Increased perinatal mortality
Increased infant mortality
Neurological cretinism
Myxoedematous cretinism
Psychomotor defects

Neonate : Neonate goiter
Neonate chemical hypothyroidism

Infancy : Goiter, thyroid deficiency (loss of energy)
Impaired school performance
Retarded physical development

Adults : Goiter with its complications
Hypothyroidism
Impaired mental functions.

Goiter

Goiter is a term applied for an enlargement of the thyroid gland, which, if is due to iodine deficiency is also termed endemic goiter. In this condition, the thyroxin level in the blood is lower than normal, which stimulates the thyroid gland to greater action, tending to cause it to enlarge as seen in Fig. 18.2.[3] This condition is characteristically associated with children. The rate of incidence of goiter increases with age and reaches the maximum level by adolescence. The prevalence rate is more among girls as compared to boys. A large percentage of children in a population could be

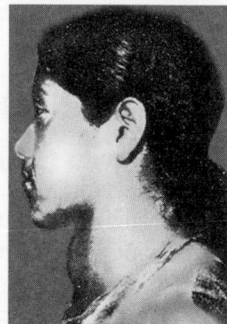

Fig. 18.2: A young woman showing endemic goiter
Source: Scrimshaw NS. Endemic goiter. Nutr Rev. 1957;15:161.

suffering from iodine deficiency leading to lethargy, which in the long run can cause irreparable losses due to fall in output in households and in the work place.

These can ultimately have its toll on high costs of medical and institutional care. Mental disability leads to poor school performance by children thus, producing long-term effects in their lives.[5]

Cretinism

Cretinism is a term used to denote severe iodine deficiency during intrauterine life. This includes a wide range of disorders like mental deficiency, deaf mutism and spastic paralysis of legs in varying degrees are associated with this condition. There are two types of cretinism which are known clinically:

1. Neurological cretinism: This involves mental retardation, deaf mutism, squint and spastic rigidity affecting the lower limbs.
2. Myxoedematous cretinism: In this condition, sings of hypothyroidism are observed, e.g. coarse, dry skin, swollen tongue, deep horse voice, apathy and mental deficiency. Signs like, sluggish bowel sounds and weak abdominal muscles may also be observed.

Hypothyroidism

This condition is characterized by signs like course dry skin, husky voice and delayed tendon reflexes.

Psychomotor Defects

Low or inadequate iodine levels in school children have shown poor scholastic performance and lower IQ levels, besides poor motor coordination.

Imparied Mental Function

Reduced mental functions have been observed in populations with low iodine levels. They have low intelligence levels and high degree of apathy which is evident by lack of initiative and decision making capacity in people.

ASSESSMENT OF IDD IN A COMMUNITY

The parameters helpful in assessing the extent of prevalence of IDD in a community can be gauged by a few simple signs and laboratory tests like:

- Prevalence of goiter
- Prevalence of cretinism
- Urinary iodine excretion
- Serum T4 levels
- Serum TSH levels
- Prevalence of neonatal chemical hypothyroidism
- Iodine levels in drinking water
- Iodine levels in the soil.

CLASSIFICATION OF IDD

Based on the severity of the problem, IDD has been graded into three categories as follows:

Mild IDD: When in an endemic area, urinary iodine level ranges from 5.0 to 9.99 µg/dL and goiter prevalence is 10–30%, it is considered as mild. At this stage mental and physical growth are not affected and the thyroid hormone levels too may be normal.

Moderate IDD: In moderate IDD, the median urinary iodine excretion level is 2.0–4.99 µg/dL and prevalence rate of goiter is about 20–50%. Thyroid hormone levels may be reduced with increased risk of hypothyroidism. Sings of cretinism however, may be absent.

Severe IDD: Areas with median urinary iodine levels of 2.0 µg/dL or less and goiter prevalence of 30–100% are considered to be severe. Here presence of marked hypothyroidism, mental retardation and cretinism are obvious.

CAUSES OF IDD (ANTITHYROID FACTORS)

Geoclimatic Factors

IDD occurs mainly due to geoclimatic factors. It is mainly the low content of soil which is responsible for the environmental iodine deficiency. This is particularly seen in hilly areas, where iodine content is lost due to years of washing of the soil by glaciers and heavy rains and in plains by recurrent flooding. These conditions tend to leech out the iodine from the soil which further result in lower levels of all vegetation grown in that soil. Deforestation and soil erosion add to compound the problem further.

Drugs

In Kerala, studies conducted by Kerala Agricultural University revealed that frequent consumptions of tapioca could be one reason for prevalence of goiter in that area. It is due to the presence of hydro-organic acid which blocks the uptake of iodine by thyroid causing gland (tapioca and goiter incidence of Kerala, 1998).[6]

A second group of drugs which appear to block thyroxin synthesis even in the presence of adequate iodine are thiourea, thiouracil, phenol derivatives and cobaltous chlorides.

Antithyroid Compounds in Foods

There are certain dietary factors which can inhibit the uptake of iodine. These are termed as 'goitergenic' due to the fact that they increase susceptibility to goiter resulting from iodine deficiency.

Cabbage is known to have an antithyroid compounds as also the seeds of most of the mustard family. The substance is known as goitrin.[7]

A precursor of goitrin, progoitrin is also present in the seeds of some plants and has been identified in plants like white turnips. Progotrin is active only when converted to goitrin. These compounds are not heat labile and hence, raw and cooked form both can be potentially goitrogenic. Continuous ingestion of small amounts of goitrin or other unidentified goitregens that may exist alter normal thyroid hormone synthesis. Polluted water with presence of *E. coli* tends to produce goitrogenic substances.[8] Organic chlorine insecticides widely used in agriculture can cause goiter. Endemic goiter is also found where sand stone type of soil which is rich in lime and calcium is present.[9]

Faulty cooking and dietary practices which reduce the bioavailability of iodine make Keralites prone to IDD.[6] Prevalence of more than 4% goiter in a given place indicates iodine deficiency in the soil and can contribute to deficiency in the foods grown in that place.

PREVENTION OF IDD

Dietary sources of iodine although exist, but are too small in amounts to present deficiency in endemic areas.

The WHO study group on endemic goiter in the early fifties had recommended that all food salts should be iodized compulsorily in any country or area where goiter is endemic, local variations in incidence of disease being disregarded.[10]

The easiest way of prevention of goiter in an endemic area is found to be fortification of food items with iodine or iodine supplementation.

IODINE FORTIFICATION

Fortification of salt has been the most successful way of preventing goiter. Other food items like wheat flour, methi, sugar or drinking water have also been practiced in different parts of the world.

The reason why salt has been widely used is due to the fact that it is universally consumed by all sections of the community irrespective of economic status and is consumed in the same level throughout the year. Production of salt is confined to a few production centers. By adding a dose of fixed iodine to salt at centralized locations, the majority of the population can have access to adequate amounts of iodine. The mixing of salt is simple with no adverse chemical reactions. Nor is there any change in color, taste or odor, besides being cost effective also.

Certain studies have shown that nonvegetarians have higher levels of iodine as compared to vegetarian though there are other reports which have not been consistent with these findings.[11]

Salt can be fortified either with potassium iodate or potassium iodide. Fortification with potassium iodide is more stable, hence commonly used. Daily consumption of 10 g of iodate salt (25 ppm of potassium iodate), provides about 150 µg of iodine. This level of fortified salt if used on regular basis can help prevent mild to moderate degree of deficiency disorders.

Certain Points to be Considered While Using Iodized Salt

* According to Nutrition Advisory Ministry of Family Welfare of the Govt. of India, the date of manufacturing should be stamped on salt packets, which must be moisture proof. This is done, since iodized salt needs to be consumed within one year of iodization. According to NIN Hyderabad, under standard conditions including transportation by rail or road, 25–30% of iodine is lost within 3 months and 40–60% within one year of iodization
* Salt should not be stored in open space or damp places and never beyond 6 months. It should be protected from moisture, sunlight and high temperature. Containers should be air tight and prevent from humidity in the air. The moisture content in the salt, humidity in the air, acidity of the salt and chemical form of iodine are important factors limiting the stability of iodine[12]
* Salt should be added to the food after cooking to reduce the loss of iodine. Addition of salt before cooking hastens the loss of other nutrients including iodine. Cooking losses and extent of absorption are some of the factors, which determine the availability of iodine to the body.

Noniodized salt has been banned in most of the states in the country. Therefore, only iodized salt alone should be used.

Iodized Oil Injections

Oil injections of iodine can provide iodine for 4 years but is used only in selected populations. But this practice had been strongly opposed by Goplan since thousands of disposable syringes would be used and a whole array of 'injectors'.[13]

Iodine Tablets

Although iodine tablets of 100–500 µg of potassium iodate are available for daily use, it is difficult to implement their use regularly and ensure its proper utilization regularly. Oral administration needs direct target contact therefore, their method has not been very popular.

Iodized Water

Fortification of water by iodine was introduced by Dr Rosaiuwanik of Bangkok. Since water is a daily necessity like salt, potassium iodate is added to the water stored in vessels for drinking purpose. However, again it had many limitations, like water consumed varies from day-to-day and season-to-season, the water may also not be totally safe for drinking if not stored hygienically. More over the iodine mixed in water may not be acceptable in taste and odor.[14]

IDD—THE INDIAN SCENARIO

IDD has been described as the world's single most significant causes of preventable brain damage and mental retardation. It affects about 14% of the world's population and 834 million people are affected by goiter.[15] The average goiter prevalence in Asia is about 7.3%.[16]

In India, estimate made in 1989 suggested that 150 million persons are at risk from IDD, 54 million people had goiter and 2.2 million people suffered from cretinism.[17] Table 18.1 gives an estimate of a total of 275 districts surveyed in the country in 1998, of which 235 have been found endemic for IDD.[18]

Table 18.1: Prevalence of iodine deficiency disorders in different states/ UTs of India			
State	Total number of districts	No. of districts surveyed	No. districts endemic
Andhra Pradesh	23	7	6
Arunachal Pradesh	10	10	10
Assam	18	18	18
Bihar	38	22	21
Goa	02	02	02
Gujarat	19	16	08
Haryana	16	09	08
Himachal Pradesh	12	10	10
Jammu and Kashmir	15	14	11
Karnataka	20	17	06
Kerala	14	14	11
Madhya Pradesh	45	16	16
Maharashtra	31	29	21
Mizoram	04	04	04
Manipur	08	08	08
Meghalaya	05	02	-
Nagaland	07	07	07
Orissa	30	02	02
Punjab	12	03	03
Rajastan	27	03	03
Sikkim	04	04	04
Tamil Nadu	21	12	12
Tripura	03	03	03
Uttar Pradesh	67	34	29

Source: Govt. of India, (NGCP) 1998.

Nearly 90,000 still births or neonatal deaths occur in India due to IDD. The Himalayan goiter belt is the worlds' greatest IDD affected area, and spread to 2400 km from Jammu in the North West and Kashmir to Manipur in the North East. As per estimate in 1997 no state in India was found to be IDD free.[19]

Biochemical hypothyroidism has been reported up to 10% among neonates in northern India.[20]

The National Goiter Control Program (NGCP) which was initiated in 1962 by the Government of India, to survey the magnitude of this problem was redesignated as National Iodine Deficiency Disorder Control Program (NIDDCP) in 1992. In 1996, the WHO declared 90% iodization of edible salt in its member countries.

The objective of this project was to reduce the prevalence of goiter in the age groups of 10–14 years to less than 5% and to bring down to zero, the number of cretin born by the year 2000. It was aimed to provide iodized salt to 100% population by strengthening the monitoring system from production to consumption level.[21]

The effects and benefits of iodine intervention indicated were as follows in Table 18.2.

Table 18.2: Effects and benefits of iodine intervention

Effects	Benefits
Reductions in: 1. Mental deficiency 2. Deaf mutism 3. Spastic diplegia	1. Higher work output in the household and in work place 2. Reduced cost of medical care and custodial care 3. Reduced education. Cost from reduced absenteeism and grade repetition and higher academic achievement by students
4. Squint 5. Dwarfism 6. Motor deficiency	

DIETARY SOURCES OF IODINE

Iodine content from dietary sources depends to a large extent on the soil and fertilizer conditions from soil of one region to that of another. Marine or deep-sea fish and shellfish are high in iodine content. Sea water contain about 0.05 mg/L (0.05 ppm) of iodine. People consuming sea weed which is grown along the coastal areas can get adequate quantities of iodine.

The leaves and flower of plants (spinach, turnip green and broccoli) appear to have higher iodine concentration than the root vegetables.

Drinking water provides about 10%, and about 90% comes from the food consumed depending upon the soil on which the crop is produced.

Although fish is rich in iodine, but since the thyroid gland which is rich in it, is located in the head, it is of little value if the head part of the fish is discarded. Sea salt is also considered rich in iodine, containing 0.28 ppm of iodine.[22]

REFERENCES

1. Hetzel BS. Iodine deficiency disorders (IDD) and their eradication. Lancet. 1983;11:1126.
2. Brahmam GNV. Iodine deficiency disorders. In: Textbook of Nutrition, Eds. Bamji MS, Prahlad Rao N, Reddy V. New Delhi: Oxford & IBH Publishing Co. Pvt. Ltd; 1996. pp.278-86.
3. Scrimshaw NS. Endemic goiter, Nutr Rev. 1957;15:161.
4. World Health Organization 1998, Iodine deficiency Disorders. In: J Trop Pediatr. 1998;44(5):270-4.
5. Jayakrishna T, Jeeja MC. Iodine deficiency disorders in school children in Kannur Dist. (2002), Kerala Research Level Development Center for Development Studies, Thiruvanthapuram. Iodine deficiency disorders in school children in Kannur Dist. (2002), Kerala Research Level Development Center for Development Studies, Thiruvanthapuram.
6. Kerala Sastra Sahihtya Parishat, Keralathile Samakaika Arogya Prasnangal. KSSP, 1998.
7. Greece MA. The significance of naturally occurring antithyroid compounds in the production of goiter in man. Border's Rev Nutr Res. 1960;21:61.
8. Kulkarni AP, Bharath JP. Textbook of Community Medicine. 1998.
9. Mahajan BK, Gupta MC. Textbook of Preventive and Social Medicine. New Delhi: Jaypee Brothers; 1995.
10. WHO Study Group on Endemic Goiter. Bull Wrld Hlth Orgn. 1953;9:293.
11. Remer T, Neubert A, Manz F. Increased risk of iodine deficiency with vegetarian nutrition. Br J Nutr. 1999;81(1).
12. Narsingha Rao BS. Fortification of salt with iron and iodine to control anemia and goiter: Development of a new formula with good stability and bioavailability of iron and iodine, National Institute of Nutrition, ICMR Bulletin 1996, Hyderabad.
13. Gopalan C. Micro nutrient malnutrition, SAARC. The need for food based approach. Nutrition Foundation of India (NFI) Bull, 1998, New Delhi.
14. Dunn JT. Iodine supplementation and the prevention of cretinism. Annals of the New York Academy of Sciences. 1993;678(1):158-68.
15. World Health Organization Report,1998,1999.
16. World Health Organisation,1985; Iodine Deficiency Disorders in South East Asia, WHO/SEARO Regional Health papers, No. 10, WHO, New Delhi.
17. Kochupillai N. Organisation and Implementation of neo natal hypothyroid screening program in India. A primary health care approach. Ind J Ped. 1985;52:223.
18. Government of India, National Iodine Deficiency Control Program. Ministry of Family Welfare. 1998.
19. Park K. Textbook of Preventive and Social Medicine, 1997, Bonarside's Bhanot Publishers.
20. Kochupillai N, Pandav CS. Neonatal chemical hypothyroidism in iodine deficient environments. In: The Prevention and Control of Iodine Deficiency Disorders. Hetzel BS, Dunn JT, Stanbury JB (Eds). Amsterdam: Elsevier.
21. International Council for Control of iodine deficiency disorders (ICCIDD), Proposed guidelines for assessment of progress towards IDD elimination. IDD Newsletter. 1995;1192:19.
22. Pandav CS, David P, Hunton, Viswanathan H. Partnership to end hidden hunger, Collaboration of the stakeholders in sustaining elimination of iodine deficiency disorders. SOS a Billion 1997.

Role of Other Micronutrients in Children

POTASSIUM

Potassium in the human body constitutes almost 98% within the cells, most of which is in the skeletal muscle. After calcium and phosphorous, it is the third most common mineral in the body.[1] It is involved in many body processes like fluid balance, protein synthesis, nerve conduction, energy production, muscle contraction, synthesis of nucleic acids and control of heart beat. In many of its roles, potassium is opposed by sodium and the two positive ions are jointly balanced by the negative ion chloride.

Functions

Potassium has an important role in various functions:
- It plays an important role in energy production in the cells in the body
- It helps maintain blood pressure at normal levels
- Essential for protein and nucleic acid synthesis
- Maintains fluid balance
- Involved in normal nerve function—Nerve transmission, muscle contraction and hormone secretion from endocrine glands
- Converts glucose into glycogen (muscle fuel)
- It is involved in kidney functions
- It helps in elimination of carbon dioxide from lungs
- It helps in maintaining acid/alkali balance
- It helps in rhythmic contractions of the heart muscle.

Potassium Deficiency

Deficiency of potassium can lead to fatigue and muscle weakness. Severe potassium deficiency can lead to electrolyte imbalance affecting all muscles, nerves and many other body functions. The main risks of potassium deficiency are as follows:
- Diarrhea/vomiting, e.g. in inflammatory bowel disease

- Chronic renal failure sharply increases potassium excretion
- Change in body pH (metabolic acidosis/alkalosis)
- Many diuretics may increase potassium losses in urine leading to depletion of the mineral
- Deficiency of magnesium also can contribute to depletion of body stores of potassium.

Signs and Symptoms of Potassium Deficiency

Deficiency of potassium may manifest in the form of any of the following signs and symptoms:
- Fatigue, lethargy
- Delayed gastric emptying
- Decreased blood pressure
- Muscle weakness
- Constipation
- Cardiac arrhythmias.

Certain factors can lead to increased potassium accretion like
- Sweating can account for loss of almost 3 g/d
- Vomiting
- Diarrhea.

Potassium is excreted mainly by the kidneys. In renal disorders, potassium may be reduced which can lead to toxicity.

Requirements

The recommended dietary allowance (RDA) as per ICMR, 2010, for infants and children which are considered as safe and adequate is as given in Table 19.1.[2]

Sources of Potassium

Plant foods are the major dietary sources of potassium. In fact they contain more potassium as compared to sodium. Good sources are cereals, pulses, fruits, green leafy vegetables, nuts and oilseeds. A normal mixed diet can provide approximately 4–7.5 g of potassium per day. Processed foods are poor sources of potassium due to its being leached out during the processing.[2]

Table 19.1: RDA for potassium in infants and children	
Age group (years)	mg/d (potassium chloride, g)
0–0.5	350–925 (1.8)
0.5–1	475–1275 (2.5)
1–3	550–1650 (3.2)
4–6	775–2325 (4.5)

Refer. ICMR, 2010

CALCIUM

The role of calcium in a growing child cannot be over stressed. Maintaining adequate levels of calcium during childhood is essential for the development of a maximum peak bone mass, which has future implications in adulthood by reducing the risk of osteoporosis.[3]

In children with chronic illnesses, fracture may occur during childhood secondary to mineral deficiency associated with the disease process or the effects of therapeutic interventions (e.g. corticosteroids) on calcium metabolism.[4]

Functions of Calcium

Bone and tooth structure: Calcium with phosphorous forms hydroxyapatite crystals which give strength and rigidity to the bones and tooth enamel: 99% of the calcium in the body is in the skeleton.[5]

Blood clotting: Calcium is an important component of the blood coagulation cascade.

Muscle contraction: In skeletal and heart muscles cell, calcium is an intercellular messenger that triggers contraction of the muscle fibers.

Nerve transmission: Calcium plays a vital role in nerve cells through depolarization of membranes and nerve transmission.

Risk Factors of Calcium Deficiency

Low levels of calcium in children over a prolonged period can lead to various long-term problems like:
- Demineralization of the skeleton and increased risk of osteoporosis, resulting in poor mobilization from skeleton to maintain adequate circulating levels
- Chronic use of certain drugs like antacids, laxatives, steroids, etc. produce a negative calcium balance by decreasing absorption and increasing excretion
- Gastrointestinal disorders like malabsorption drastically decreases fat absorption which inturn decreases the bioavailability of calcium from dietary sources, making it unavailable for absorption from the diet. Vitamin D deficiency especially in dark winter months, reduces absorption of calcium from the diet
- The common signs and symptoms of calcium deficiency are summarized in Table 19.2.

Role in Infants

Premature infants have higher calcium requirements than full-term infants. These may be met by using human milk fortifier (HMF) with additional minerals or with specially designed formula for premature infants,[6] while in

Table 19.2: Signs and symptoms of calcium deficiency[3]

- Osteoporosis
- Dental caries with poor quality enamel
- Muscle cramping and spasm
- Increased irritability of nerve cells
- Abnormal blood clotting and increased bleeding after trauma

the hospital. On discharge, also, it is advised to provide formula fed premature infant formula with higher concentration than those of routine cow's milk-based formula.

The optimum primary nutritional source of calcium during the first year of life is human milk. It has been demonstrated that the bioavailability of calcium from human milk is relatively greater than that from infant formula or cow's milk. It is therefore considered justifiable to increase the concentration of calcium in all infant formulae like soya and casein hydrolysates, to account for the potential lower biovailability of the calcium from these formula relative to cow's milk-based formula.

Role in Children

Calcium retention is relatively low in toddlers and gradually increases with approach of puberty. It is observed that calcium intake levels of 800 mg/d are associated with adequate bone mineral accumulation in prepubertal children. It is important that children be encouraged to develop eating patterns that will be associated with adequate calcium intake later in life.

Role in Preadolescence and Adolescence

There is enough data to show that efficiency of calcium absorption is increased during puberty and the majority of bone formation occurs during this stage. An intake of 1200–1500 mg/d is shown to achieve maximal net calcium balance and intakes beyond this level is excreted and hence, wasted. Studies have shown that supplementing calcium only for a short duration of say 1–2 years, may not exert long-term benefits in establishing and maintaining a maximum peak bone mass.[7] This emphasizes the importance of diet in achieving adequate intake and in establishing dietary patterns consistent with a calcium intake near recommended levels throughout childhood and adolescence.

Calcium Requirements

The calcium requirements for children of various age groups and sexes are as shown in Table 19.3.[8]

Dietary Sources of Calcium

Milk is one of the richest sources of calcium which is bioavailable. In general, calcium bioavailability from milk products and most calcium supplements

Table 19.3: Calcium requirements of infants and children

Category	Age (years)	Calcium (mg/d)*
Children	1–3	600
	4–6	600
	7–9	600
Boys/Girls	10–12	800
	13–15	800
Boys/ Girls	16–17	800

*A minimum of 200 mL/d of milk is essential to maintain this level on a cereal legume diet
Source: ICMR, 2010.[6]

is approximately 25–35%. Calcium from plant sources tends to be less bioavailable due to the presence of fiber, phytic acid and oxalates. But milk also being a good source of protein, phosphorous and sodium, there is a tendency of increased losses from the body as these are known to increase losses. Other dietary sources are ragi among cereals, legumes (gram, soybean), green leafy vegetables, certain nuts and oilseeds, dry fruits. Factors which could inhibit calcium absorption from dietary sources are as follows:

• Protein intake >20% total calories
• Phosphorous (milk products, meat, colas)
• Phytic acid (whole grains)
• Sodium
• Coffee and black tea.

For children who are lactose intolerant or allergic to milk, other alternatives need to be considered, like soya-based milk, tofu and other products. In case of children who are mildly lactose intolerant, a combination of milk with cereal or yoghurt can be attempted as it is known that the lactose load or concentration in the diet can also influence the tolerance.

Children may not always be inclined to consume milk in which case parents can try to incorporate more calcium in their diets by:

• Making custard, pudding, rice kheer, etc.
• Adding milk to cooked cereal, soups and gravies
• Making a smoothie with milk and fruit
• Altering the flavors by adding strawberry, chocolate or making eggnog, cocoa, milkshakes, etc.

MAGNESIUM

Magnesium is an essential mineral for human nutrition, and serves several important metabolic functions:

• It plays a role in the production and transport of energy. The breakdown and oxidation of glucose, fat and proteins all require magnesium-dependent enzymes[9]
• It regulates calcium triggered contraction of heart and muscle cells and is a physiologic calcium channel blocker

- It has a preventive role in management of hypertension by causing vasodilation of the coronary and peripheral arteries
- In combination with calcium and phosphorous, it is important for the structure of the bones and teeth
- It is involved in the synthesis of nucleic acids and proteins (cell reproduction)
- It can help prevent kidney and gall stones by its effect on calcium levels
- It is also known to have a role in prevention of diabetes mellitus.

Deficiency of Magnesium

- Magnesium deficiency can be caused by a lack of magnesium in the diet, by an excess of calcium or by other factors which may increase excretion or limit absorption
- Athletes and children involved in sports activities and doing strenuous activities have increased requirements[10]
- Intestinal malabsorptive conditions like chronic diarrheas, pancreatic diseases, etc. tend to reduce absorption of dietary magnesium
- Certain drugs or medicines can inhibit magnesium absorption by way of increased retention like diuretics, laxatives and chemotherapy.

Signs and Symptoms of Magnesium Deficiency

Magnesium can manifest in the form of following signs and symptoms:
- Muscle cramps and spasms, trembling
- Increased potassium and calcium losses leading to hypocalcemia and hypokalemia
- Fatigue, tiredness
- Anorexia, vomiting and nausea
- Sodium and water retention
- Impaired action of vitamin D
- Anemia
- Hypoglycemia
- Childhood hyperactivity (attention deficit behavior).
  The above deficiencies could be due to either low intake or as a result of increased absorption or decreased absorption.

Requirements

The recommended dietary allowances (RDA) as laid down by Indian Council of Medical Research (ICMR), 2010 for magnesium in children are as given in Table 19.4.[3]

Dietary Sources of Magnesium

The main dietary sources of magnesium are nuts and seeds like peanuts, almonds, raisins, seafoods like habitude, legumes and wheat cereals.

Table 19.4: RDA for magnesium in children

Group	Age	mg/kg/d	mg/d
Infants	0–6 months	6.0	30
	6–12 months	5.5	45
Children	1–3 years	4.0	50
	4–6 years	4.0	70
	7–9 years	4.0	100
Boys	10–12 years	3.5	120
Girls	10–12 years	4.5	160
Boys	13–15 years	3.5	165
Girls	13–15 years	4.5	210
Boys	16–17 years	3.5	195
Girls	16–17 years	4.5	235

Source: ICMR 2010.

VITAMIN D

Vitamin D is the only vitamin whose biologically active form is a hormone. The term 'vitamin D' refers to a family of related compounds. It is a fat-soluble vitamin that is naturally present in very few foods. It is also produced endogenously when ultraviolet rays from sunlight strike the skin and trigger vitamin D synthesis. Therefore, exposure to Sun for sometime is recommended to meet the requirements. However, it is biologically inert and has to undergo two hydroxylations in the body for activation. The first occurs in the liver and converts vitamin D to 25 hydroxy vitamin D [25(OH)D] also termed as 'calcidol'. The second occurs in the kidney and forms the physiologically active 1, 25, dihydroxy vitamin D also termed as 'calcitriol'.[11]

Functions of Vitamin D

Calcium regulation: It promotes calcium absorption in the gut and maintains adequate serum calcium phosphate concentration, thereby enabling mineralization of bone and also prevent condition of hypocalcemic tetany. A fall in blood calcium will trigger production of active vitamin D which will then stimulate calcium absorption from the diet, increases release of calcium from the bone and slows renal excretion.

Skeletal health : It is essential for normal bone growth during childhood and for maintaining bone density and strength during adulthood. Adequate levels of vitamin D in children helps prevent deficiency states like rickets in children and osteomalacia in adults.[11]

Cell growth and development: Vitamin D has an important role in the body including modulation of cell growth, neuromuscular and immune functions and reducing inflammatory conditions.[11-13] Many genes encoding proteins that regulate cell proliferation, differentiation and apoptosis are modulated in part by vitamin D.[11]

Immune system: Vitamin D enhances the activity and immune response to white blood cells in the body and therefore, also considered to play a role in prevention of cancers in the body.

Vitamin D Deficiency

Deficiency of vitamin D can occur consequent to dietary inadequacy, impaired absorption and use, increased requirement or increased excretion. Rickets and osteomalacia are classical vitamin D deficiency states. In children, vitamin D deficiency causes rickets, characterized by failure of bone tissue to mineralize adequately resulting in soft bones and skeletal deformities.[14] Prolonged exclusive breastfeeding without any vitamin D supplements is a significant cause of deficiency in children, especially in dark-skinned infants breastfed by mothers with low levels of vitamin D.[14]

Some common signs and symptoms of deficiency of the vitamin in children are listed in Table 19.5.[14]

Deficiency of vitamin D can be assessed using serum concentrations as given in Table 19.6.[15]

Requirements of Vitamin D

The recommendation of 400 IU (10 µg) as a daily supplement (only under situations of minimal exposure to sunlight) has been made by the Expert Group Committee.[15] In view of the increasing trend of limited outdoor physical activity by children leading to inadequate exposure to sunlight and obesity, it was felt that outdoor physical activity is the best means of achieving both adequate vitamin D status and controlling overweight and obesity in the population. Increasing the recommended daily intake was not a solution, neither food

Table 19.5: Signs and symptoms of deficiency of vitamin D[14]

Children	Adolescents
• Delayed growth and development (delayed crawling and walking) • Irritability and restlessness • Rickets: Softening of bones, spinal deformities • Bowed legs and knock knees, enlargement of rib sternum joints • Delayed tooth eruption and poorly formed tooth enamel • Impaired immune response with increased risk of infection	• Impaired growth of bones and musculature • Swelling and pain at the end of long bones, especially the knees • Impaired immune response with increased risk of infection

Table 19.6: Serum 25 hydroxyvitamin D concentrations as in health[14]

ng/mL*	Health status
<12	Associated with vitamin D deficiency leading to rickets in infants and children and osteomalacia in adults
12–20	Generally considered inadequate for bone and overall health in healthy individuals
≥20	Generally considered inadequate for bone and overall health in healthy individuals
>50	Emerging evidence links potential adverse effects to such high level, especially >150

*Serum concentrations of vitamin D are reported in nanograms/mL

supply can be considered as a substitute for the vitamin D available from exposure to sunlight.

Sources of Vitamin D

Food: Dietary sources of vitamin D are limited. Fish liver oil and flesh of certain fish, like salmon, tuna and mackerel. Liver, cheese and egg yolk also contain small amounts of the vitamin D. Dairy milk as also certain oils are fortified with vitamin D.

Sunlight: Exposure to sunlight is one of the commonest sources of vitamin D.[11] Ultraviolet (UV) B radiation with a wavelength of 290–320 nanometers penetrates the skin and converts cutanous 7 dehydrocholesterol to previtamin D3 which in turn becomes vitamin D3.[11] It is suggested that approximately 25–30 minutes of exposure between 10 am to 3 pm at least twice a week to the face, legs, arms and back without sunscreen usually can provide adequate synthesis of the vitamin.[12]

REFERENCES

Potassium

1. Luft K. Potassium and its regulation. In: Ziegler EE, Filer LJ (Eds). Present knowledge in Nutrition. 7th edn. Washington DC: ILSI Press; 1996.
2. ICMR. Nutrient Requirements and Recommended Dietary Allowances for Indians. A Report of the Expert Group of the Indian Council of Medical Research. 2010.

Calcium in Children

3. Institute of Medicine, Food and Nutrition Board National Research council. Recommended dietary reference intakes for calcium, phosphorous, magnesium, vitamin D and fluoride. Washington DC: National Academy Press; 1977.
4. Abrams SA. Studies of calcium metabolism in children with chronic illnesses. In: Wastney Me, Siva Subramanian KN (Eds). Kinetic models of trace element

and mineral metabolism during development. Boca Raton FL: CRC Press; 1995. pp.159-70.

5. Weaver CM, Heaney RP. Calcium. In: Shills ME, Olson JA, Shike M, Ross AC (Eds). Modern nutrition in Health and Disease. Baltimore: Williams and Wilkins; 1999.

6. Schanler RJ, Abrams SA. Postnatal intrauterine macromineral accretion rates in low birth weight infants fed HMF. J Pediatr. 1995;126:441-7.

7. Lee WT, Leung SS, Leung DM, et al. A follow-up study on the effects of calcium supplement withdrawl and puberty on bone acquisition of children. Am J Clin Nutr. 1996;64:71-7.

8. Indian Council of Medical Research. Nutrient Requirements and recommended Dietary Allowances for Indians. A report of the Expert Group of the Indian Council of Medical Research. 2010.

Magnesium in Children

9. Shils M. Magnesium. In: Ziegler EE, Filer LJ, et al. (Eds). Present knowledge in nutrition. 7th ed. Washington DC: ICSI Press; 1996.

10. Clarkson PM. Minerals: Exercise performance and supplements in atheletes. J Sports Sci. 1991;9:91.

Vitamin D

11. Institute of Medicine, Food and Nutrition Board. Reference intakes for calcium and vitamin D. Washington DC: National Academy Press; 2010.

12. Holik MF. Vitamin D In: Shils ME, Shike M, Ross AC, Callabero B (Eds). Modern Nutrition in Health and Disease, 10th edn. Philadelphia: Lippincott: Williams and Wilkins; 2006.

13. Norman AW, Henry HH. Vitamin D. In: Bowman BA, Russel RM (Eds). Present knowledge in nutrition. 9th edn. Washington DC: ISLI Press; 2006.

14. Wharton B, Bishop N. Rickets. Lancet. 2003;47:107-13 (PubMed abstract).

15. Nutrient Requirements and Recommended Dietary allowances for Indians; A Report of the Expert Group of the Indian Council of Medical Research. ICMR. 2010.

Probiotics—Role in Child Health

INTRODUCTION

The role of probiotics is generally considered as a functional food capable of altering or modifying the gut flora for beneficial effects in the human gut. The origin of use of probiotics, dates back to the 20th century, when it was first introduced by a Russian scientist and Nobel laureate Elj Metcnikoff, who suggested its possible role in modifying the gut flora by replacing harmful microbes with useful ones.[1] He suggested that the aging process results from the activity of putrefactive microbes, producing toxic substances in the large bowel. He attributed this effect to 'intestinal autointoxication' which caused the physical changes associated with old age.

The practice of fermenting milk with lactic acid bacteria (to inhibit the growth of proteolytic bacteria due to the low pH produced by fermentation of lactose) was prevalent in that era too in certain rural populations of Europe, e.g. Bulgaria and Russia. People who lived largely on milk fermented by this process also had an exceptionally long life. Based on this theory it was proposed that consumption of 'fermented milk' would 'seed' the intestine with harmless lactic acid bacteria and decrease the intestinal pH, which would further suppress the growth of proteolytic bacteria. This 'sour' milk was consumed by Methnikoff himself which called 'Bulgarian bacillus' and found that his health benefited.

The term probiotic was first introduced in 1953, by Kollath, which was described as microbially derived factors that stimulate growth of other microorganisms.[2] The definition used widely now was suggested by Roy Fuller in 1989, which is 'a live microbial food supplement which beneficially affects the host animal by improving its intestinal microbial balance.'[3] On the other hand, another term 'prebiotic' is also used which is described as nonabsorbable food components that beneficially stimulate one or more of the gut beneficial microbial groups and thus, have a beneficial effect on human health.[4]

The most commonly used prebiotics are carbohydrate substrates, e.g. dietary fiber, which has the ability to promote the components of the normal intestinal microflora which may evince a health benefit to the host.

Table 20.1: Definitions[2-4]

Probiotics	A live microbial food ingredient which is beneficial to health
Prebiotics	A nondigestible food ingredient which beneficially affects the host by selectively stimulating the number of bacteria in the colon having the potential to improve host health
Synbiotic	A mixture of pre- and probiotics which beneficially affects the host by improving the survival and implantation of live microbial dietary supplements in the gastrointestinal tract (GIT), thereby improving host health and well being

When probiotics and prebiotics are administered in combination, it is termed as 'synbiotics'. The combined effect has a definitive benefit by synergestic action (Table 20.1).

SOURCE OF PROBIOTICS

The microbiota of a newborn develops rapidly after birth. It is initially dependent on the mother's microbiota, mode of delivery, birth environment and rarely genetic factors.[5,6] The maternal vaginal and intestinal flora constitutes the source of bacteria, which colonizes the intestine of the newborn, the dominative strains being facultative anaerobes like the enterobacteria, coliforms and lactobacilli. By the time the child is weaned, the microflora alters gradually and begins to resemble that of an adult. Although there are almost 500 different microbial species in the GIT, the ones with beneficial properties include mainly bifidobacteria and lactobacilli. Others include bacteroides, *Clostridium*, *Bifidobacterium*, *Escherichia* and *Veillonella*. The initial compositional development of the gut microflora is considered a key determinant in the development of normal gut barrier functions.[7]

Intestinal mucosal defense mechanisms acting in the lumen and mucosa restrict colonization by pathogenic bacteria by interfering with the adherence of microorganisms to the mucosal surface. The normal gut microbiota can prevent the overgrowth of potential pathogens in the GIT.

PROBIOTICS—CRITERIA

For organisms to be considered as probiotic the criteria needed to be fulfilled are as follows:[8]
- Should be isolated from the same species as its intended host
- Should have a demonstrable beneficial effect on the host
- Should be nonpathogenic
- Should be able to survive transit through the GIT
- On storage, large number of viable bacteria must be able to survive prolonged periods.

MECHANISM OF ACTION

The mechanism of the beneficial effects of probiotics is broadly based on:

1. Those arising from colonization and inhibition of pathogenic bacteria.
2. Those effects which arise from enhancement of the host immune response and intestinal barrier function.
3. Those which suppress growth or epithelial binding/invasion by pathogenic bacteria and production of antimicrobial substances.
4. Those which control transfer of dietary antigen.
5. Those which stimulate mucosal and systemic host immunity.

There are known to be more than 400 bacterial species, both resident microbiota as well as a variable number of transient species existing in any given specific region of the intestine. The intestinal bacteria are controlled by the epithelial cells which form a physical barrier and are also capable of discriminating between resident flora and enteric pathogens. Specific glycoconjugates are released by the epithelium in response to the presence of bacteria which act as receptors for the attachment of bacteria. The intestinal epithelium completely inihibits the adherence of pathogens by increased production of bacteriocins, hydrogen peroxide, biosurfactants, mucin and defensin-β 2, an antimicrobial peptide. This antagonism of the pathogenic bacteria are most effective when the probiotic themselves adhere to the intestinal epithelium. The number of viable bacteria colonizing the intestine depends on factors like:

- Probiotic formulation
- Coadministration with food or milk
- Gastric pH
- Intestinal motility
- Composition of intestinal microbiota.

Probiotics are also known to modulate cytokine release from cells of the GIT, thereby providing immunity. By its interaction with epithelial cells, T cells and dendritic cells of the gut, produce anti-inflammatory and immune regulatory effects.

The action of one probiotic is also affected by the presence of another strain of probiotic and they also exhibit host specific and strain specific difference in action, ability to colonise the gut and clinical efficacy.[9]

The prebiotic acts as an alternative for probiotics or their cofactors. Complex carbohydrates pass through the lower gastrointestine where that become available for some colonic bacteria, but are not utilized by the majority of bacteria present in the colon. The commonly used prebiotics in human nutrition are galacto-oligosaccharides, fructo-oligosaccharides, inulin and its hydrolysates, malto-oligosaccharides and resistant starch.[8] Figure 20.1 presents the concept of synergistic mechanism of pre- and probiotics.

The probiotics have the ability to dampen inflammation of the gut which may require anti-inflammatory mediators. Chronic diseases like allergies and other autoimmune and inflammatory diseases are known to benefit

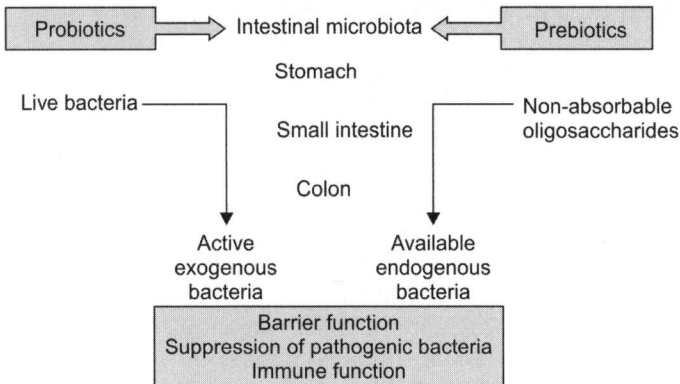

Fig. 20.1: The probiotic and prebiotic concepts: Altering the composition of intestinal microbiota by viable bacterial supplements versus nonabsorbable bacterial substrates[8]

from probiotics. The rationale of probiotic therapy involves normalization of the properties of unbalanced indigenous microflora by specific strains of the healthy gut microflora.[8]

CLINICAL USES

In Infants

It is well known that breastfeeding has a protective role in preventing infectious diseases which is done by multiple mechanisms. It is believed that there are certain components in breast milk which can modulate the composition of intestinal flora amongst which bifidobacteria comprise a significant number in the normal intestinal flora in breastfed infants.[10]

It is postulated that a combination of increased bifidobacterial counts and decreased concentration of other enterobacteria and luminal host factors may play a role in protecting premature babies and newborns from diarrheal diseases.[8]

Necrotising enterocolitis is one of the common devastating intestinal diarrhea occurring in 10–25% of the premature infants and very low birth babies with a mortality of 20–30%. Babies given supplements of lactobacillus GG daily is known to show reduction of this entity in some trials, which suggest a co-relation between the reduction of lactobacilli and the increased risk of necrotizing enterocolitis.[11,12]

Diarrheal Diseases

Infective diarrhea: Acute infantile diarrhea due to rotavirus is the most common type of diarrhea encountered in infants worldwide for which oral rehydration solution (ORS) is the primary treatment. A systematic review of the results of various trials has revealed an overall reduction in the duration of diarrhea by 17–30 hours.[13-15]

Traveler's diarrhea: Travelers visiting high-risk areas are prone to have acute episode of diarrhea, though most of them are self limiting. Several studies using probiotics (*Saccharomyces boulardii*) for treating such diarrhea confirmed a significant beneficial effect on the duration of the diarrhea.[16,17] It is observed that *S. boulardi* which is more effective on bacterial diarrhea compared to lactobacillus GG (LGG) has proven to be more beneficial in viral or idiopathic bacteria.

Allergy

Atopic disease, a manifestation of food hypersensitivities is generally due to the intestinal microflora which contributes to the processing of food antigens in the gut. It is believed that probiotics have a role in modifying the structure of potential antigens, reducing the intestinal permeability and the generation of proinflammatory cytokines that are elevated in patients with a variety of allergic disorders.[8]

A number of studies have evaluated the efficacy of probiotics in allergenic conditions like rhinitis, atopic dermatitis and food allergy in children, which are promising but their definitive role in any of these conditions is still not clear.[18,19]

Lactose Intolerance

Probiotics have been shown to have a positive role in the management of lactose intolerance, a condition widely prevalent in various sections of the population. The effect is observed by its action on lactose digestion by reducing the symptoms of intolerance and also slowly orocecal transit.[20]

The mechanism involved is that during fermentation the pathogenic bacteria, e.g. *Lactobacillus* (e.g. *L. bulgaricus*) and *Streptococcus thermophilus* produce lactase, which hydrolyses the lactose in dairy products to glucose or galactose. Their effect exerted on the lactase activity in vivo in the gut lumen facilitates digestion and decreases intolerance; this phenomenon has been demonstrated in children and adults.[21,22]

There are other clinical uses of probiotics, e.g. in prevention of colon cancer, pouchitis, liver disease and sepsis, all of which are more applicable in adults, rather than in children.

Probiotic Food Supplements

Probiotics in the form of food are widely available, some of which are as follows:
- Live yoghurts containing *Lactobacillus*, *Streptococcus*, etc.
- Ferments dairy products
- Cheese
- Freeze-dried supplements
- Fruit juices

- Infant weaning foods
- Jelly
- Fructooligosaccharides as biscuits and powdered chocolate drinks.

DISADVANTAGES OF PROBIOTICS

Despite their benefits, probiotics have not proven beneficial in some conditions in various trials. In case of childhood allergies, a trial designed to show the effectiveness of probiotics, in fact showed that the group given the good bacteria were more likely to develop sensitivity to allergens. There are reports indicating that yogurt could be a possible cause for obesity, but this theory was contested on the ground that the obesity could be linked to the dairy products which may be high fat rather than the yoghurt per se. There is a possible risk of antibiotic resistance transfer by the use of probiotics to more pathogenic bacteria. Some strains of lactobacillus were found to be resistant to vancomycin, which can be of serious concern. Almost 68.4% of the isolates have been found to be resistant against multiple antibiotics.[9]

REFERENCES

1. Metchnikoff E. Essais optimists. Paris. The prolongation of life. Optimistic Studies. Translated and edited by P. Chalmers Mitchell. London. Heineman. 1907.
2. Hamilton—Miller JM. The role of probiotics in the treatment and prevention of *H. pylori* infection. Int J Antimicrobial Agents. 2003;22(4):360-6.
3. Fuller R. Probiotics in man and animals. J Appl Bactriology. 1989;66(5):365-78.
4. Gibson GR, Roberfroid MB. Dietary modulation of the human colonic microflora: introducing the concept of prebiotics. J Nutr. 1995;125:1401-12.
5. Fravier CF, Vaughan EE, De Vos WM, et al. Molecular monitoring of succession of bacterial communities in human neonates. Appl Environ Microbiol. 2002;68(1):219-26.
6. Bennot Y, Mitsuoka T. Development of intestinal microflora in human and animals. Bifidobacteria Microflora. 1986;5:13-25.
7. Hooper LV, Wong MH, Thelin A, et al. Molecular analysis of commensal host microbial relationships in the intestine. Science. 2001;291:881-4.
8. Harish K, Verghase T. Probiotics in humans – evidence based review. Calicut Med J. 2006;(4):e 3.
9. Kumar K. Probiotics In: Basics of Clinical Nutrition, 2nd Edn. Ed Joshi YK. New Delhi: Jaypee publishers; 2008.pp.397-403.
10. Yoshita M, Fujita K, Sakata H. Development of the normal intestinal flora and its clinical significance in infants and children. Bifido Microflora. 1991;10:11-27.
11. Sticker T, Braegger CP. Oral probiotics prevent necrotizing enterocolitis. J Pediatr Gastroenterol Nutr. 2006;42:446-7.
12. Hoyos AB. Reduced incidence of necrotizing enterocolitis associated with enteral administration of *Lactobacillus acidophilus* and bifidobacterium in infants to neonates in an intensive care unit. Int J Infect Dis. 1999;3:197-202.
13. Allen SJ, Okoko B, Martinez E, et al. Probiotics for treating infectious diarrhea. Cochrane Database Syst Rev. 2004;2:CD003048.
14. Szajewska H, Mrukowiez JZ. Probiotics in the treatment and prevention of acute infectious diarrhea in infants and children: a systematic review of published

randomized, double blind placebo controlled trials. J Pediatr Gastroenetrol Nutr. 2001;33(2):S17.

15. Van Neil CW, Feudtners C, Garrison MM, et al. Lactobacillus therapy for acute infectious diarrhea in children: a meta analysis. Pediatrics. 2002;109:678.

16. Katelaris PH, Salam I, Farthing MJ. Lactobacilli to prevent traveler's diarrhea. N Engl J Med. 1995;333:1360-1.

17. Bleichener G, Blehaut H, Mentec H, et al. *Sacchromyces boulardii* prevents diarrhea in critically ill tube fed patients. A multi centre, randomized, double blind placebo controlled trial. Intens Care Med. 1997;23:517-23.

18. Miralgia del Giudice M, De Luca MG. The role of probiotics in the clinical management of food allergy and atopic dermatitis. J Clin Gastroenterol. 2004;38:S84-5.

19. Isolauri E, Arvola T, Sutas Y, et al. Probiotics in the management of atopic eczema. Clin Exp Allergy. 2002;30:1604-10.

20. Sandres ME. Summary of the conclusions from a consensus panel of experts on health attributes on lactic cultures: significance to fluid milk products containing cultures. J Dairy Sci. 1993;76:1819-28.

21. Saltzman JR, Russel RM, Golner B, et al. A randomized trial of *Lactobacillus acidophilus* BG2F04 to treat lactose intolerance. Am J Clin Nutr. 1999;69:104-6.

22. Shermack MA, Saavedra JM, Jackson TL, et al. Effect of yoghurt on symptoms in hydrogen production in lactose malabsorbing children. Am J Clin Nutr. 1995;62:1003-6.

Diet in Constipation

Constipation in children is a very common disorder and is responsible for up to 25% of all pediatric gastroenterological consultations and up to 3% of all pediatric outpatient visits. It is estimated that in 90% of the cases, the problem is functional in origin while about 10% of them might have some latent organic cause.[1]

A systematic review of literature reveals a prevalence of constipation ranging from 7–29.6% both in Western and non Western countries.[2] According to Baker,[3] most of the time there does not seem to be any obvious anatomic, biochemical or physiologic abnormalities. A majority of them seem to be associated with functional factors resulting due to probable improper toilet training. Children usually have a tendency to withhold stool, either due to laziness, or preoccupation with playing or even after a painful experience of stool passage on earlier occasions.

Parents generally keep a keen track of the stooling pattern of their child, since this reflects his status of well being, rather a healthy digestive system. This is particularly true for most mothers with children especially in their first 2 years of life.

The normal frequency of bowel movements varies with age. Infants pass a mean of four stools per day, which progressively decreases on an average, to two stools per day at 1 year and one stool every 2–3 days. But as long as the stools are soft and passage is painless, it cannot be termed as constipation. It may be defined as a delay or difficulty in defecation present for 2 or more weeks or as passing less than three stools per week.

Based on the type of presentation of symptoms,[4] etiology of constipation can be broadly divided into:
- Medical cause
- Surgical cause.

IDIOPATHIC/FUNCTIONAL CONSTIPATION

This is perhaps the most common causes of constipation observed among children. The gastrointestinal tract undergoes changes in its physiological forms as the child grows from infancy to older age. The frequency of stool passage can be as frequent as one stool after every feed to almost 1–2 stools every 2–3 days in a breastfed child. As the child is introduced to complementary cereal based diet, the frequency and the consistency of the child also alters to 1–2 stools per day. To a large extent this may depend on how effective toilet training received by the child from the first year of his life. To term constipation as functional, certain criteria need to be fulfilled.[5] These are as follows:

1. Two stools or less per week.
2. At least one episode of incontinence per week.
3. History of stool withholding behavior.
4. Abdominal pain.
5. Fecaloma in the rectum.
6. Presence of bulky stools tending to clog toilets.

Management

Children with such type of constipation require timely and prompt action on the part of the parents and the health care givers. Proper toilet training at an age when the child is able to sit without support can help prevent such situations. A great deal of patience may be required to deal with toddlers as they tend to be restless and easily distractible. Training from an early age can help the child form a habit, so that by the time he reaches the school going stage, he is completely habituated to a set time to pass stool.

It is equally important to maintain a fixed routine for the child regarding his eating and sleeping pattern. Erratic timings of waking and sleeping also influence the gastrointestinal reflex to conform to a regular normal cycle of evacuation.

Stress is another factor which could cause functional constipation. It could be pressure on the child to get ready for school or in older children, the fear of an approaching examination or just disinterest in attending school.

The key to management lies in disciplining the child's routine in such a way that it does not impact the normal physiological functions like sleep hours, meal timings and bowel functions. Waking up late and consequently rising late can affect the eating pattern of the child thus disturbing the normal physiological cycle. An adequate diet with a good amount of fiber and residue can help maintain the normal bowel movements. Encouraging consumption of green leafy vegetables and liberal amounts of fruits, whole grain cereals and pulses from the early years will help them develop taste for these foods, and thus, develop healthy eating habits. Excess consumption of milk and milk products, processed or tinned foods need to be curtailed in the schedule of the child's diet. Excess of milk in the diet also should be avoided as it can compensate for the solid cereal based food intake, thereby depriving adequate fiber in the diet. Apart from this cow's milk allergy has also been reported to present like features of Hirschprung's disease.[4,5] Plenty of fluids in the form of water are equally important to maintain hydration, thus helping in maintaining the motility of the gut and softening of stools.

MEDICAL CAUSES OF CONSTIPATION

Apart from functional factors, occasionally certain other factors can affect the normal bowel movement of children. Among them hypothyroidism is a well known cause.

At times just electrolyte imbalance can also alter the normal functioning as in case of hypercalcemia. Dehydration is an important nonfunctional factor affecting bowel functioning.

Some other factors like medicines used for any other problems can cause constipation like anticholinergics, antispasmodics and certain resins (chloestyramine).

Finally, dietary factors as already mentioned earlier have a definitive role in causing constipation. These may be summed up as follows:

- Malnutrition
- Anorexia
- Dehydration[6]
- Excess cow's milk intake
- Residue insufficiency (especially in older children)
- Celiac disease
- Cystic fibrosis (pancreatic enzyme related)
- Meconium ileus (at birth).

SURGICAL CAUSES OF CONSTIPATION

Certain infrequent causes of constipation could be:

- Hirschprung's Disease
- Colonic or ileal atresia
- Meconium ileus related to cystic fibrosis
- Chronic intestinal pseudo obstruction syndrome
- Anorectal malformations
- Medullar and sacral malformations.

All of the above require surgical interventions where dietary support can help post surgery

MANAGEMENT OF CONSTIPATION

Management of constipation in a child calls for prompt dietary intervention and education of the parents. The primary goal of dietary management is aimed at;

- Providing relief to the child
- Modifying diet as per the age and requirement of the child
- Education of the parents
- Behavioral therapy and lifestyle modifications.

Most of the problems of constipation among children are a chronic one thus, requiring long-term management. Approximately 30% of the children even beyond puberty continue to struggle with symptoms of constipation like infrequent and partial stool evacuation and fecal incontinence.[7]

This can have a long-term debilitating affect on the overall growth and development of the patient, besides affecting his morale. It is therefore important to focus on the management in terms of diet and lifestyle to prevent significant morbidity.[8]

Treatment of chronic constipation involves 4 phases as recommended by NAPSGHAN (North American Society for Pediatric Gastroenetrology, Hepatology and Nutrition.[1] These are as follows:

1. Education.
2. Dissipation.
3. Prevention of reaccumulation of feces.
4. Follow-up.

Parents need to be educated, reassured and counseled regarding the normal stooling pattern of children which varies from that at birth or early infancy when the child is exclusively breast fed to older children when they are weaned off to a full 'family pot' diet.

They should be advised to refrain from blaming the child for his/her bowel habits. On the contrary, they should try to inculcate prompt toilet training, so that the child is accustomed in terms of his eating and sleeping habits.

Adequate and the right type of diet is no doubt one factor which can influence the bowel habits by a good proportion of dietary fiber, but it may not always be the sole cause for chronic constipation in certain children. Dietary fiber given in therapeutic doses may not always be acceptable by the child due to the high bulk form and difficulty in consuming it, besides not being very palatable. Therefore, it would be wise if parents do not insist or pressurize the child to consume fiber in this form. Rather the use of laxatives will help the child in passage of soft stools besides regulating the intestinal motility. Fears of side effects of prolonged or recurrent use of laxatives are unfounded since studies have not revealed any such evidence against them.[9]

Parents need to be reassured about the safety of such medicines used as laxatives in prescribed doses offered. The myth of osmotic laxatives having long-term side effects is in fact unfounded. However, a balanced diet with a good helping of whole cereals, pulses, green leafy vegetables and fruits still need to be complied with for long-term healthy gut motility, but of course without forceful implementation of fiber in the diet.[1]

Another factor commonly recommended is a liberal intake of fluids or water to improve bowel function with a view that increased amounts will help in smoother stool output. Actually, this again is another myth as indicated by various studies.[10,11] It is in fact the solutes and not the water which contributes to ileal effluents; therefore minor increase in liquid intake will not help in altering stool consistency. Hence, it is recommended that unless there is evidence of dehydration, children with constipation should not be forced to drink more than normal amounts of water.

Disimpaction

This is done to remove large fecal mass present usually in children with constipation, to relieve the child of pain and discomfort. Rectal disimpaction is done with phosphate soda enemas, saline enemas or mineral oil enemas.

Recently use of PEG (polyurethane glycol) at the doses of 1–1.5 kg/d has been found to be very effective and acceptable by both children and parents.

Maintainence Therapy

Use of laxatives to maintain soft stools and prevent constipation is usually recommended initially to prevent recurrence of impaction. Osmotic laxatives and PRG are used intermittently to prevent constipation.

Behavioral Therapy

Along with maintenance therapy, behavioral therapy also is initiated for long-term results and maintaining regular bowel movements. Toilet training is encouraged by allowing the child to get on the toilet for 5–10 minutes daily at a fixed time after every meal. This stimulates the gastro colic reflex allowing for an attempt to defecate. The child is asked to strain actively while placing his feet on the foot rest, thus avoiding holding back the urge to defecate. Children failing to respond to any of the combined above therapies are then referred to for psychological counseling.

Follow-up

Studies have shown that even after successful intervention in a child with constipation, relapse within the first 5 years was found in 50% of the treated children, while 30–50% of them persisted to have symptoms after 5 years of follow-up, even beyond age 18 years.[7]

To summarize successful management of children with constipation lies in:

- Education of parents and children about normal bowel habits and long-term adherence to treatment program
- Use of PEG as first-line drug in childhood constipation close and long-term follow-up in children with constipation to monitor relapse or persistence of symptoms.

REFERENCES

1. Constiption Guidelines Committee of the North American Society for Pediatric Gastoenterology, Hepatology and Nutrition: Evaluation and treatment of constipation in infants and children: recommendations of the North American Society for Pediatric gastroenterology, Hepatology and Nutrition. 2006;43:e1-e13.
2. Van den Berg MM, Benning MA, Di Lorenzo C. Epidemiology of childhood constipation: a systematic review. Am J Gastroenterol. 2006;101:2401-9.

3. Baker SS, Liptak GS, Colletti RB, et al. A medical position statement of the North American Society for Pediatric Gastroenteroogy, Hepatology and Nutrition. J Pediatr Gastroenterol Nutr. 1999;29:612-26.

4. Singh SJ, Arbuckle S, Little D, et al. Mortality due to constipation and short segment Hirschprung's disease. Pediatr Surg Int. 2004;20:289-91.

5. Kawai M, Kubota A, Ida S, et al. Cow's milk allergy presenting as Hirschprung's disease mimicking symptoms. Pediatr Surg Int. 2005;21:850-2.

6. Manz F, Weatz A. The importance of good hydration for prevention of chronic diseases. Nutr Rev. 2005;63:S2-S5.

7. Van Ginkel R, Reitsma JB, Buller HA, et al. Childhood constipation: longitudinal follow up beyond puberty. Gastroenterology. 2003;125:357-63.

8. Loening-Baucke V. Constipation in early childhood: patient characteristics, treatment and long term follow up. Gut. 1993;34:1400-04.

9. Muller-Lissner SA, Kamn MA, Scarpignato C, Wald A. Myths and misconceptions about chronic constipation. Am J Gastroenterol. 2005;100:232-42.

10. Schlessinger M, Fordtran JS (Eds). Gastroenterology,ed 6. Philadelphia: Saunders; 1998.pp.1451-71.

11. Debongnie JC, Phillips SF. Capacity of the human colon to absorb fluid. Gastroenterolgy. 1978;74:698-703.

Food Allergies and Intolerances

"What is food for one, is to others bitter poison"

—**Lucretius**

Food allergy is an immune system response to a food that the body mistakenly believes is harmful. Once the immune system decides that a particular food is harmful, it creates specific antibodies to it. The next time one eats that food, the immune system releases massive amounts of chemicals, including histamine, in order to protect the body. These chemicals trigger a cascade of allergic symptoms that can affect the respiratory system, gastrointestinal tract (GIT), skin or cardiovascular system.

Symptoms range from a tingling sensation in the mouth, swelling of the tongue, or throat, difficulty in breathing, vomiting, abdominal cramps, diarrhea, hypotension and also loss of consciousness to death. Symptoms typically appear within minutes to 2 hours after consumption of food which is allergenic to the individual.

Food allergies are usually mediated by IgE antibody directed to specific food proteins. However, other immunological mechanisms can also play a role. Foods most commonly causing these reactions in children are milk, egg, peanuts, soya and fish.

Adverse reactions to food may be toxic or nontoxic:

1. Toxic reactions are not related to individual sensitivity but occur in anyone who ingests a sufficient quantity of tainted food, e.g. reactions to histamine in scombeoid fish poisoning. On the other hand, nontoxic adverse reactions to food depend on individual susceptibility and are either nonimmune mediated, i.e. food intolerance[1] as shown in Table 22.1, or immune mediated, i.e. food allergy.

PATHOGENESIS

Allergic reactions to food are either IgE mediated or non IgE mediated[2] as given in Table 22.2. The role of IgE mediated reactions in food allergy is well

Table 22.1: Some conditions related to food intolerance[1]

- Gastrointestinal disorder
- Structural abnormalities, hiatal hernia, pyloric stenosis, Hirschsprung's disease, tracheoesophageal fistulas
- Disaccharide deficiencies—Lactose, sucrase, iso-maltose complex, glucose–galactose complex
- Pancreatic insufficiency, cystic fibrosis
- Gallbladder disease
- Peptic ulcer disease
- Malignancy
- Galactosemia
- Phenylketonuria
- Jitteriness (caffine)
- Pruritis (histamine)
- Headache (tyramine)
- Disorientation (alcohol)
- Psychologic disorder
- Neurolologic disorder
- Auriculotemporal syndrome (facial flush from tart food)

Table 22.2: Food allergy; target organs and disorders[2]

Target organs	IgE mediated disorder	Non Ig E mediated disorder
Skin	Uriticaria and angioedema atopic dermatitis	Atopic dermatitis Dermatitis herpetiforms
GIT	Oral allergy syndrome Gastrointestinal "Anaphylaxis" Allergic eosinophillic gastroenteritis	Proctocolitis Enterocolitis Allergic eosinophill Gastroenteritis Enteropathy syndrome Celiac disease
Respiratory tract	Asthma Allergic rhinitis	Heiner syndrome
Multisystem	Food-induced anaphylaxis, food assoc., exercise-induced anaphylaxis	

established. Persons who are genetically prone to atopy produce specific IgE antibodies to certain proteins to which they are exposed.

The symptoms of IgE mediated reactions typically involve the skin, respiratory system and GIT.[3]

A schematic picture of the pathogenesis is depicted in Fig. 22.1.[4] As mentioned above, when the food enters the GIT and undergoes protein digestion, the antigen (Ag) processing begins. As the antigen presenting cells present Ag to the T cells, specific cytokines are produced. In the allergic individual, the T-cells will secrete increased amounts of IL-4, IL-5 and IL-13, among the mediators and reduced amounts of IFN-a and TNF-a when compared to that in an individual who is not allergic. The T-cell in turn regulates

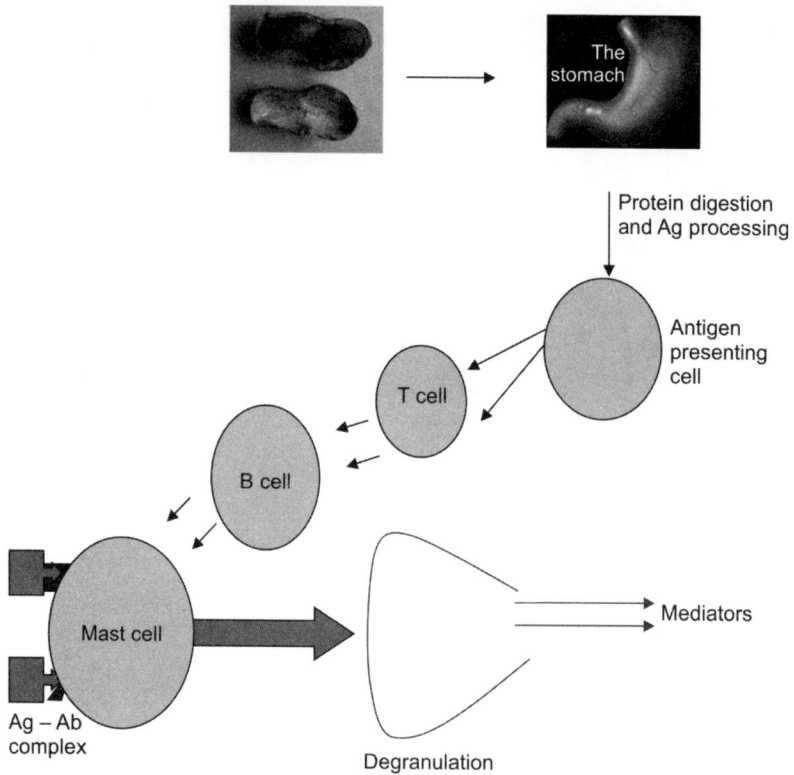

Fig. 22.1: Pathogenesis of food allergy[4]

eventual specific Ig E production by B cells. This specific Ig E is attached to mast cells with mediator release at the mucosal site. Thus, the clinical symptoms follow.

The usual protective mechanisms—Gastric pH, digestive enzymes, mucosal glycoproteins and peristalsis prevent this transmission to a certain extent. But the gut may not be able to effectively exclude intact antigens because of immaturity (infants), injury, malabsorption or infection. Agents causing increased intestinal permeability like alcohol, tobacco or asprin and exercise immediately after food intake may hasten the process.

During the first year of life, the infant diet is the most powerful determinant of the growth and development of the child and food allergy is the most common health problem. It is well established that the feeding of solids is best delayed up to 6 months to reduce the risk of allergy.

In infancy, food allergy is expressed as crying colic, vomiting, diarrhea, rashes, eczema and cold like respiratory congestion. Some infants with food allergy can become seriously ill and fail to thrive unless their allergy is recognized and corrected.

Infants, who develop food allergy in their first year of life, may 'outgrow' the first effects but tend to grow into children with more pervasive health, behavior and learning problems unless their diet is properly managed.

COMMON FOOD ALLERGENS

Over 90% of IgE mediated food allergies in childhood are caused by eight foods: Cow's milk, hen's egg, soy, peanuts, tree nuts (and seeds), wheat, fish and shellfish.[5] In children, milk (casein, lactoglobulins and egg ovalbumin, conalbumin) are the common agents causing food allergy. Prevalence wise, most common food allergens at all ages in western countries are citrus fruits, tomato, egg, strawberry, soy, wheat and fish. Among Indians, common food allergens are cashew nut, coconut, wheat, fish (esp. shellfish), peanut, milk, egg, meat. Amongst spices, mustard and garlic are known to cause allergic reactions.

SKIN MANIFESTATIONS OF FOOD ALLERGY

Skin is one of the most commonly targeted organs in food hypersensitivities. Clinical manifestations of food hypersensitivity range from symptoms of atopic dermatitis, to urticaria and angiodema and herpetiformins.

Dermatitis herpetiformis is typically associated with gluten-sensitive enteropathy, which involves a chronic papulovesicular skin manifestations involving pruritis as a hallmark of the disease.[6]

RESPIRATORY MANIFESTATION OF FOOD ALLERGY

Acute respiratory manifestation of food allergies involves either cutanous or GI symptoms. Egg, milk, peanut, soy, fish, shell fish and tree nuts are the most common food allergens confirmed to elicit respiratory reactions.[7]

It is observed that food-induced allergic reactions are more common in young pediatric patients than in older children and adults. Allergic sensitization or clinical reactions to foods in infancy predict the later development of respiratory allergies and asthma.

Food-induced allergies may increase airway hyper responsiveness in patients with moderate to severe asthma and may do so without inducing acute asthma symptoms.

Respiratory symptoms, especially asthmatic reaction, induced by food allergens are considered risk factors for fatal or near fatal reactions. Following features indicate the need for evaluation of food allergy in patients with asthma.

- Asthma triggered after ingestion of particular foods
- Unexplained acute, severe asthma exacerbations
- Patients with asthma that is accompanied by other manifestation of food allergy (e.g. anaphylaxis, moderate to severe atopic dermatitis).

MANIFESTATIONS OF GIT

The GIT is a very common target organ for IgE mediated reactions to foods. Symptoms of GI "anaphylaxis" occur shortly after ingestion of the offending food and include nausea, vomiting, abdominal pain and diarrhea.

DIAGNOSIS OF FOOD ALLERGY

Once food allergy is identified as a likely cause of symptoms, confirmation of diagnosis and identification of implicated food(s) needs to be done.

Diagnosis becomes easier when history implicates a particular food like in patients with acute reactions, e.g. urticaria or anaphylaxis. In patients with atopic dermatitis or asthma the causative factors are more difficult to pinpoint the causal foods.

MAINTENANCE OF FOOD DIARY

A regular maintenance of food diary indicating all the foods taken and occurrence of symptoms, the frequency of incidence or the severity can all help the physician come to definite conclusion.

ELIMINATION DIET

Once there is suggestion of food-related illness and tests for IgE antibody to food are positive, elimination of the particular food from the diet is the first step. Disappearance of symptoms on elimination can be highly indicative of that particular food as causative agents. Challenge with the same food once improvement is achieved, can justify the elimination of the food if symptom reoccur.

ORAL FOOD CHALLENGES

Double-blind placebo controlled food challenges are considered the gold standard for diagnosing food allergy.[3,8]

In this procedure, the patient avoids the suspected food for at least 2 weeks, antihistamine therapy is discontinued and doses of asthma medications are decreased as much as possible. After intravenous access is obtained, graded doses of either a challenge food or a placebo food are administered. The food is hidden either in another food or in opaque capsules. However, this procedure is done under medical supervision strictly, so that any severe reactions if occur can be handled immediately.

PRICK PUNCTURE SKIN TESTING

This method involves determining the presence of specific IgE antibody, when the patient is not on antihistamines. The skin is punctured through glycerinated extract of a food. A local wheal and flare response indicates the presence of food specific IgE antibody, with a wheal diameter of more than 3 mm indicating a positive response.

The predictive value of this test is over 95% and hence, of more value when they are negative. On the other hand the positive predictive value is only 50%, therefore this test cannot be considered in isolation. Intradermal allergy skin tests are not very reliable as they are highly false positive. Fresh extracts of fruits and vegetables are recommended for this test since the protein in commercial extracts of most fruits and vegetables are prone to degradation.[9]

IN VITRO TESTING (RAST)

This test is more practical than prick test for screening of food allergy in primary care office setting. As with skin tests this test too is highly sensitive for confirming negative result, i.e. ruling out an IgE mediated reaction. But when highly sensitive assays are used, the levels of food specific IgE antibody correlate with clinical reactivity to only certain foods (milk, egg, peanuts and fish).

Tests are Positive

1. Eliminate food.
2. If the patient has multiple sensitivities or an unclear history, perform open or single blind food challenges.
   a) If the challenge test is positive, challenge.
1. Eliminate foods (if only a few foods).
2. If multiple foods are implicated, consider double blind, placebo-controlled food challenges.
   a) If challenge is positive, eliminate food.
   b) If challenge is negative, reintroduce food.
3. Diagnosis established
   a) Educate patient about treatment and avoidance.
   b) Re-evaluate at appropriate intervals if tolerance is likely.[10]

ORAL ALLERGY SYNDROME

As the name denotes, symptoms are limited to the oral cavity. They are characterized by pruritis and edema of the oral mucosa occurring after ingestion of certain fresh fruits and vegetables.[11]

The reaction occurs primarily in patients with allergic sensitivity to pollens and is caused by Ig E antibodies directed toward cross reacting proteins found in pollen fruits and vegetables. A characteristic feature of this syndrome is that patients are usually not symptomatic to cooked foods since the causative allergens are heat labile.

CHINESE RESTAURANTS SYNDROME

As the name denotes, reaction occurs after ingestion of Chinese food. The manifestations may be in the form of sensation of warmth and burning over head and shoulders, headache, stiffness and weakness of limbs. The culprit attributed is the monosodium glutamate (MSG) or ajinomoto, the essential ingredient of any Chinese cuisine.

SULFITE SENSITIVITY

Sulfite-based compounds containing sodium bisulphate which are present in wines, vinegar, beverages, dried fruits and even medicine and eye drops, TPN and dialysis fluids can also cause hypersensitivity. Asthma, anaphylaxis and cutanous reactions are common manifestation. Cross sensitivity can also occur with MSG and aspirin.

AURICULOTEMPORAL SYNDROME (FREY SYNDROME)

This syndrome is often misdiagnosed as a food allergy. It is manifested immediately as unilateral rarely bilateral flushing, sweating or both, localized to the distribution of the auriculotemporal nerve, in response to gustatory or tactile stimuli.[12]

In children, the flushing usually begins within seconds after eating and subsides approximately 30–60 minutes later.

HEINER SYNDROME

This is a non IgE mediated adverse pulmonary response to food. It is not a very common manifestation but can present in infants by an immune reaction to cow's milk protein with precipitating antibody IgG, resulting in pulmonary infilterates, pulmonary hemosiderosis, anemia, recurrent pneumonia and failure to thrive.

ANAPHYLAXIS

This refers to a dramatic multiorgan reaction associated with IgE mediated hypersensitivity. Foods commonly associated with anaphylaxis are peanuts, tree nuts (walnuts, almonds, cashew, hazel nuts) and shell fish. This is more common in patients with underlying asthma.[13]

Anaphylaxis may be induced in two forms, food associated or exercise induced. It may occur when exercise follows the ingestion of a particular food to which IgE mediated sensitivity is usually demonstrable (e.g. celery) or less commonly may occur after the ingestion of any food.

CELIAC DISEASE

This is actually an example of non IgE mediated disease. In this the causative factor is the gliadin fraction of the protein gluten in wheat. It presents over a period of time, may be months or years with steatorrhea, flatulence and failure to thrive. The characteristic diagnostic feature is extensive flattening of villi of the jejunal mucosa.

ALLERGIC EOSINOPHILIC GASTROENTERITIS

This is an IgE mediated disease, but many patients do not exhibit specific IgE antibody to foods. Manifestations are severe reflux, post prandial abdominal pain, vomiting, early satiety and diarrhea. The diagnosis is suggested by presence of inflammation and significant eosinophilic infilteration of the esophagus, stomach or small intestine.

INFANTILE PROCTOCOLITIS

This involves the lower GI tract and is of short duration. The ingestion of the responsible food (usually cow's milk protein or breast milk from mothers who are consuming cow's milk) causes diarrhea with blood in the stool.

MIGRAINE

Migraine headaches have been associated with food allergies/ hypersensitivity. Studies on children with migraine showed that 93% of 88 children recovered on oligoantigenic diets. The causative foods were identified by sequential reintroduction, and the role of the foods provoking migraine was established by a double blind controlled trial in 40 children. Most patients responded to several foods. Many foods were involved suggesting an allergic rather than metabolic pathogenesis. Associated symptoms which improved in addition to headache included abdominal pain, behavior disorder, fits, asthma and eczema. In most of the patients in whom migraine was provoked by nonspecific factors like blows to the head, exercise and flashing lights, this provocation did not occur while they were on oligoantigenic diet.[14]

TREATMENT/MANAGEMENT

Management of food allergies are best done by 'avoidance'. Dietary elimination of the offending food(s) is the simplest methods to manage allergies/ intolerances. Other modalities include medical management and in case of emergencies, injectable epinephrine and oral antihistamine should always be readily available at hand. Prompt administration of epinephrine at the first signs of a severe reaction must be stressed since delayed attention has been associated with fatal and nonfatal food allergic reactions.[13]

Identification of the offending food(s) is very crucial since successful management involves life long avoidance of foods in any form, directly or indirectly. Following points need to be considered in the dietary management of any food allergy/intolerance.

1. Elimination of the offending food.

2. Read all the labels on food products carefully and the ingredients mentioned there in. Any word indicating any close resemblance to the offending food should be checked, e.g. in a milk-free diet, not only milk in any visible form should be avoided but any indication of words like 'casein', 'whey', lactose, or 'flavoring colors', etc. should also be kept in the mind since these are also indirect signs of milk protein being present in some form. It may be a part of ingredient in recipes like in bakery products; chocolates, etc. Egg protein may be present in a number of commercial products available over the counters, all of which may not necessarily indicate its inclusion.

In case of protein allergy, where, peanut-based products like butter is used along side with any nonpeanut product, but the spatula used or the bowls used may not be separate for these products, chances of allergic reactions can be possible.

Some of the hidden allergens which can go unnoticed are as follows:
   - Eggs—Baked foods, noodles, puddings
   - Milk—Pies, cheese, bakery products
   - Soy—Baked foods, candy
   - Wheat—Soups, snacks, savories
   - Fish—Seafood flavors.
3. It is safer to avoid use of all artificial foods or dining out.
4. In case of infants and toddlers, avoiding of any such food in the maternal diet is advisable, e.g. eggs, cow's milk, peanut, etc. Continuation of exclusive breastfeeding at least till 6 months is encouraged. Solid foods should be introduced only after 6 months.
5. Introduction of known hyperallergic foods can be delayed, e.g. cow's milk can be delayed till about 10–12 months, eggs till about 2 years and peanuts/nuts/fish can be delayed even up to 3 years.
6. Smoking should be refrained by elders in and around the periphery of the child's environment, since smoking increases the risk of recurrent wheeze and asthma. This is also known to lead to life threatening food allergy.
7. If traveling take specially packed foods.
8. When dining out ask for information on ingredients.
9. In case of a child does react to any allergenic food, give medication immediately/ seek medical help, keep injectable epinephrine at hand.
10. In case of peanut allergy, if any peanut containing food is handled by the mother or caregiver or cutlery, etc. used, they should be washed thoroughly.
11. Roasting of peanut has been known to increase allergic properties.

Probiotics have been also considered to have beneficial effects on the host by improving its intestinal microbial balance, e.g. yogurt which contains Lactobacillus and bifidobacterium species.[15]

RECOGNIZING ALLERGIES IN CHILDREN

Generally most allergies can be detected by visible signs or symptoms in children. They may give indirect 'feelers' which should not be ignored since these may well be warning signals of some allergy. Commonly described signs by children could be

- Putting hands to mouth, pull or scratch tongue or voice may change
- Food is too spicy
- My tongue is hot or something is pricking it
- My mouth is tingly, itches or feels funny
- My tongue feels full or my throat feels thick.

REFERENCES

1. Bruijinzeel-Koomen C, Irtolani C, Aas K, Bindslev-Jenson C, Bjorksten B, Moneret-Vautrin D, et al. Adverse reactions to food. Allergy. 1995;50:623-35.
2. Geha RS. Regulation of Ig E synthesis in humans. J Allergy Clin Immunol. 1992;90:143-50.
3. Bock SA, Atkins FM. Patterns of food hypersensitivity during sixteen years of double blind, placebo- controlled challenges. J Pediatr. 1990;117:561-7.
4. Burks W. J Peanut Allergy: a growing phenomenon. Clin Invest. 2003;11(7):950-2.
5. Allen KJ, Hill DJ, Heina RG. Food allergy in childhood. MJA. 2006;185(7):394-400.
6. Scott H, Schierer MD. Clinical aspects of gastrointestinal food allergy in childhood. Pediatrics. 2003;111(6):1617-24.
7. Burks W. Respiratory manifestations of food allergy. Pediatrics. 2003;111(6):1625-30.
8. Sampson HA, Albergo R. Comparison of results of skin test, RAST and double blind placebo controlled food challenges in children with atopic dermatitis. J Allergy Clin Immunol. 1984;74:26-33.
9. Block SA, Lee WT, Remingio L, Holst A, May CD. Appraisal of skin tests with food extracts for diagnosis of food hypersensitivity. Clin Allergy. 1978;8:559-64.
10. Stcherer SH. Manifestations of food allergy. Evaluation and Management, Mount Sinai School of Medicine, New York. American family physician, Pub. By the American academy of family physician. Jan 15, 1999.
11. Irtolanic C, Ispano M, Pastorello E, Bigi A, Ansaloni R. The oral allegy síndrome. Ann Allergy. 1988;6112:47-52.
12. Beck SA, Burks AW, Woody RC. Auriculotemporal syndrome seen clinically as food allergy. Pediatrics. 1989;83:601-3.
13. Sampson HA, Mendelson LM, Rosen JP. Fatal and near fatal anaphylactic reactions to food in children and adolescents. N Engl J Med. 1992;327:380-4.
14. Eqqer J, Carter CM, Wilson J, Turnor MW, Soothill JF. Is migraine food allergy? A double blind controlled trial of oligoantigentic diet treatment. Lancet. 1983;2(8355):865-9.
15. Majamaa H, Isolauri E. Probiotics: a novel approach in the management of food allergy. J Allergy Clin Immunol. 1997;99:179-85.

Index

Page numbers followed by *f* refer to figure and *t* refer to table.